Atlas of
Cardiovascular Pathology

To A.S.G.

Current Histopathology

Consultant Editor
Professor G. Austin Gresham, TD, ScD, MD, FRC Path.
Professor of Morbid Anatomy and Histology, University of Cambridge

Volume Twelve

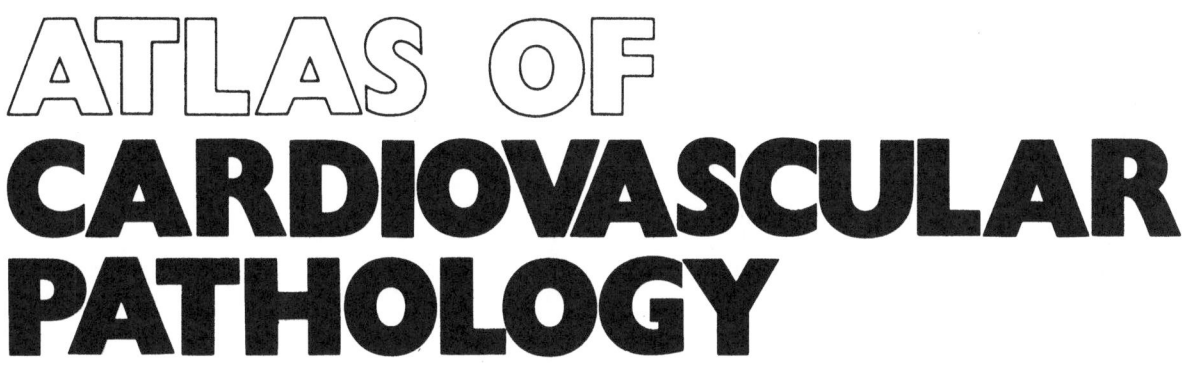

ATLAS OF CARDIOVASCULAR PATHOLOGY

BY

E. G. J. OLSEN, MD, FRC Path., FACC
Consultant Pathologist
National Heart Hospital, London

assisted by
R. A. FLORIO, FIMLS
National Heart Hospital, London

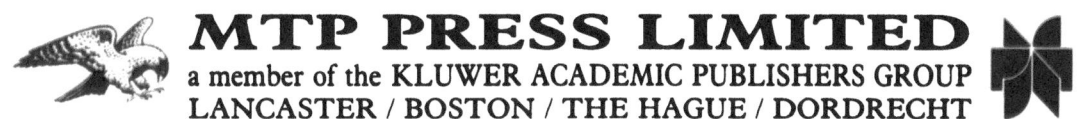

MTP PRESS LIMITED
a member of the KLUWER ACADEMIC PUBLISHERS GROUP
LANCASTER / BOSTON / THE HAGUE / DORDRECHT

Published in the UK and Europe by
MTP Press Limited
Falcon House
Queen Square
Lancaster, England

British Library Cataloguing in Publication Data
Olsen, E. G. J.
    Atlas of cardiovascular pathology. — (Current histo-
    pathology; v.12)
    1. Cardiovascular system — Diseases — Atlases
    I. Title   II. Florio, R. A.   III. Series
    616.1'0022'2   RC669
    ISBN-13: 978-94-010-7940-2   e-ISBN-13: 978-94-009-3209-8
    DOI: 10.1007/978-94-009-3209-8

Published in the USA by
MTP Press
A division of Kluwer Academic Publishers
101 Philip Drive
Norwell, MA 02061, USA

Library of Congress Cataloging in Publication Data
Olsen, E. G. J. (Eckhardt G. J.)
    Atlas of cardiovascular pathology

    (Current histopathology; v. 12)
    Includes bibliographies and index.
    1. Heart—Diseases—Atlases.   2. Histology,
    Pathological—Atlases.   I. Florio, R. A. II. Title.
    III. Series.   [DNLM: 1. Heart—pathology—atlases.
    WI CU788JBA v.12 /WG 17 052a]
    RC682.9.047   1987   616.1'207   86-27533

Phototypesetting by Titus Wilson, Kendal.
Colour origination by Laserscan, Stretford, Manchester.
Bound by Butler and Tanner Ltd., Frome and London.

Contents

Current Histopathology Series

Consultant Editor's Note

At the present time books on morbid anatomy and histology can be divided into two broad groups: extensive textbooks often written primarily for students and monographs on research topics.

This takes no account of the fact that the vast majority of pathologists are involved in an essentially practical field of general Diagnostic Pathology providing an important service to their clinical colleagues. Many of these pathologists are expected to cover a broad range of disciplines and even those who remain solely within the field of histopathology usually have single and sole responsibility within the hospital for all this work. They may often have no chance for direct discussion on problem cases with colleagues in the same department. In the field of histopathology, no less than in other medical fields, there have been extensive and recent advances, not only in new histochemical techniques but also in the type of specimen provided by new surgical procedures.

There is a great need for the provision of appropriate information for this group. This need has been defined in the following terms.

(1) It should be aimed at the general clinical pathologist or histopathologist with existing practical training, but should also have value for the trainee pathologist.
(2) It should concentrate on the practical aspects of histopathology taking account of the new tech-

niques which should be within the compass of the worker in a unit with reasonable facilities.
(3) New types of material, e.g. those derived from endoscopic biopsy should be covered fully.
(4) There should be an adequate number of illustrations on each subject to demonstrate the variation in appearance that is encountered.
(5) Colour illustrations should be used wherever they aid recognition.

The present concept stemmed from this definition but it was immediately realized that these aims could only be achieved within the compass of a series, of which this volume is one. Since histopathology is, by its very nature, systemized, the individual volumes deal with one system or where this appears more appropriate with a single organ.

This atlas of cardiovascular pathology is a valuable addition to the *Current Histopathology* series. It reflects the increasing use of new methods in diagnostic work and illustrates the importance of proper preparation of specimens together with a detailed clinicopathological correlation in order to enhance diagnostic success.

Cardiovascular disease confronts every pathologist. This well illustrated comprehensive volume will be a useful bench manual in pathology laboratories.

G. Austin Gresham
Cambridge

Acknowledgements

I gratefully acknowledge the co-operation of The Macmillan Press Limited who have permitted me to reproduce previously published illustrations and tables.

My thanks are also due to those colleagues who have supplied me with material for illustration.

I am gratefully indebted to Miss P. J. Higham for typing the entire manuscript and to Mr B. Richards for his help with the photographs.

Preface

Pathology in general is closely linked with clinical medicine and in cardiovascular pathology this interdependence is, perhaps, greater than in most other specialities.

In recent years great advances in investigatory procedures have taken place, including the examination of fresh endomyocardial tissue obtained by bioptome, permitting not only clinico-pathological correlation but also examination at histochemical and ultrastructural levels. Angiography has gained wider usage and two-dimensional echocardiography is no longer the preserve of specialized units. Percutaneous coronary transluminal angioplasty is a relatively new approach to relieving obstructive coronary artery disease. Cardiac pathology has therefore moved apace, providing not only a background to clinical manifestations but also visual proof for other investigations such as immunology and virology. Such investigations have played an essential role in establishing pathogenetic mechanisms for diseases such as cardiomyopathies.

Changes in the pattern of disease have also taken place with, for example, a decrease in rheumatic heart disease in industrialized countries. Portals of entry and infective agents in infective endocarditis have also changed. However, despite sophisticated techniques of recognition and up-to-date therapeutic approaches, endocarditis has remained a world problem. Separate chapters have been dedicated to these topics.

The aim of an atlas is to link the written word with pictorial representation of disease but, in this volume, the text also includes a summary of the background and advances made and, where appropriate, a classification. Key references are cited so that this short volume is a complete overview of the topics under discussion.

A large section has been devoted to the normal heart. Detailed knowledge of the anatomy, microscopy and ultrastructure is essential to understand and interpret the changes which occur in diseases and which, more often than not, can be subtle. There is no routine procedure for opening the heart as this is dependent on the possible future procedures that are planned, such as morphometric analysis. The conventional procedure, that of 'following the blood stream', is however detailed.

Pathological correlation and the interpretation of echocardiographic changes may be desired and therefore a short section has been included on cutting the heart according to conventionally used echocardiographic planes.

The heart can only react to physiological changes or damage in a limited way and therefore a separate chapter on hypertrophy and dilatation and another chapter dealing with changes in the endocardium, which reflect haemodynamic alteration and may additionally show diagnostic features, are also included. Degeneration together with changes in connective tissue and ischaemic heart disease are separately presented. Atherogenesis, recognition of myocardial infarction and the earliest morphological changes discernible at histochemical and ultrastructural levels of investigation, which are within the scope of modern routine laboratories, are emphasized.

Recently, great advances have been made in our understanding of myocarditis, facilitated by the evaluation of sequential biopsies. This has permitted diagnostic criteria to be established, a new definition to be formulated and a classification to be proposed. The intimate relationship of myocarditis with dilated cardiomyopathy has been detailed and additional reference to investigatory studies using molecular virological techniques has been made. Similar advances in endomyocardial disease related to eosinophilia have been highlighted.

Chapter 10 deals with neoplasms of the heart and pericardium and Chapter 11 with common and rare diseases of the arteries. A chapter on pulmonary hypertension combining angiographic and morphlogical changes, and also incorporating a large section on the normal pulmonary vasculature, completes this book.

The topics of this Atlas have been carefully chosen and, in order to avoid repetition of other publications, congenital heart disease and the changes following surgery have been omitted.

This Atlas is principally directed to pathologists in practice or in training but it is also hoped that it will be of value to physicians and surgeons and other workers engaged in the study of the heart. It is also hoped it will be of help to teachers, at both postgraduate and undergraduate levels.

The Normal Heart

1

It is not the purpose of this atlas to detail the various techniques of postmortem examination for which the reader is referred to specialized texts, but to concentrate on the removal of the heart from the lungs after the rib cage has been opened. The heart can be removed following removal of the thoracic viscera (Figure 1.1a). It is appropriate to follow the time-honoured dictum 'never touch or cut before inspection'.

Inspect the outer surfaces of the pericardium. Identify the pulmonary veins.

In cases of suspected pericarditis, it is advisable to secure a swab for bacterial (or viral) investigation. Any fluid accumulation should be carefully measured; 5–10 ml of clear, pale, yellow fluid is normal but pericardial effusion is usually deemed to be present if the fluid accumulation in the pericardial cavity exceeds 50 ml of fluid. The pericardium should then be opened fully by fashioning an inverted T-incision (Figure 1.1b). Separation of any adhesions may require sharp dissection. Once the pericardium has been deflected, further inspection can now be undertaken.

The coronary arteries should then be gently palpated. If extensive calcification is present it is often wiser not to proceed further but, after separation of the heart from the lungs, large segments of the affected coronary arterial tree can be removed and decalcified and further examination can then be undertaken. The pulmonary trunk should be incised with care to avoid dislodgement of any possible pulmonary embolus. The heart can now be removed.

The pericardium should then be fully opened and the aorta and pulmonary trunk are now displayed (Figure 1.1c). The pericardium is then trimmed around the inferior vena cava. Place the index finger and middle finger in close apposition into the transverse sinus of the pericardial cavity and divide the aorta and pulmonary trunk between these two fingers. If this simple technique is followed a uniform length of great vessels for the particular examiner is assured. To identify the pulmonary veins the apex of the heart should be firmly gripped and pulled up so that the pulmonary veins are under slight tension (Figure 1.1d). By retaining the grip on the cardiac apex the atria should be gently freed from adhesions and the pericardial reflection should be divided. Working towards the right side of the heart taking care not to damage the bronchus or right pulmonary artery, the superior vena cava and right pulmonary veins should be identified, freed from surrounding tissue and should then be divided. The last cut through the inferior cava is then made if the heart is removed *in situ*, or after organs have been removed *en bloc* according to the Rokitansky method. The heart is now free[1].

External Landmarks

Ventral View

Place the heart in the normal anatomical position. Identify the following structures: the aorta, the pulmonary trunk, right and left atrial appendages, right and left pulmonary veins, anterior longitudinal sulcus, right coronary sinus, acute margin, obtuse margin, apex and incisura apicis cordis and the superior vena cava. See Figure 1.2.

Dorsal View

Identify the orifice of the inferior vena cava, right and left atria, pulmonary veins, coronary sinus and posterior longitudinal sinus, right and left ventricles (Figure 1.3).

It will be noted that anteriorly the heart is mainly composed of the right atrium and right ventricle with only a small portion of the left ventricle showing, whereas, posteriorly equal portions of right and left atria and ventricles can be identified.

Examination of Coronary Arteries

Reference has already been made to dealing with the coronary arteries in which calcification can be felt. If no abnormalities are observed sectioning at half centimetre intervals along the course of the arteries at right angles to the lumen can now be undertaken at this stage or deferred after opening the cardiac chambers.

If ischaemic heart disease or cardiac infarction is suspected the coronary arteries should be injected with radio-opaque material before opening the heart. This can be achieved by manual injection or by an adaptation of the apparatus designed for injecting pulmonary vasculature (Figure 1.4). The bottles containing water and formal saline can be raised or lowered to the diastolic pressure during life. A normal coronary arteriogram is illustrated in Figure 1.5.

It may be necessary to study individual coronary arteries in detail. The heart is then opened as follows: the origins of the right and left coronary arteries are identified and for the apex a cut is made as close as possible to the interventricular septum anteriorly through the ventricles and as close as possible to the origin of the coronary arteries. The right ventricle is then unfolded and the right coronary artery can then be X-rayed (Figure 1.6). The left ventricle and vessels of the interventricular septum can be separately evaluated.

Opening of the Heart

There is no 'routine' procedure for opening the heart. Abnormalities such as stenosed valves should be left intact and adaptations are necessary, depending on the

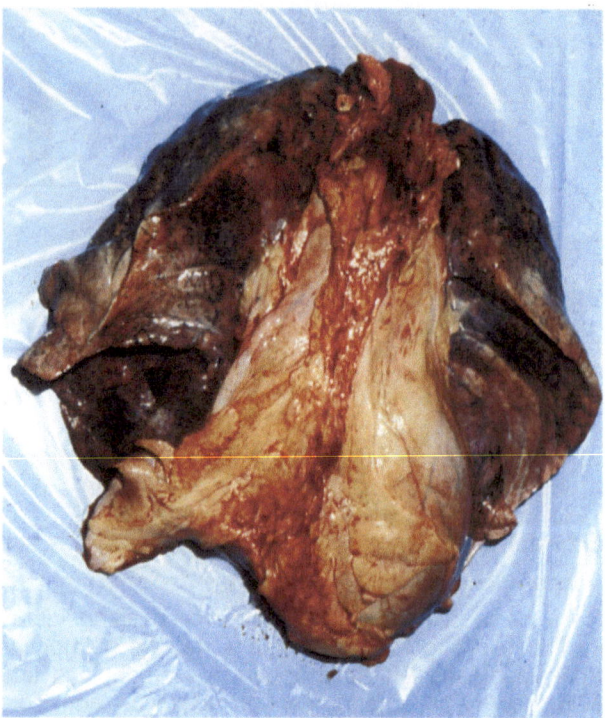

Figure 1.1a General view of the heart and lungs having been removed *en bloc*

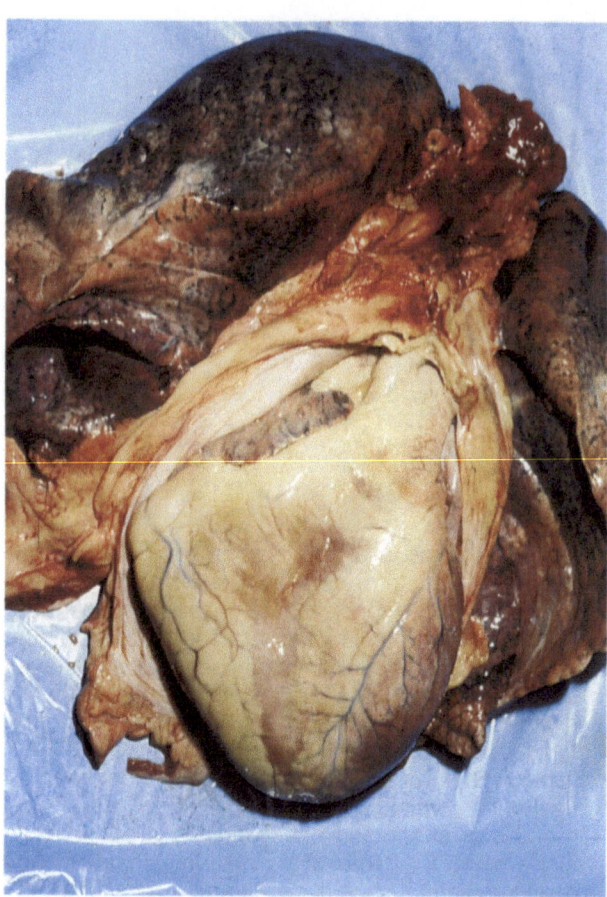

Figure 1.1b The pericardium has been partially opened to permit inspection of the epicardium and gentle palpation of the coronary arteries

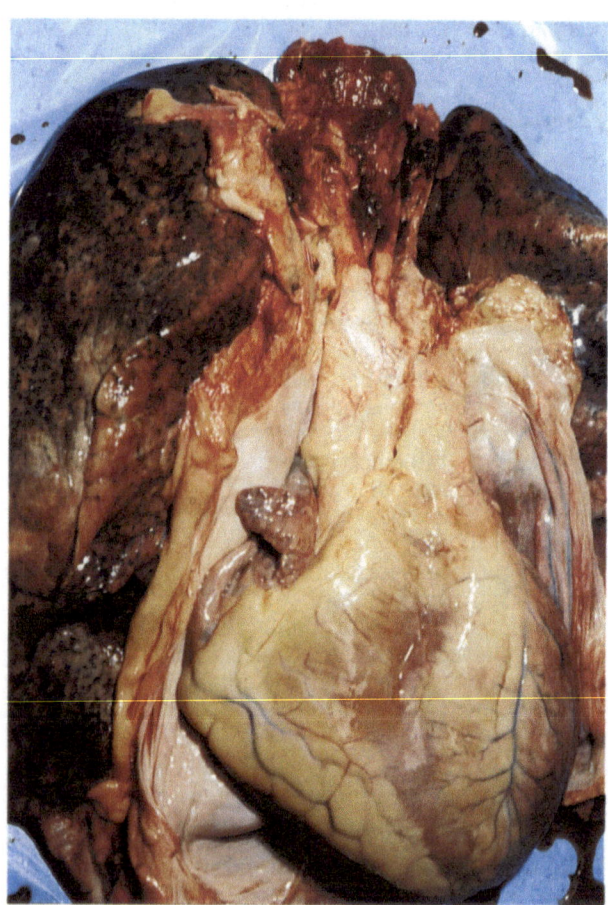

Figure 1.1c The great vessels are now exposed and should be divided between index and middle finger

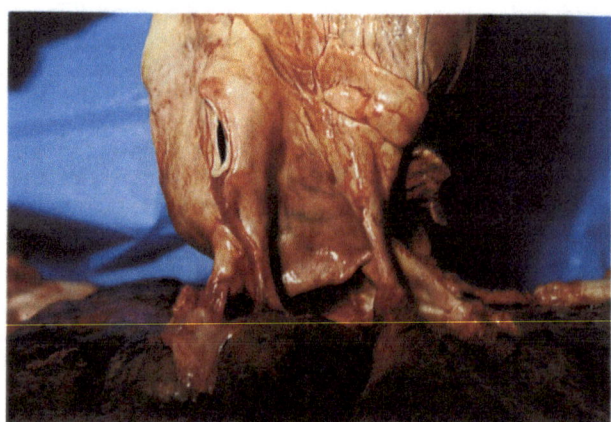

Figure 1.1d The apex has been pulled upwards, revealing the pulmonary veins

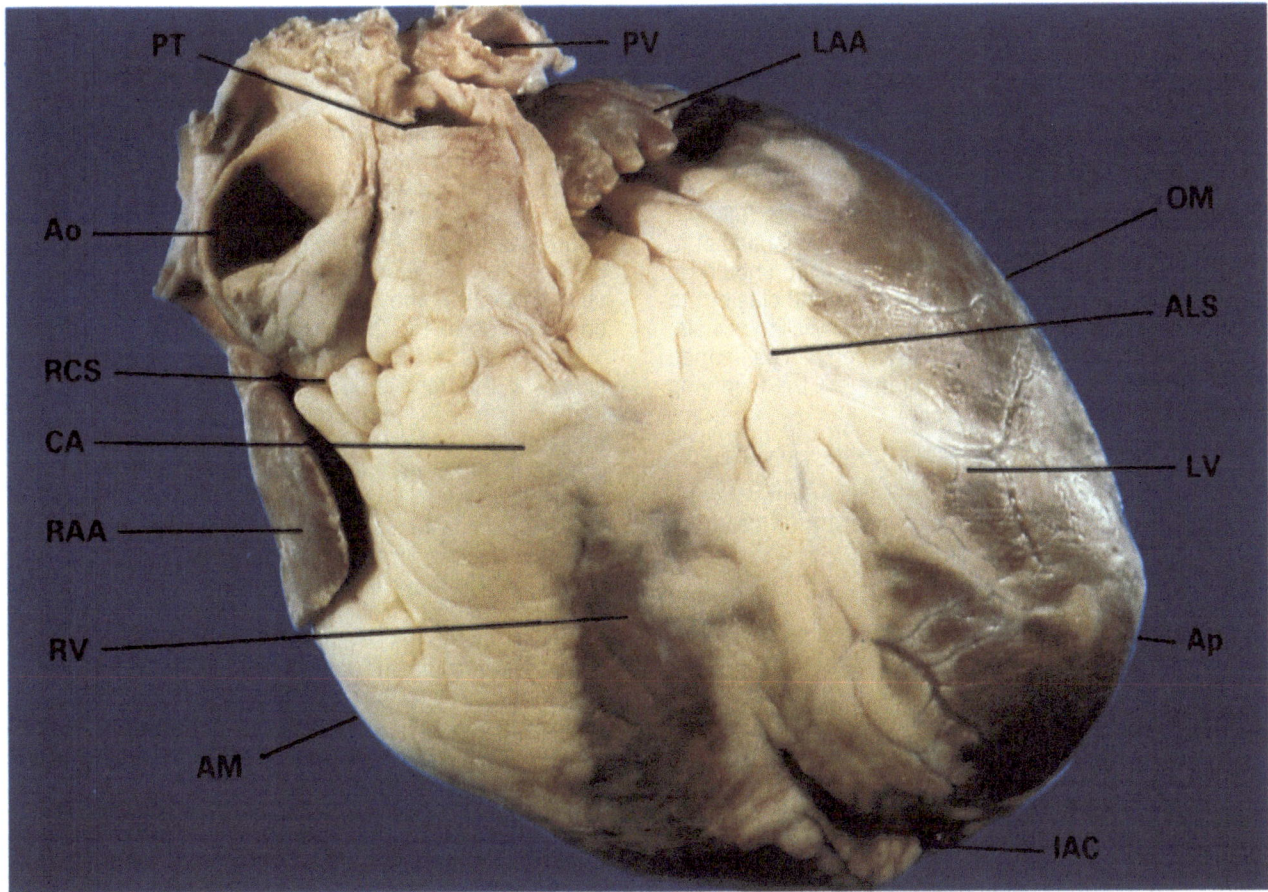

Figure 1.2 Ventral view of the heart: PT = Pulmonary trunk; Ao = Aorta; RCS = Right coronary sulcus; CA = Conus arteriosus; RAA = Right atrial appendage; RV = Right ventricle; AM = Acute margin; IAC = Incisura apicis cordis; Ap = Apex; LV = Left ventricle; ALS = Anterior longitudinal sulcus; OM = Obtuse margin; LAA = Left atrial appendage; PV = Pulmonary vein

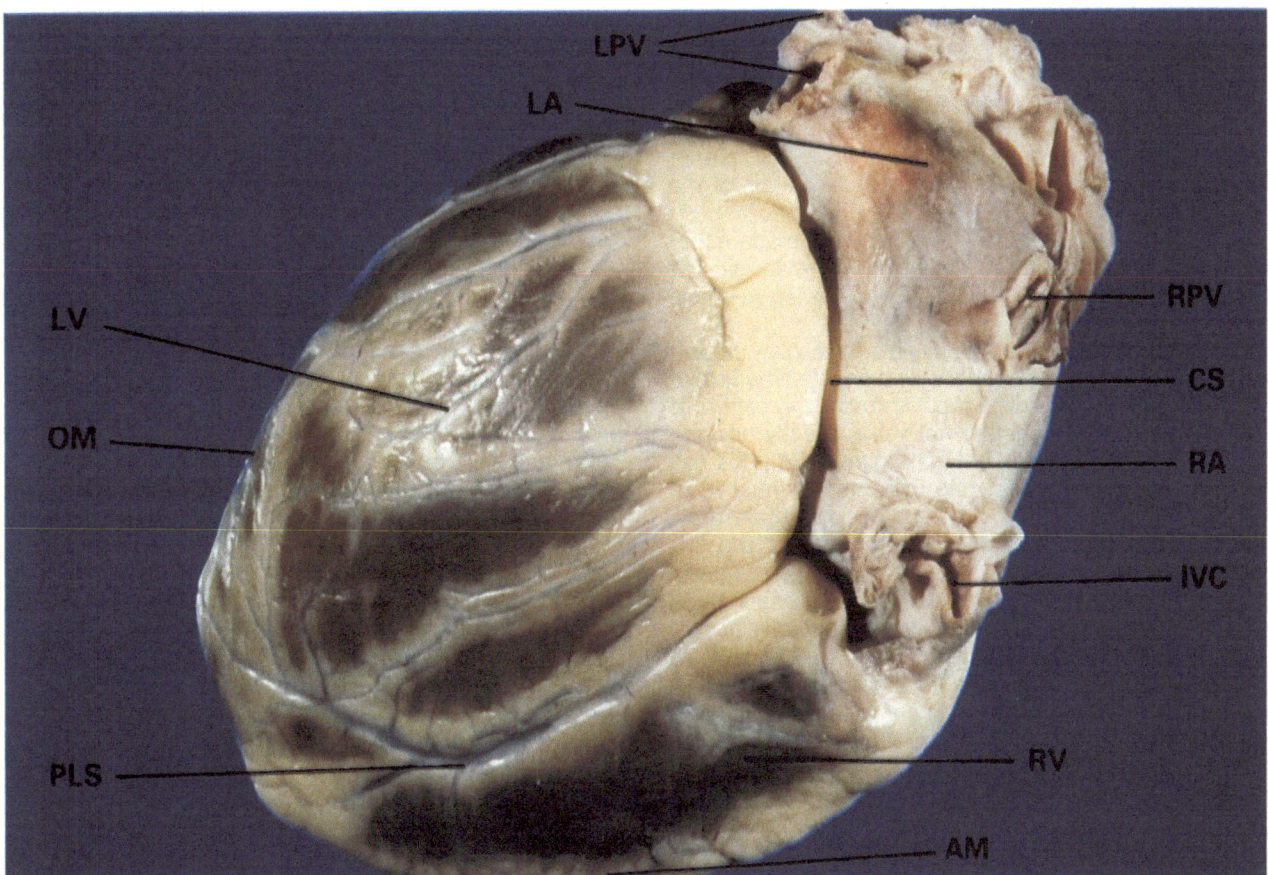

Figure 1.3 Dorsal view of the heart: LPV = Left pulmonary veins; LA = Left atrium; LV = Left ventricle; OM = Obtuse margin; PLS = Posterior longitudinal sulcus; AM = Acute margin; RV = Right ventricle; IVC = Inferior vena cava; RA = Right atrium; CS = Coronary sulcus; RPV = Right pulmonary vein

investigation one wishes to undertake. For example, in cases of myocardial infarction the ventricles can be cut transversely at 1 cm intervals for morphometric assessment of the damaged myocardium.

A convenient way of opening the heart is as follows: The first cut is made 3–4 cm above the apex parallel to the atrio-ventricular groove (Figure 1.7). Care should be taken not to extend the cut through the ventricles but to allow a thin rim of muscle at the posterior wall to remain, acting as a hinge so that the apical portion can be flapped back into position. By undertaking this cut the following can be assessed:

(1) whether or not two ventricular cavities are present;

(2) the presence or absence of asymmetric hypertrophy of the interventricular septum (in cases of hypertrophic cardiomyopathy);

(3) subendocardial infarction.

The second cut is made to open the right atrium 0.5 to 1 cm in front of the opening of the inferior vena cava. This cut should be extended 0.5 cm above and parallel to the atrio-ventricular junction to the tip of the right atrial appendage (Figure 1.8). For better display, a vertical cut towards the inferior vena cava can be made. The right atrium is now open. A cut is now made along the acute margin of the right ventricle avoiding cutting through commissures of the tricuspid valve. This cut joins cut one (Figure 1.8). The right atrium and the inflow portion of the right ventricle are now open (Figure 1.9). A cut displaying the outflow tract of the right ventricle (to the right of the anterior papillary muscle) and close to the interventricular septum should be made extending through the pulmonary valve (Figure 1.10a and b).

The left atrium is best displayed by incising the left atrial appendage. The cut is extended posteriorly across the roof of the left atrium between the opening of the right and left pulmonary veins and extended towards the atrio-ventricular groove (Figure 1.11). The cut is then redirected in such a manner as to encircle the inferior left pulmonary veins to reach the obtuse margin of the left ventricle.

A cut through the obtuse margin is now made either anteriorly or posteriorly to the mitral valve to join cut one. The left atrium and inflow tract of the left ventricle can now be displayed (Figure 1.12).

Two procedures are now possible to display the left ventricular outflow tract and the aortic valve. The first of the procedures is to make a cut through the centre of the anterior leaflet of the mitral valve directly into the aortic valve (see dotted lines on Figure 1.12). This has the disadvantage of destroying the anterior mitral valve leaflet. Alternatively – and a procedure to be preferred – is to cut a segment of the anterior wall of the left ventricle which includes the anterior papillary muscle and this cut is extended behind the pulmonary trunk (which may require some freeing from connective tissue) into the aorta (Figure 1.13).

All the chambers are open for inspection in detail.

By opening the heart in this manner the various open chambers can now be repositioned to the original position and is ready for future examination without having distorted the anatomy[1] (Figure 1.14).

Dissection of the Heart According to Echocardiographical Planes

M-mode and two-dimensional (2D) echocardiography is a well-recognized adjunct to clinical diagnosis. Correlation between the changes observed with this method of examination and morphology may be necessary in which case a different approach to dissection to that described above is necessary.

Long and short axis planes are conventionally used, the long axis view is illustrated in Figure 1.15a. The entire heart (fresh or fixed) is bisected with a long sharp knife in the longitudinal axis from the anterior mitral valve leaflet to the aortic valve (Figure 1.15b), which corresponds to the 2D long axis view.

Short axis echocardiographical views correspond closely to the transverse sections through the ventricles (cut 1, Figure 1.7). Frequently, however, a cut higher than this cut, i.e. midway through the apex to the ventricular groove, is conventionally used (Figure 1.16a).

The apical four-chamber view is another plane frequently used in clinical practice. To correspond with this view the heart is also cut along the long axis but at right angles to the view illustrated in Figures 1.15a and b. This view permits visualization of all four chambers of the heart and is particularly useful in congenital heart disease. Although the specimen cannot be as well repositioned as with the dissection described above, provided that the coronary arteries and valves have been inspected prior to sectioning, this plane also permits examination at a future date if required.

Examination of Atrial and Ventricular Chambers

The Right Atrium (Figures 1.17 and 1.18)

In the right atrium the crista terminalis is usually a well-formed muscle bundle which encircles the right atrial appendage, separating the posterior part, the 'sinus venarum cavarum', from the anterior trabeculated part of the atrial appendage. From the crista the trabecular or pectinate muscles emanate at right angles and sweep towards the opening of the inferior vena cava. The wall of the atrial appendage between the wall of the pectinate muscles can be extremely thin.

In the interatrial septum a rounded depression, the *fossa ovalis*, the floor of which is formed by the embryonic septum primum, can be identified. The fossa is surrounded by a prominent muscular ridge, the *limbus of the fossa ovalis*, which forms a concentric margin superiorly and anteriorly of varying prominence. The opening of the coronary sinus is often guarded by a well-formed valve termed the *Thebesian valve* or *valve of the coronary sinus*. Not infrequently fenestration may be seen.

Similarly, around the inferior vena cava, a valvular structure can be identified which is, however, often vestigial. This is the *Eustachian valve* or *valve of the inferior vena cava*. (Continuation of the valve constitutes the tendon of Todaro.) (Figure 1.18).

Chiari's net Fenestration of the valves of the inferior vena cava and coronary sinus may be excessive (Figure 1.19) which may result in lace-like fibrous strands involving also the crista terminalis. In some instances these strands may criss-cross the right atrial cavity to which the term Chiari's net is applied. This represents remnants of the embryonic right valves of the sinus venosus. Not infrequently some small opening of venous channels can be identified in the interatrial septum.

Probe patency of the fossa ovalis In up to 25% of normal hearts the floor of the fossa ovalis has failed to fuse with the limbus of the foramen ovale anteriorly permitting a probe to be passed between these two structures (Figure 1.20).

Morphological identification of the right atrium In many

complex congenital anomalies the cardiac chambers may not be in their normal position and it is therefore essential that, morphologically, the chambers are identified. During life the blunt shape of the right atrial appendages is helpful. Postmortem, two additional features characterize the right atrium:

(1) the crista terminalis; and

(2) the limbus of the fossa ovalis.

All other structures are variable. Vessels normally entering the chamber may drain into another chamber or may be absent.

The floor of the right atrium is formed by the *tricuspid valve* (Figure 1.21).

Right Ventricle

The tricuspid valve The valve consists of three leaflets, the anterior, septal and posterior leaflets or, when considered *in situ*, septal, antero-superior and inferior leaflets. The three commissures (antero-septal, antero-inferior and inferior) are best identified by fan-shaped chordae tendineae. The three leaflets can each be divided into three zones: the *rough zone* which is the line of closure of the valve, usually 1 mm or so away from the thin free edge: the *clear zone* characterized by the thin translucent portion of the valve leaflet occupying the greatest area and the *basal zone* a few millimetres in width between the clear zone and the annulus or valve ring which is often not well defined (Figure 1.21). On average 25 chordae tendineae of variable length and thickness have been identified[2].

The right ventricle Three papillary muscles can be identified. The anteriorly sited muscle is usually the largest whilst the posteriorly situated papillary muscle often consists of a variable number of small projections; see Figure 1.21.

The septal papillary muscle exhibits great variability and in view of this may be referred to as the 'medial papillary complex'[3] (Figure 1.22).

Another important structure which identifies the right ventricle morphologically is the *crista supraventricularis*, separating superiorly the inlet portion from the outlet portion. This is often a prominent muscular ridge[4]. Its horizontal portion lies just beneath the pulmonary valve. Two limbs can be identified, the parietal part is formed by the right ventricular wall and the septal limb merges with the interventricular septum between the limbs of the trabecula septomarginalis or merges directly with that structure. The trabecula septomarginalis form a prominent ridge on the septal wall of the right ventricle. Towards the apex the trabecula split and become continuous with the papillary muscles. One structure is usually prominent: this is the *moderator band* which crosses the right ventricular cavity. Occasionally several less prominent bands are found (Figure 1.17).

The term 'crista supraventricularis' has in recent years caused much confusion and should be reserved for the normal heart[5].

The *membranous portion of the interventricular septum* can be identified beneath the septal leaflet of the tricuspid valve, best see by translumination or by raising the heart towards the light.

The pulmonary valve (Figure 1.22) This consists of three semilunar-shaped leaflets separated by three commissures. When the heart is *in situ*, valve leaflets are designated posterior, right and left anterior leaflets. In the centre of each semilunar valve along the line of

closure a small fibro-cartilaginous nodule (corpus Arantii) is found from which thin fibrous strands radiate, affording strength to the valve leaflets. The leaflets are attached to the infundibulum of the right ventricle along their convex margin.

Morphological identification of the right ventricle The morphological characteristics which permit identification of the right ventricle are:

(1) the crista superventricularis; and

(2) the medial papillary complex.

The Left Atrium

The morphology of this chamber differs from the right atrium in several important respects. The atrial appendage which also consists of trabeculated muscle is smaller and not demarcated by a muscular ridge. The small opening of the appendage and the large smooth-walled portion of the chamber can easily be identified. Furthermore, the limbus of the fossa ovalis is absent. At the site of the fossa ovalis some fibro-muscular strands can sometimes be observed (Figure 1.23). The pulmonary veins drain into the left atrium, usually as four separate channels, the right and left superior and right and left inferior veins. They enter the chamber usually at the site of the superior rounded portion (Figure 1.23). Occasionally, variations of the veins are observed.

Morphological identification of the left atrium The morphological characteristics permitting identification of the left atrium are, apart from the smaller atrial appendage:

(1) absence of the crista terminalis; and

(2) absence of the limbus of the fossa ovalis.

Left Ventricle

The mitral valve The mitral valve consists of two leaflets, the larger anterior leaflet and the narrow posterior leaflet, separated by two commissures: the postero-medial and the antero-lateral (Figure 1.24). The anterior leaflet is triangular in shape and has been likened to a curtain, whilst the posterior leaflet is flatter and characteristically subdivided by clefts into scallops. Usually, three scallops can be identified: the postero-medial, the middle and the antero-lateral, but great variation exists. The posterior leaflet, like all the leaflets of the tricuspid valve are subdivided into rough, clear and basal zones. The anterior leaflet, in contrast, consists of rough and clear zones only, being continuous with the aortic valve.

On average, like the tricuspid valve, 25 chordae have been found including two fan-shaped chordae identifying the site of the commissures[6].

Two papillary muscles, the postero-medial and antero-lateral are identified (Figure 1.25). Considerable variation is found, particularly in the postero-medial muscle. This may be represented by a single pillar-like structure or be composed of several smaller heads of differing size.

The left ventricle is cone-shaped and its inner wall shows fine trabeculation. The wall thickness diminishes towards the apex, at which level it may only be 1 to 2 mm thick. The apex and part of the interventricular septum of the outflow tract are also trabeculated but as the aortic valve is approached the wall becomes smooth. In contrast to the right ventricle, no muscular bands akin to the crista superventricularis or papillary conus are present.

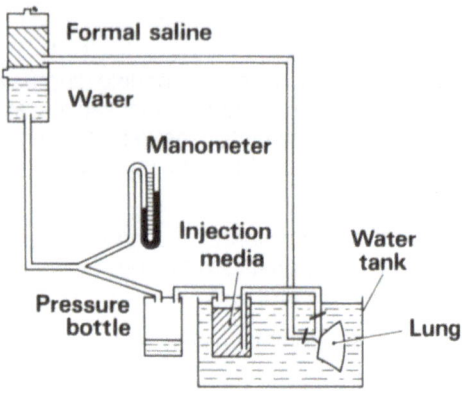

Figure 1.4 Diagrammatic representation of the apparatus for injection of pulmonary or coronary vessels

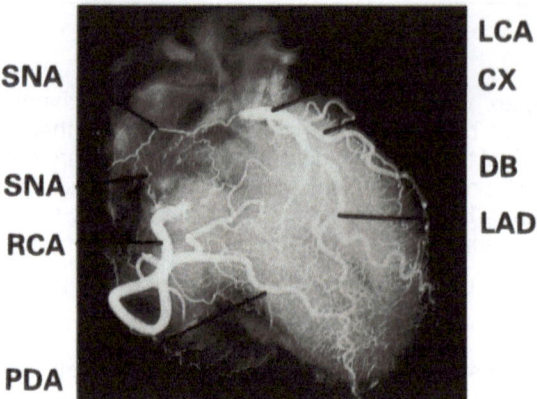

Figure 1.5 Normal coronary arteriogram; SNA = Sinus node artery (arising from right and left coronary arteries); RCA = Right coronary artery; PDA = Posterior descending artery; LAD = Left anteror descending branch of the left coronary artery; DB = Diagonal branch; CX = Circumflex artery; LCA = Left coronary artery

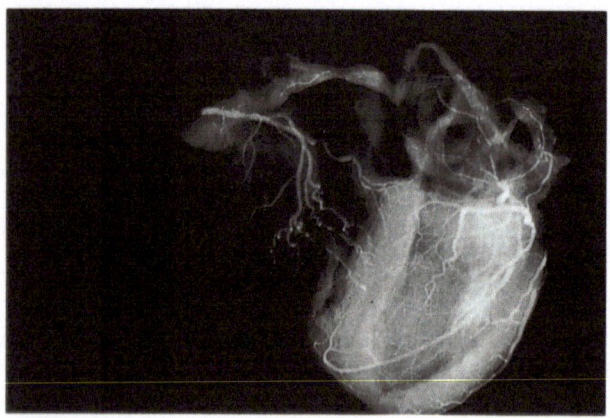

Figure 1.6 The right ventricle has been opened anteriorly close to the interventricular septum after injecting the coronary arteries. The coronary artery has been cut close to its origin from the aorta. The cut has been extended through the right atrium. The entire right side of the heart has been unfolded to allow visualization of the right coronary artery

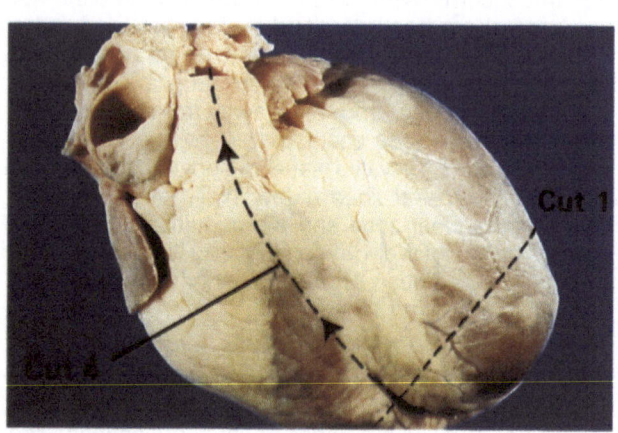

Figure 1.7 Anterior (ventral) view of the heart. The first cut should be made 3–4 cm above the apex, parallel to the atrio-ventricular groove

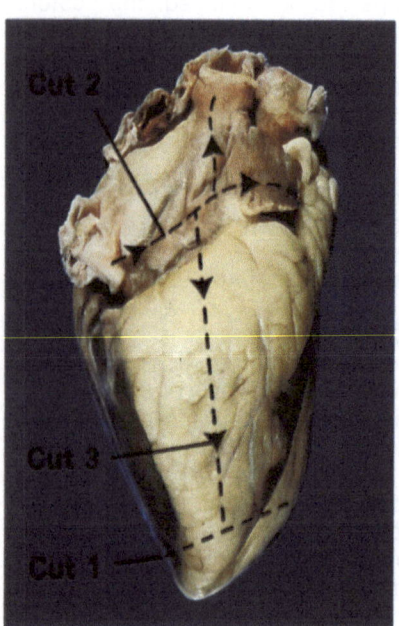

Figure 1.8 The heart viewed from the acute margin. The second cut is made 0.5–1 cm in front of the opening of the inferior vena cava and extended 0.5 cm above and parallel to the atrio-ventricular junction. For better visualization a vertical cut towards the superior vena cara can be made, avoiding the region of the sinuatrial node. The third cut is then made along the acute margin to join up with cut 1

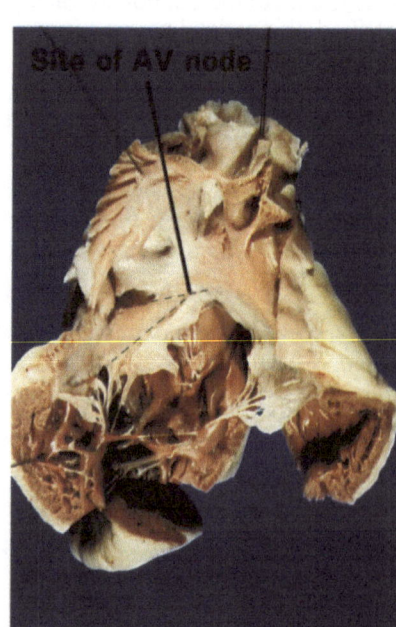

Figure 1.9 The right atrium and inflow part of the right ventricle are now open. The dashed lines localize the atrio-ventricular node (see text)

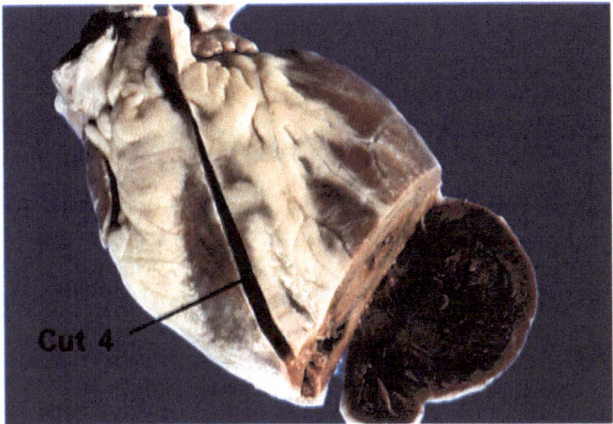

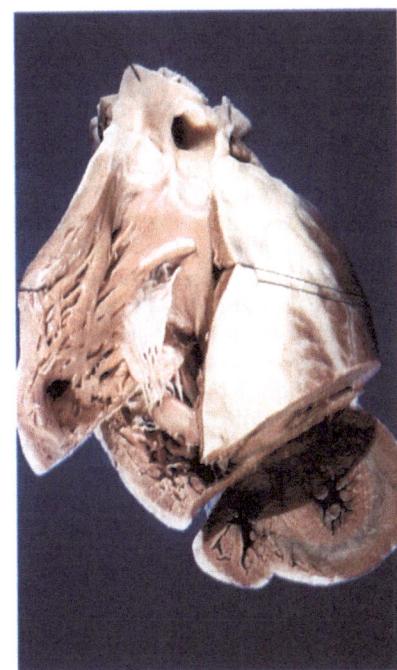

Figure 1.10b The out-flow part of the right ventricle and pulmonary valve are now open

Figure 1.10a To display the outflow part of the right ventricle a cut close to the interventricular septum is made extending from cut one through the pulmonary valve and pulmonary trunk

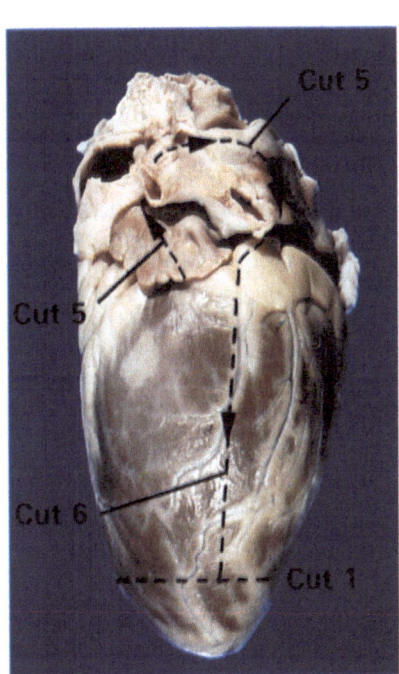

Figure 1.11 The heart viewed from the obtuse margin. The left atrial appendage is incised and a cut is made across 'the roof' of the left atrium between left and right pulmonary veins and directed in such a way as to reach the obtuse margin which is then cut to join cut one

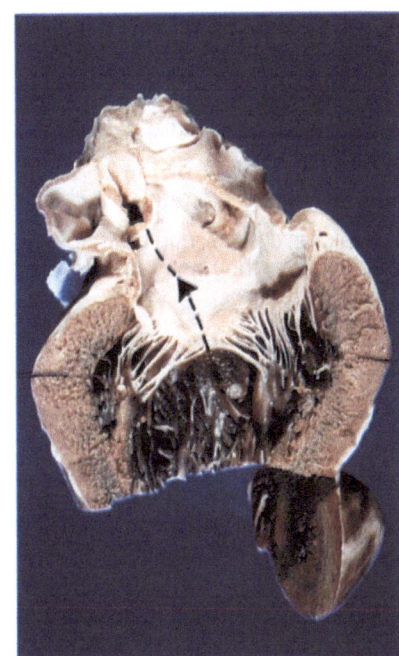

Figure 1.12 The left atrium and mitral valve and inflow part of the left ventricle are now open ready for closer inspection

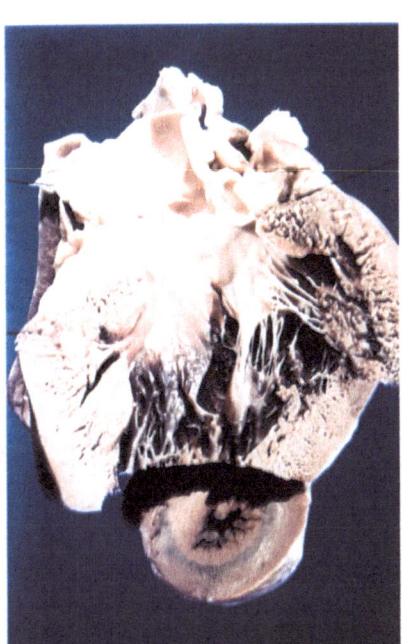

Figure 1.13 A wedge of the anterior wall of the left ventricle has been made to include the chordae tendineae of the mitral valve and extended to the aorta displaying the outflow tract of the left ventricle

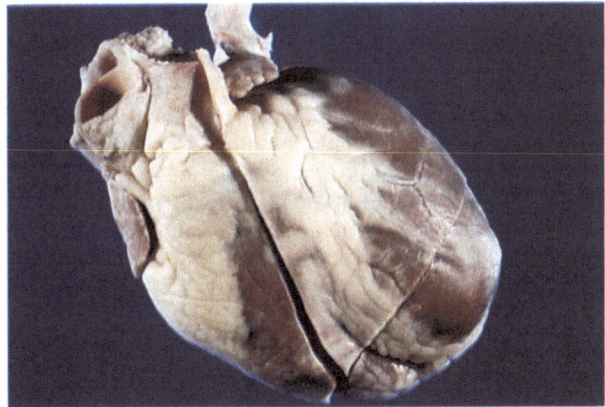

Figure 1.14 All opened chambers have been repositioned; the anatomy of the heart has not been distorted

The aortic valve The aortic valve, like the pulmonary valve, is composed of three leaflets and nowadays these are referred to as the right and left coronary and non-coronary cusps according to the ostia of the coronary arteries arising from the sinuses. The valve leaflets vary in size. In the majority of cases the right coronary cusp is most frequently the largest, followed in frequency by the non-coronary cusp. Only rarely are the three leaflets identical in size. The structure of the semilunar valves is similar to the pulmonary valve and corpora Arantii and fibrous strands can be identified (Figure 1.26).

Parts of the non-coronary and left coronary cusps are in fibrous continuity with the anterior leaflet of the mitral valve. The non-coronary cusp is in fibrous continuity with the central fibrous body and the membranous septum. Anteriorly the non-coronary cusp and posteriorly the left coronary cusp are anchored to the muscular portion of the aortic outlet and the annulus (forming part of the fibrous skeleton of the heart). The aortic sinuses are part of the root of the aorta. When the aortic valve leaflets are open a line can sometimes be identified, the so-called aortic bar.

Morphological identification of the left ventricle The morphological characteristics which identify the left ventricle are:

(1) absence of the crista supraventricularis; and

(2) absence of the papillary muscle of the conus or chordae tendineae straddling the outflow portion.

In addition, the shape, which is conical, and the trabeculation, which is finer compared to the right ventricle, also form positive identifiable features.

Muscle Bundles of the Heart

Most workers studying the arrangement of the muscle bundles of the heart are agreed that superficial, middle and deep layers can be defined. Methods of investigation have included boiling of the heart in acetic acid and 'unfolding' the bundles, injection of plastic material and dissection. It has been found that no two hearts are the same.

The diagrammatic presentation of Wartman and Souders[7] is convenient (Figure 1.27). The apex is composed of spirally arranged superficial fibres which are split into superficial and deep layers by the deep bulbo-spiral muscle in the left ventricle and the deep sino-spiral muscle in the right ventricle. Superficial fibres also make up the papillary muscles.

A different approach was made by Rodbard in 1973[8] who, by injecting intramuscularly monomeric liquid methyl methacrylate, was able to define sets of concentric bands of muscle fibres arranged as incomplete discs. Numerous discs constituted a compartment (the ventricular muscle was made up of nine such discrete compartments) and three suborgans:

(1) inlet or cushion (mitral and tricuspid valve rings, valves and papillary muscles);

(2) pump or ventricle;

(3) outlet or infundibulum (spirally arranged) and origin of the pulmonary artery and aorta.

More recently Anderson *et al.* in 1980, by dissecting a single heart, largely confirmed the arrangement of muscle bundles described by previous workers earlier this century, but various points of different emphasis have emerged. These include that separation into superficial, middle and deep layers is not distinct and that the role of the fibrous skeleton of the heart in affording support for the muscle mass has previously been overstated. The integration of the right ventricular papillary muscle into the left ventricular fibre system was also emphasized. The left ventricular fibre arrangement was actually spiral superficially and circular in the main muscle mass but with a tendency for fibres to run in the ventricular long axis in the deep layers, particularly in the papillary muscles[9].

Localization of the Main Components of the Conduction System

Sinus Node

This structure is situated beneath the summit of the right atrium and is most easily located by identifying the superior vena cava and the crest of the right atrial appendage. At the junction of these two structures the sulcus terminalis is found and the node is often sited slightly towards the lateral aspect of the superior vena caval/atrial junction (Figure 1.28)[10]. Identification with the naked eye of the nodal artery and tissue is possible.

Atrio-ventricular Node

This node is situated in the right atrium in the base of the interatrial septum at the apex of the triangle of Koch (at the central fibrous body). This triangle is formed by the tendon of Todaro (continuation of the Eustachian valve) and the annulus of the tricuspid valve. A convenient way to localize the node is to draw an imaginary line from the opening of the coronary sinus to the centre of the septal leaflet of the tricuspid valve, at that point is the site of the node which corresponds to the apex of the triangle of Koch (Figure 1.29).

The Bundle of His

This is a continuation of the atrio-ventricular node and entering the central fibrous body becomes the penetrating atrio-ventricular bundle. On leaving the central fibrous body it reaches the crest of the muscular septum beneath the membranous septum. A quick method for inspecting the bundle at autopsy is to make an incision in the left ventricle through the lower part of the membranous septum into the muscular crest (Figure 1.30).

Bundle branches As soon as the bundle has left the central fibrous body, branches arise on the left in a series of flat bands over a distance of approximately 2 cm. The bands are situated subendocardially and can often be identified with the naked eye. Three major radiations can usually be identified, the posterior, middle and anterior radiations, but great variation is present. Occasionally, a small branch of a muscle bundle leaves the subendocardial position and crosses the ventricular cavity (Figure 1.30). The bundle continues as the right bundle, initially subendocardial, then continues in an intramuscular position near the medial papillary muscle complex and within the trabecula septomarginalis to reach the moderator band where it again becomes subendocardial in position.

The Coronary Arterial System and Venous Drainage

Two main arteries supply the myocardium (Figure 1.31).

Left Coronary Artery

The vessel arises from the left coronary sinus of Valsalva and passes to the left across the root of the aorta to reach the interventricular sulcus. The main stem is usually short, rarely exceeding 2.5 cm; it divides usually into two or, occasionally, three branches.

(1) Left anterior descending branch. This vessel runs into the interventricular sulcus to the apex. Several branches arise from this vessel, the largest of which is the diagonal artery; its origin is variable but not infrequently it arises proximally.

(2) The circumflex artery courses to the left to reach the atrio-ventricular sulcus. Its extent varies greatly, depending on the dominance of vascular supply (please see below). If large, it reaches the posterior interventricular sulcus and may form the posterior descending artery.

One of the largest branches of the circumflex artery is termed the marginal artery which courses anteriorly and diagonally towards the obtuse margin and apex.

(3) In about a third of cases a third branch arises from the main stem of the left coronary artery between the left anterior descending branch and the circumflex artery, coursing obliquely across the anterior left ventricle.

The Right Coronary Artery

This vessel arises from the sinus guarded by the right coronary cusp, courses behind the pulmonary trunk to reach the right atrioventricular groove where it continues to form the posterior descending artery in the posterior interventricular sulcus in cases of right dominant vascular supply. In the region of the acute margin the marginal artery frequently arises. Other branches include:

(1) the conus artery;

(2) the artery to the sinus node; and

(3) the artery to the atrioventricular node which arises from a U loop formed by the right coronary artery after the posterior descending branch has been given off (in cases of right dominance). In its course the right coronary artery supplies innumerable branches to the right atrium and, depending on the dominance, the posterior aspect of the left atrium also.

Dominance of the Coronary Arterial Blood Supply

This is determined by the vessel which forms the posterior descending artery. Data of dominance vary. For right dominance an incidence of 48–85% has been reported but for left dominance between 9.5 and 19.4%. Balance of blood supply is present when both the right and left circumflex coronary arteries form parallel channels around the posterior interventricular sulcus. An incidence of between 3.5 and 34% has been reported[1].

Blood Supply of Other Areas to the Heart

The diaphragmatic surface of the left ventricle receives dual blood supply in about 70% of cases, in 20% from the right and 10% from the left coronary artery only. The interventricular septum is predominantly supplied by the left anterior descending branch of the left coronary artery.

Anastomoses between Left and Right Coronary Arteries

These occur frequently and are widely distributed throughout the myocardium. An important anastomosis between the right and left coronary arteries is the so-called Kugel's artery[11], coursing in the interatrial septum.

Venous Drainage

The coronary veins accompany the coronary arteries. The great cardiac vein accompanies the anterior descending artery of the left coronary artery. It reaches the left atrioventricular sulcus and receives venous channels from the obtuse margin forming the coronary sinus.

The middle cardiac vein runs in the posterior longitudinal sulcus accompanying the artery in that site, opening near the proximal part of the coronary sinus (Figure 1.32). The small cardiac vein accompanies the right coronary artery draining near the opening of the coronary sinus in the right atrium.

Numerous unnamed venous channels course posteriorly over the left ventricle, the longest of which is called the posterior vein of the left ventricle. Anteriorly, several venous channels can also be identified, emptying either into a small coronary vein or into the right heart directly.

The oblique vein of the left atrium can sometimes be identified at the posterior aspect of that chamber. It represents the left common cardinal vein of the embryo.

The coronary sinus is formed by the confluence of great cardiac vein and those channels draining the obtuse margin. It runs in the atrio-ventricular groove parallel to the circumflex artery of the left coronary artery. It receives the vessels named above.

Lymphatic Drainage

This consists of two networks: the endocardial and the epicardial.

Small capillary-sized channels form in the subendocardial region and in the myocardium and drain towards the subepicardium. These networks are densely and evenly distributed. Five orders, according to their size in ascending order, have been described[12]. Two main collecting trunks pass into the mediastinum.

Nerve Supply of the Heart

The heart receives its innervation by both sympathetic and parasympathetic components of the autonomic nervous system.

Sympathetic System

Efferent nerves arise from the lateral grey columns of the upper four or five dorsal segments and reach, as myelinated fibres, adjacent ganglia. From these ganglia they relay into thoracic nerves to reach the cardiac plexus or reach cervical ganglia (upper, middle and inferior) and relay as unmyelinated posterior ganglionic fibres passing in three cervical cardiac nerves to the cardiac plexus.

Afferent impulses reach the dorsal root ganglia of the upper four or five spinal nerves and via synapses in the posterior and lateral grey matter of the spinal cord, reach the hypothalamus or cortex.

Parasympathetic System

Fibres arise in the vagal nuclei, the nucleus ambiguus, and run in the vagi as preganglionic myelinated fibres to

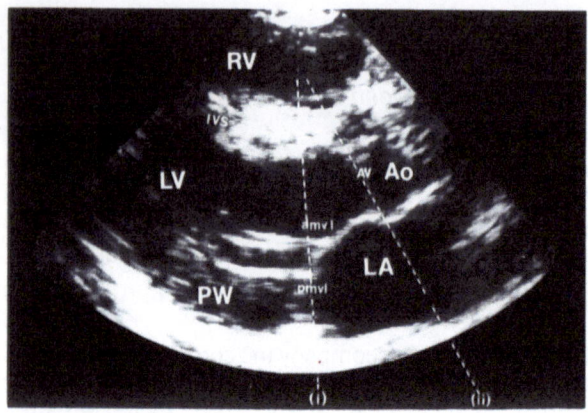

Figure 1.15a Echocardiograph of the parasternal long axis view of the left ventricle: RV = Right ventricle; IVS = Interventricular septum; LV = Left ventricle; PW = Posterior wall; pmvl = Posterior mitral valve leaflet; amvl = Anterior mitral valve leaflet; AV = Aortic valve; AO = Aorta; LA = Left atrium. (By courtesy of Dr R. M. Donaldson)

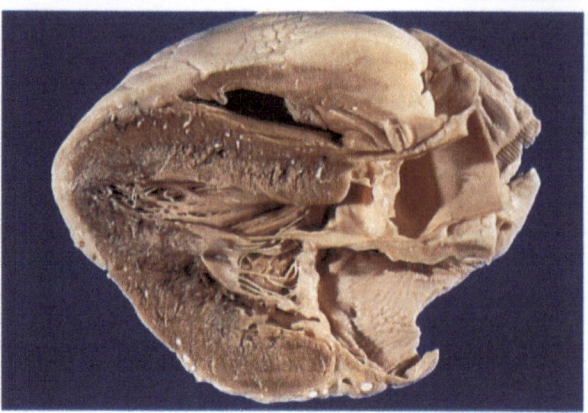

Figure 1.15b The normal heart has been dissected to correspond with the plane illustrated in Figure 1.15a. By convention, the apex is to the left of the posterior wall of the left ventricle at the lower border.

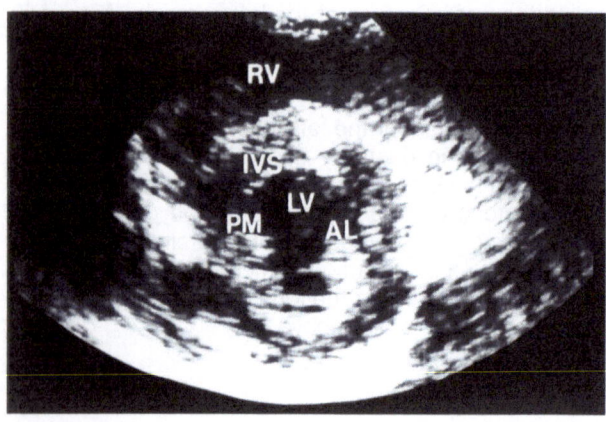

Figure 1.16a Parasternal short axis view at the level of the antero-lateral and postero-medial papillary muscles: RV = Right ventricle; IVS = Interventricular septum; PM = Postero-medial papillary muscle; LV = Left ventricle; AL = Anterolateral papillary muscle. (By courtesy of Dr R. M. Donaldson)

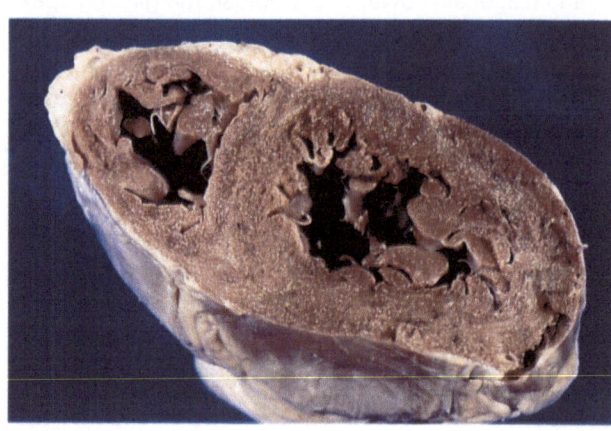

Figure 1.16b Cross-section of the heart view from below corresponding with Figure 1.16a

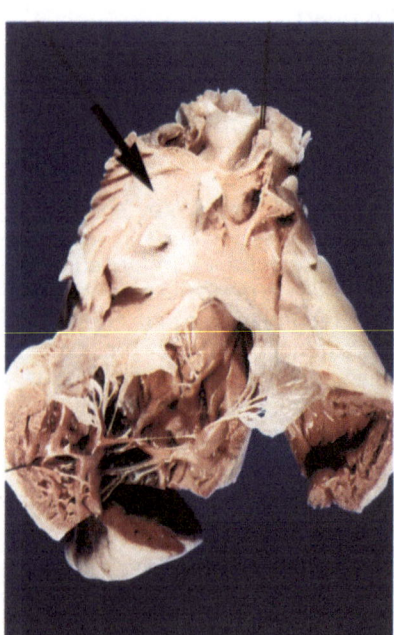

Figure 1.17 General view of the right atrium. The crista terminalis (arrowed) separating the smooth from the trabeculated part is a muscular ridge from which the pectinate muscles emanate

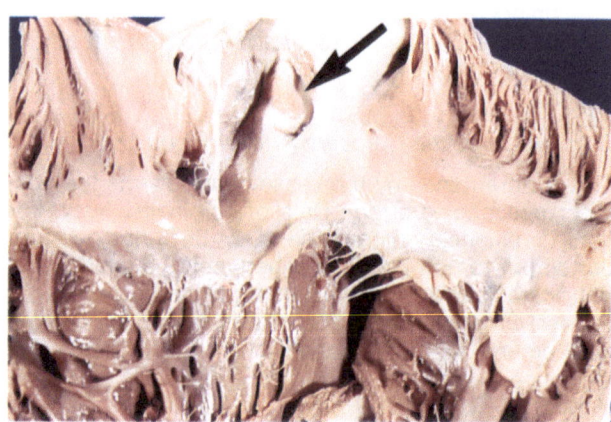

Figure 1.18 The valve guarding the sinus venosus (Thebesian valve) is fenestrated. The limbus (arrowed) of the fossa ovalis encircles the fossa. The valve guarding the inferior vena cava (Eustachian valve) can be seen at the upper border of the illustration

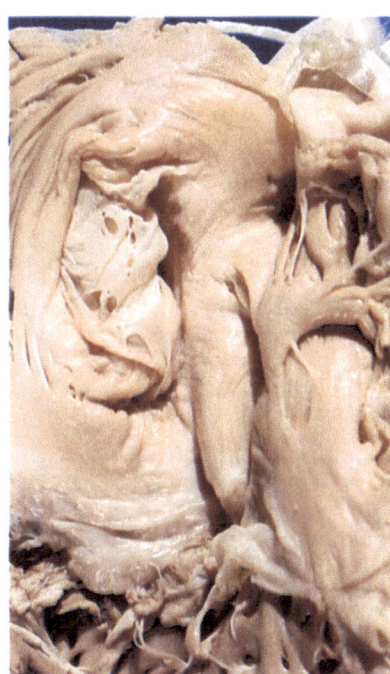

Figure 1.19 Fenestration of the valve guarding the inferior vena cava and coronary sinus is shown. If a lace-like pattern is noted, criss-crossing the right atrium, the term 'Chiari's net' applies

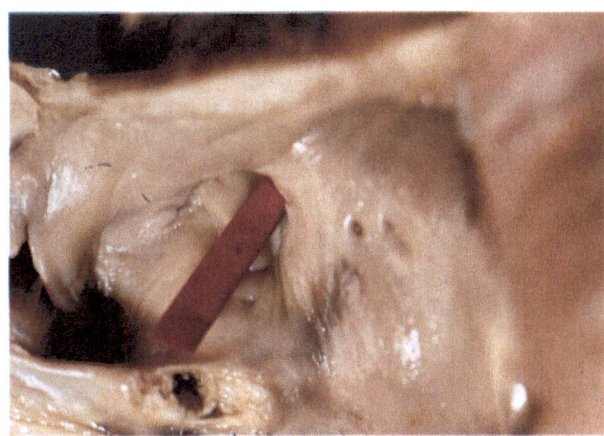

Figure 1.20 Probe patency is present. The red tape passes between the limbus of the fossa ovalis and the septum primum which forms the floor of the fossa ovalis

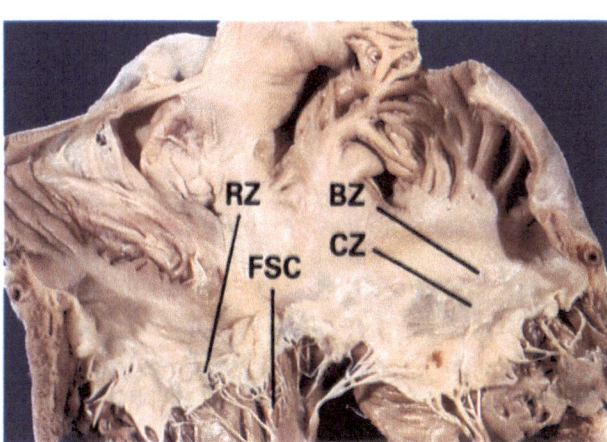

Figure 1.21 View of the tricuspid valve. The thickened band represents the line of closure, the 'rough zone'. This is followed by the clear zone, best see in the large anterior leaflet. The basal zone is a few millimetres thick, adjacent to the valve ring. The septal leaflet is ill-defined as is often the case. The fan-shaped chordae define the commissures. RZ = Rough zone; CZ = Clear zone; FSC = Fan-shaped chordae; BZ = Basal zone

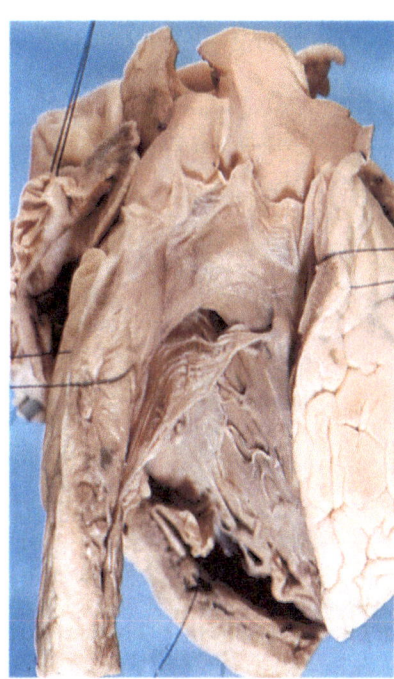

Figure 1.22 The medial papillary complex. One muscular projection can be clearly seen into which chordae insert. In addition, a minute muscular projection can also be seen as well as direct insertion of chordae tendineae into the septal muscle of the right ventricular outflow tract. Note the crista supraventricularis, the thick muscular band beneath the pulmonary valve

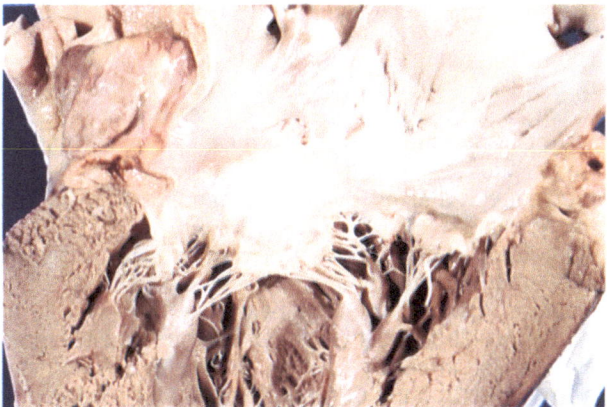

Figure 1.23 The left atrium is displayed to show the absence of the features that are found in the right atrium and opening of the pulmonary veins. In the region of the fossa ovalis some trabeculation can be seen. Note the uniform thick endocardium of the chamber

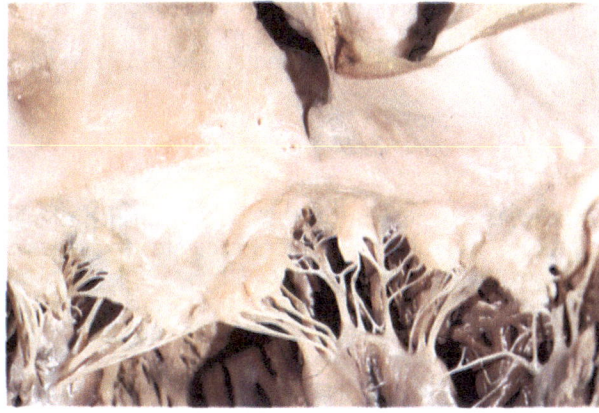

Figure 1.24 Close-up view of the mitral valve. (For full description, please see text)

the ganglia of the cardiac plexus. Short postganglionic fibres enter the heart. A variable number of parasympathetic cardiac branches, as well as superior, middle and inferior nerves, anastomose with the sympathetic nervous system.

Afferent fibres reach the inferior vagal ganglia and from there impulses reach the dorsal vagal nuclei, cardiac nucleus and formatio reticularis.

The Cardiac Plexus

Consists of a superficial part situated in the aortic arch and the deeper portion situated between the bifurcation of the trachea.

Dimensions of the Heart

Heart Weights

Tables are readily available for weights of the heart. They are calculated, among other things, according to body length or body weight. Table 1.1 is modified from Zeek[3].

Table 1.1   Adult heart weights (g)

Height		Male	Female
150 cm	(4′ 11″)	243–323	215–275
152 cm	(5′ 0″)	249–329	221–281
155 cm	(5′ 1″)	252–332	224–284
160 cm	(5′ 3″)	262–342	233–293
165 cm	(5′ 5″)	271–351	242–302
170 cm	(5′ 7″)	281–361	251–311
175 cm	(5′ 9″)	290–370	260–320
180 cm	(5′ 11″)	300–380	269–329
183 cm	(6′ 0″)	306–386	274–334
185 cm	(6′ 1″)	309–389	277–337
191 cm	(6′ 3″)	319–399	286–346

Heart weights in children have been tabulated by Roessle and Roulet in 1932[14], and by Coppoletta and Wolbach in 1933[15], and in the foetus right and left ventricular weights have been recorded by Hislop and Reid in 1972[16].

Weighing of the heart is often inaccurate and should only be undertaken after the chambers have been opened and blood clot has been removed. Up to 30 g is within the margin of error. For more accurate assessment the procedure mentioned in Chapter 3 should be followed.

Heart Wall Measurements

Atrial walls measure between 2 and 2.5 mm in thickness. Conal measurements are more accurate for assessing right ventricular wall thickness as this avoids erroneous inclusion of trabecula. Measurements are taken 1 to 1.5 cm below the pulmonary valve (along cut 3), 2 to 3 mm in thickness is deemed normal

Left ventricular wall thickness is best measured along the obtuse margin (cut 6) approximately 1 to 1.5 cm below the posterior leaflet of the mitral valve; 12 to 15 mm thickness is normal.

Measurements of the walls of diseased hearts have to be interpreted with great caution as dilatation is a frequent accompaniment of hypertrophy. In extreme cases wall measurements may be normal or thinner than normal and heart weight more than double.

Valve Measurements

It is usual to record the diameter of the valves or the circumference (by cones) prior to opening. If opened, linear measurements are as shown in Table 1.2.

Table 1.2   Heart valve measurements

	Linear (mm)	Diameter (mm)
Tricuspid valve	110–130	36
Pulmonary valve	75–85	23
Mitral valve	90–110	27
Aortic valve	70–80	20

Cardiac Chamber Volumes

Volumes of cardiac chambers can variously be assessed (see references 17 and 18). Approximate values are:

Right atrium 79 ml
Right ventricle 70 ml
Left atrium 57 ml
Left ventricle 43 ml.

Histology of the Heart

The Pericardium

The parietal part of the pericardium is lined by mesothelial cells. The outer layer is composed of interwoven bundles of collagen tissue (Figure 1.33).

The Epicardium

The epicardium is superficially lined by mesothelial cells. In addition, adipose tissue, blood and lymph vessels can be identified (Figure 1.34).

The Myocardium

Ventricular muscle fibres or cardiocytes are between 50 and 100 µm long and typically show a branching pattern (Figure 1.35). The diameter of the fibres varies between 5 and 12 µm, although up to 15 µm is considered normal by some workers. Each cardiocyte consists of a sarcoplasm in which contractile elements which are the functional units of the cell, are contained. The nucleus is usually centrally placed, fusiform or vesicular in shape. The nucleus is often surrounded by a clear zone in which lipofuchsin granules can be found. The cell is enveloped by a fine membrane, the sarcolemma, which is in direct contact with the endomysium. Cross-striation, dark anisotropic and light isotropic bands can be seen on haematoxylin and eosin preparation but are better observed in preparations stained by phosphotungstic acid–haematoxylin (Figure 1.36).

Intercalated discs can also be discerned histologically. The structures are however better seen on semi-thin or electron microscopic examination (see below).

The muscle fibres are aggregated into bundles separated by thin strands of connective tissue, the endomysium. Larger groups of myocardial fibres are separated by wider strands, the perimysium, which contain collagen fibres. The perimysium is continuous with the endocardium and the epicardium. Both the endomysium and perimysium are rich in blood supply.

Atrial muscle fibres are thinner and longer than ventricular muscle fibres (Figure 1.37). The nuclei are often vesicular and exhibit great variation in size. The perinuclear clear zone is often more prominent than in the ventricular cardiocytes. Adipose tissue is also frequent and fibro-elastic strands connecting the epicardium with the endocardium can often easily be identified.

The Endocardium

In the left atrium the endocardium measures up to 300 μm in thickness (Figure 1.38a and b) whilst the right atrial endocardium measures up to 100 μm in thickness only (Figure 1.39). The ventricular endocardium is significantly thinner. In the left ventricle the inflow tract measures only 10 μm while in the outflow tract it measures 20 μm in thickness (Figure 1.40). Right ventricular measurements are 7 μm in the inflow and 10 μm in the outflow tract[19]. The endocardium is composed of an endothelial lining, collagen tissue, elastic fibres and smooth muscle.

Valves

Irrespective of the site of the valve, each consists of a layer of collagen tissue, a layer rich in elastic tissue and an intervening zone of varying prominence, the zona spongiosa[20]. The collagen tissue layer, also referred to as the 'holding face', faces the chamber or great vessel when the valve is closed and against which pressure builds up. The elastic tissue is also known as the 'deformed face' (Figure 1.41).

Thick-walled vessels of capillary size have been clearly demonstrated[21]. They are usually confined to the bases of the valves but may on rare occasions be found elsewhere approaching the free edge. Thin-walled capillary and lymphatic channels have also been documented extending throughout the leaflets especially those of the atrio-ventricular valves and chordae tendineae[22].

Conduction Tissue

This differs in many important respects from myocardial tissue. Conduction tissue is thinner (2 to 7 μm) than myocardial tissue. It consists of loosely interwoven and anastomotic strands. Cross-striation is less prominent and the fibres stain less strongly with haematoxylin and eosin as there are fewer myofibrils present (Figure 1.42). Nuclei are oval in shape.

Within the various components of the conduction system differences in cell type exist.

The sinus node is arranged around the artery to the node and tapers distally in a carrot-shaped fashion (Figure 1.43). It is 2 to 3 mm in length. Several small arteries can additionally be identified. The nodal tissue is embedded in fibrous tissue, increasing with age. Elastic tissue and adipose tissue are also found, particularly in the elderly.

It has been suggested that fibrous tissue increases up to the age of 40 years, elastic tissue throughout life and adipose tissue after the age of 40 years[23]. These changes are however not constant[24].

Histochemistry

Glycogen is patchily distributed throughout the myocardial cells (Figure 1.44) but focal accumulation around the nuclear poles is frequently found. Succinic dehydrogenase is located in the mitochondria and is distributed focally throughout the myocardium with aggregates around the nuclear poles (Figure 1.45). Lipid droplets are usually not present in normal cells.

In valvar tissue the zona spongiosa, the layer between the collagen tissue and elastic tissue layers is rich in acid mucopolysaccharides staining blue with Alcian Blue stain (pH 2.5) (Figure 1.46).

Ultrastructure

The myocardium is considered to be a functional syncytium.

The sarcolemma (plasmalemma) envelops the myocardial cell or cardiocyte and is 8 to 9 nm thick. It frequently has a scalloped appearance, considered to be a fixation artefact. At its outer aspect the sarcolemma is invested with a 20 to 30 nm wide external lamina (basement membrane) (Figure 1.47).

The transverse tubular system (T system) is formed by invaginations of the sarcolemma penetrating transversely the cardiocytes (a longitudinal T system linking the transverse tubules is also identified).

Surface vesicles are formed by pouches of the sarcolemma.

The Intercalated Disc

This is in continuity with the sarcolemma and consists of opposing membranes, running a convoluted path if the cell meets end to end. A gap between opposing membranes is identified in which specialized regions are recognized: the fascia adhaerens, desmosomes (macula adhaerens, 200 to 400 nm in diameter) and the nexus (fascia occludens or tight junction) the region wherein the interstitial gap is at its narrowest (2 to 3 nm) (Figure 1.48).

The Sarcotubular System

This is another system, consisting of a network of fine tubules, continuous throughout the cell. Special areas of contact (coupling) with the plasmolemma or its extension which forms the T tubules is found but without communication with the extra-cellular space.

The term 'Z tubules' is applied to the tubules found in the vicinity of the Z bands (Figure 1.47).

Contractile Apparatus

The functional unit of the working cardiocyte is the sarcomere, the area between two Z bands. Each sarcomere is made up of thick (myosin, 0.1 nm × 10 nm) and thin filaments (actin, 1 nm × 5 nm) interdigitating, which results in the characteristic bands. The A band contains myosin and actin filaments. In the centre of the H zone only myosin filaments are present (seen in the relaxed state). The M band is a high density band, in which the thick filaments are held together at their mid-point. The L zone is a low density band. Each A band is flanked by a light band (I band) composed of actin filaments only. In the Z band, the I band filaments form a basket-weave and provide points of insertion of two sarcomeres (Figure 1.47).

Mitochondria

These structures provide the main energy supply of the cardiocyte and are situated between myocardial fibrils and at their nuclear poles. They are rounded or oval in shape (4 nm × 1 nm) limited by membranes, the inner layer of which is folded into cristae (Figure 1.47).

The Nucleus

This is usually centrally situated, oval or fusiform in shape and has a double-layered membrane in which

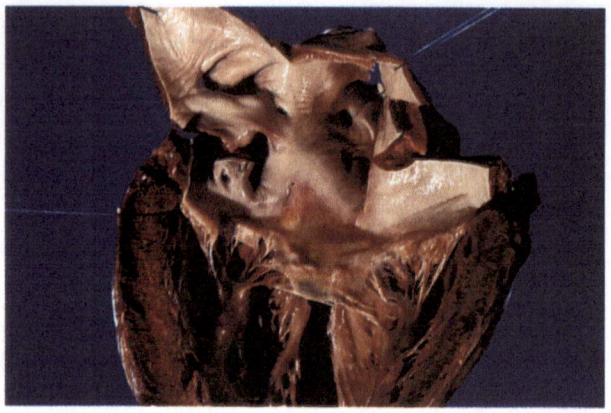

Figure 1.25   The left ventricle has been opened along the obtuse margin to show the two papillary muscles. By rotating the heart for illustration the postero-medial muscle lies at the right and the antero-lateral on the left side of the illustration

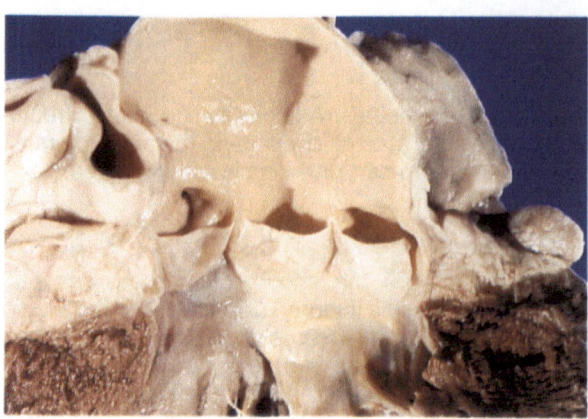

Figure 1.26   Illustration of the three leaflets of the aortic valve. The ostium of the right coronary artery can be seen

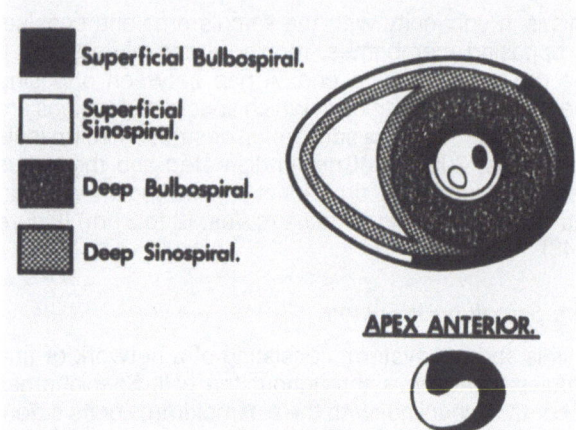

Figure 1.27   Diagrammatic representation of the arrangement of the muscle bundles, modified from Wartman and Souders[7] (By permission of The Macmillan Press Limited, London and Basingstoke)

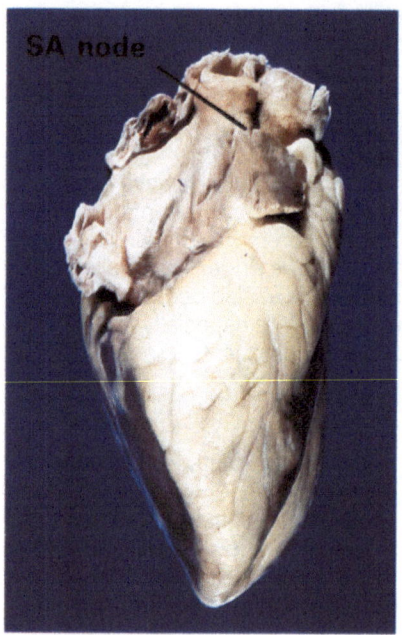

Figure 1.28   Localization of the sinus node which is located in the crest of the right atrial appendage, close to the junction of the superior vena cava but it may be slightly lateral in position

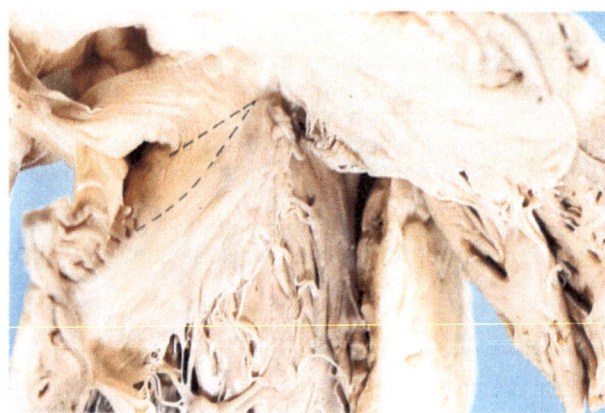

Figure 1.29   Localization of the atrio-ventricular node, sited at the apex of the triangle of Koch

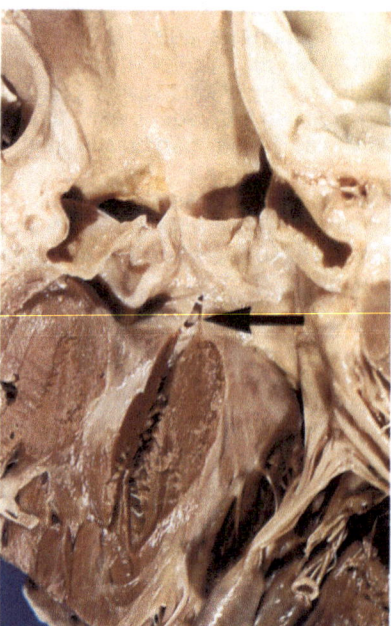

Figure 1.30   A cut has been made through the lower part of the membranous septum of the muscular interventricular septum to display the bundle of His, which is the brown triangular area surrounded by fibrous tissue (the central fibrous body) (arrowed). Three radiations of the left bundle can also be seen, two of which cross the left ventricular cavity

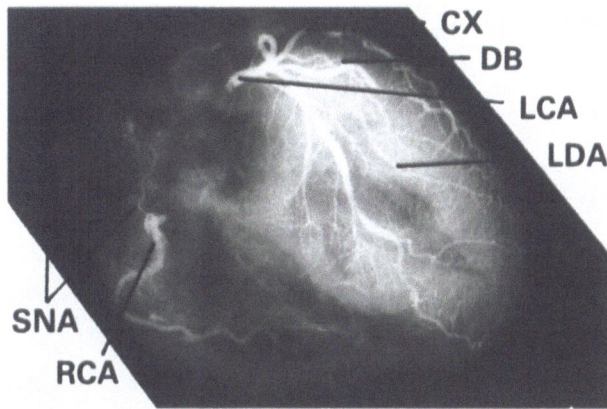

Figure 1.31 Coronary arteriogram; SNA = Sinus node artery (arising from right and left coronary arteries); RCA = Right coronary artery; LAD = Left anterior descending branch of the left coronary artery; DB = Diagonal branch; CX = Circumflex artery; LCA = Left coronary artery

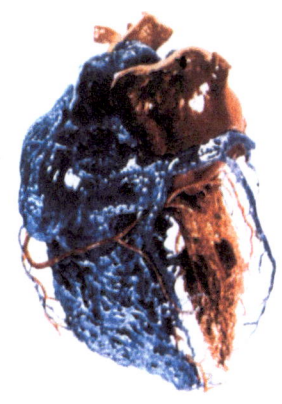

Figure 1.32 Resin-injected model of the posterior (dorsal) view. The right side of the heart is coloured blue, the left red. The coronary sinus runs in the atrio-ventricular groove encircling the left atrium. The middle and small cardiac veins are clearly seen (From the collection of the Pathology Museum of the Hammersmith Hospital, Royal Postgraduate Medical School)

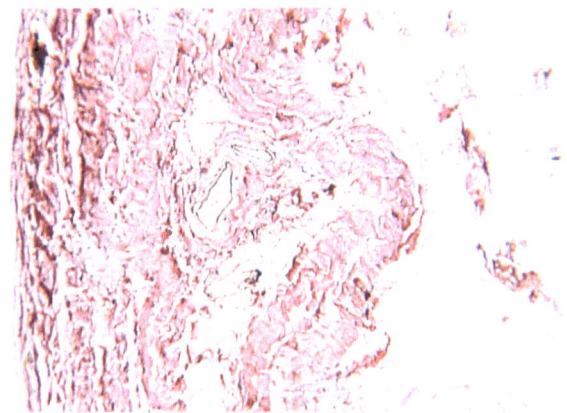

Figure 1.33 Photomicrograph of the parietal layer of the pericardium showing interwoven bundles of collagen, arterioles and an occasional focus of adipose tissue surrounded by collagen tissue. Elastic van Gieson × 50

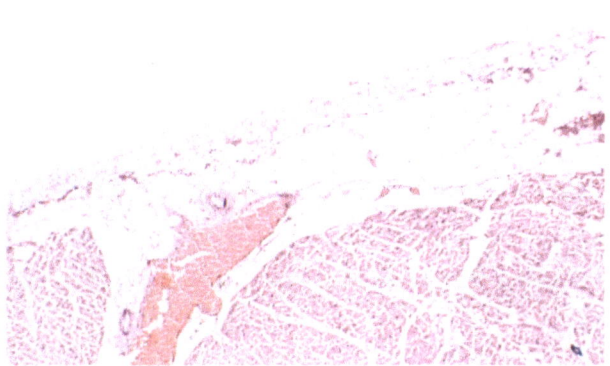

Figure 1.34 The superficial layer of the epicardium also consists of collagen tissue which is covered by mesothelial cells. A layer of adipose tissue, rich in vascular elements, intervenes between that layer and the myocardium. H & E × 25

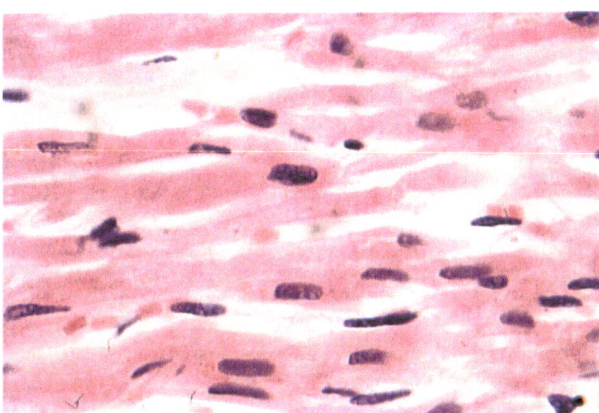

Figure 1.35 Photomicrograph of ventricular cardiocytes, the nuclei of which are fusiform in shape. They may have a more compact chromatin pattern or they may be vesicular. H & E × 200

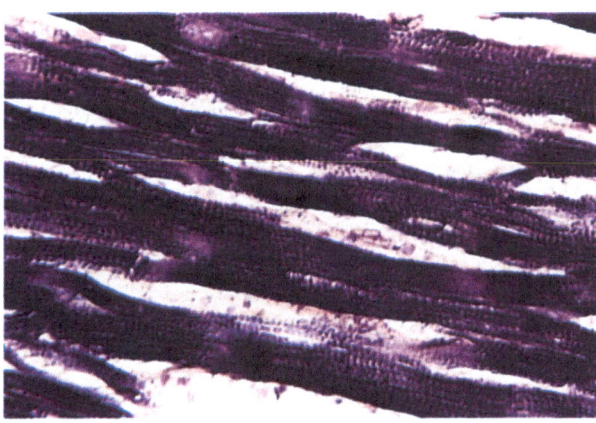

Figure 1.36 Striation of normal myocardial fibres (cardiocytes). Phosphotungstic acid–haematoxylin × 250

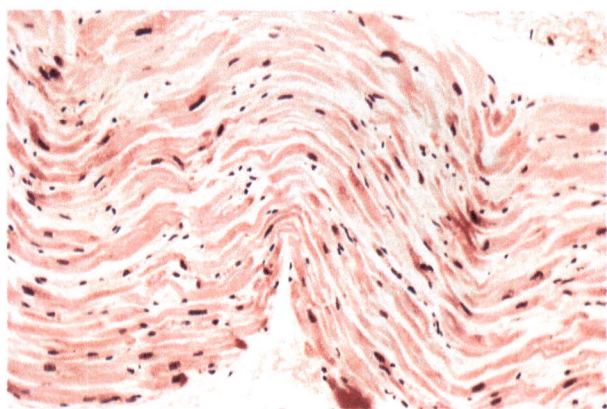

Figure 1.37   Atrial muscle fibres are thinner than ventricular muscle fibres and the fibres often show a wavy pattern.   H & E × 50

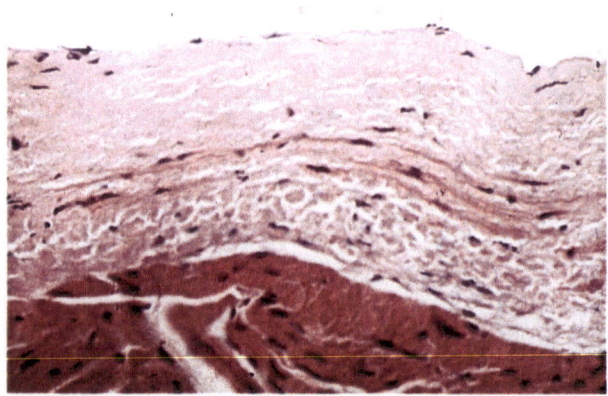

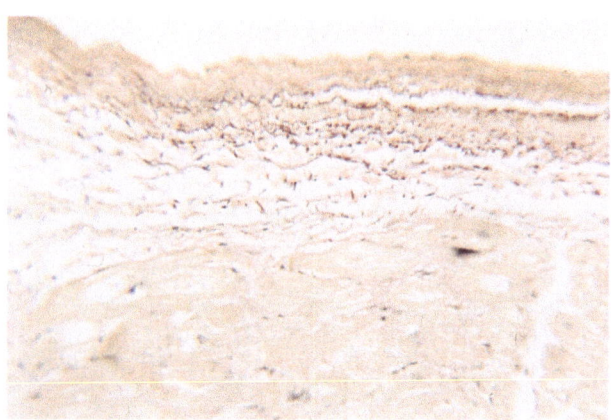

Figure 1.38a,b   The endocardium is thickest in the left atrium and is arranged in the following manner: endothelial cells, collagen tissue, internal elastic lamina, smooth muscle, external elastic lamina, collagen tissue in which there may be elastic fibres which condense as the myocardial junction is approached.   (a) H & E × 25. (b) Elastic van Gieson × 25

Figure 1.38b

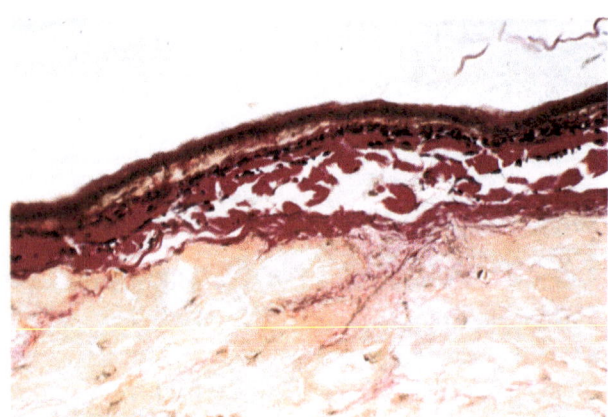

Figure 1.39   The right atrial endocardium, though considerably thinner than that of the left atrium, shows a similar arrangement. Elastic van Gieson × 50

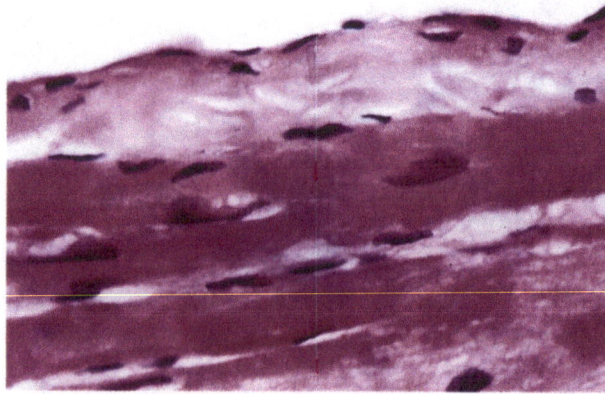

Figure 1.40   Left ventricular endocardium consists of endothelial cells and collagen tissue (and some fragmentation of elastic fibres). Only rarely is a smooth muscle fibre found.   H & E × 250

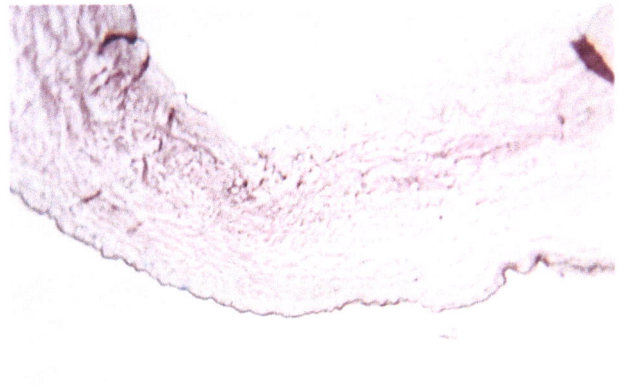

Figure 1.41 The basic structure of a valve leaflet consists of a layer in which elastic tissue can be identified and a collagen tissue layer. Between these two layers is the so-called 'zona spongiosa', rich in mucopolysaccharides, which can be of varying prominence. Elastic van Gieson × 50

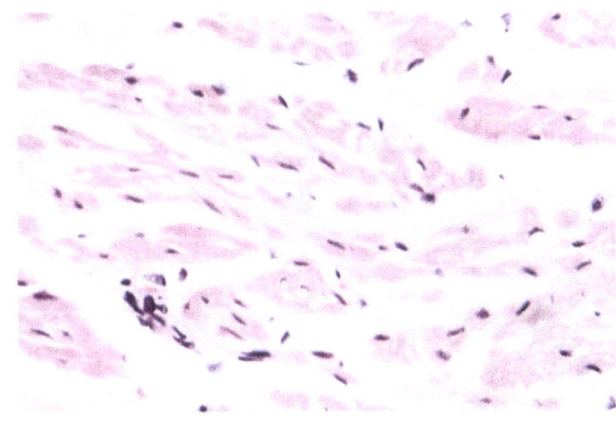

Figure 1.42 Illustration of conduction tissue which differs from cardiocytes in several ways (see text). H & E × 150

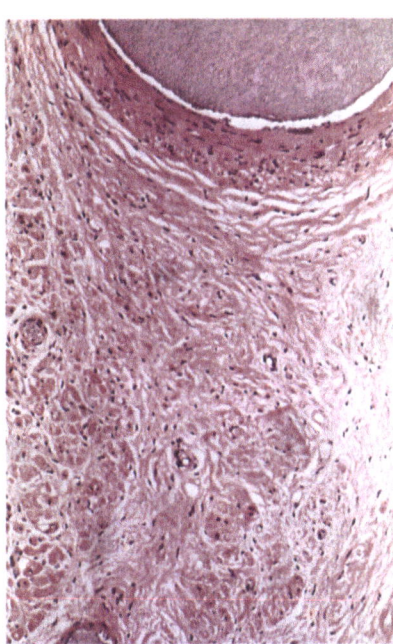

Figure 1.43 Low power view of the sinus node showing the contrast between conducting tissue and the atrial myocardium (at the left border of the illustration), in being thinner and paler. The lumen of the artery of the node is filled with contrast medium. H & E × 25

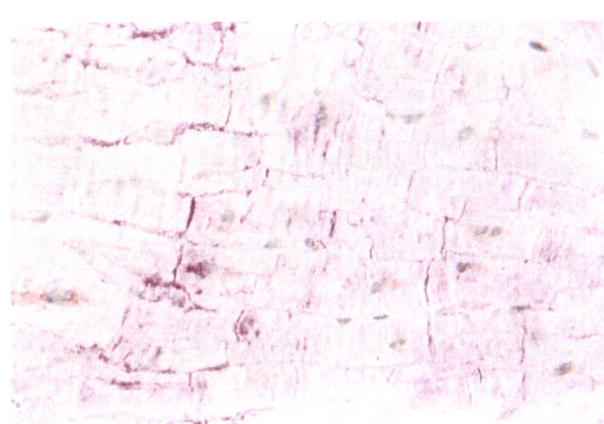

Figure 1.44 Glycogen is evenly distributed in the normal myocardium, patchily between myocardial fibrils. Varying degrees of accumulation occur at the nuclear poles. PAS × 200

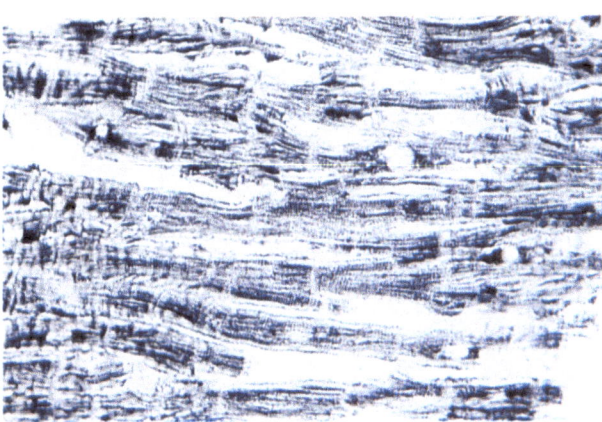

Figure 1.45 Succinic dehydrogenase distribution is illustrated. Accumulation at nuclear poles (nuclei, empty areas) again occurs. MTT × 200

Figure 1.46 The zona spóngiosa contains acid mucopolysaccharides (see also Figure 1.41). Alcian Blue × 25

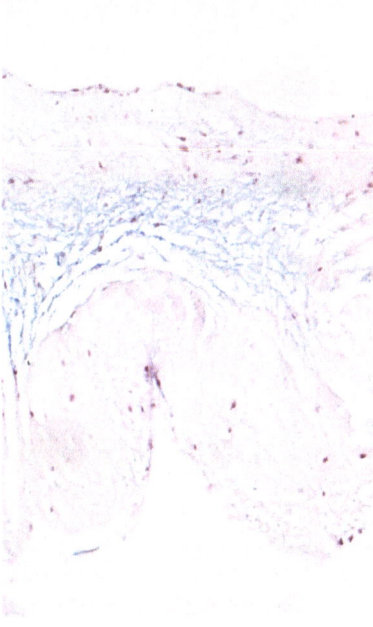

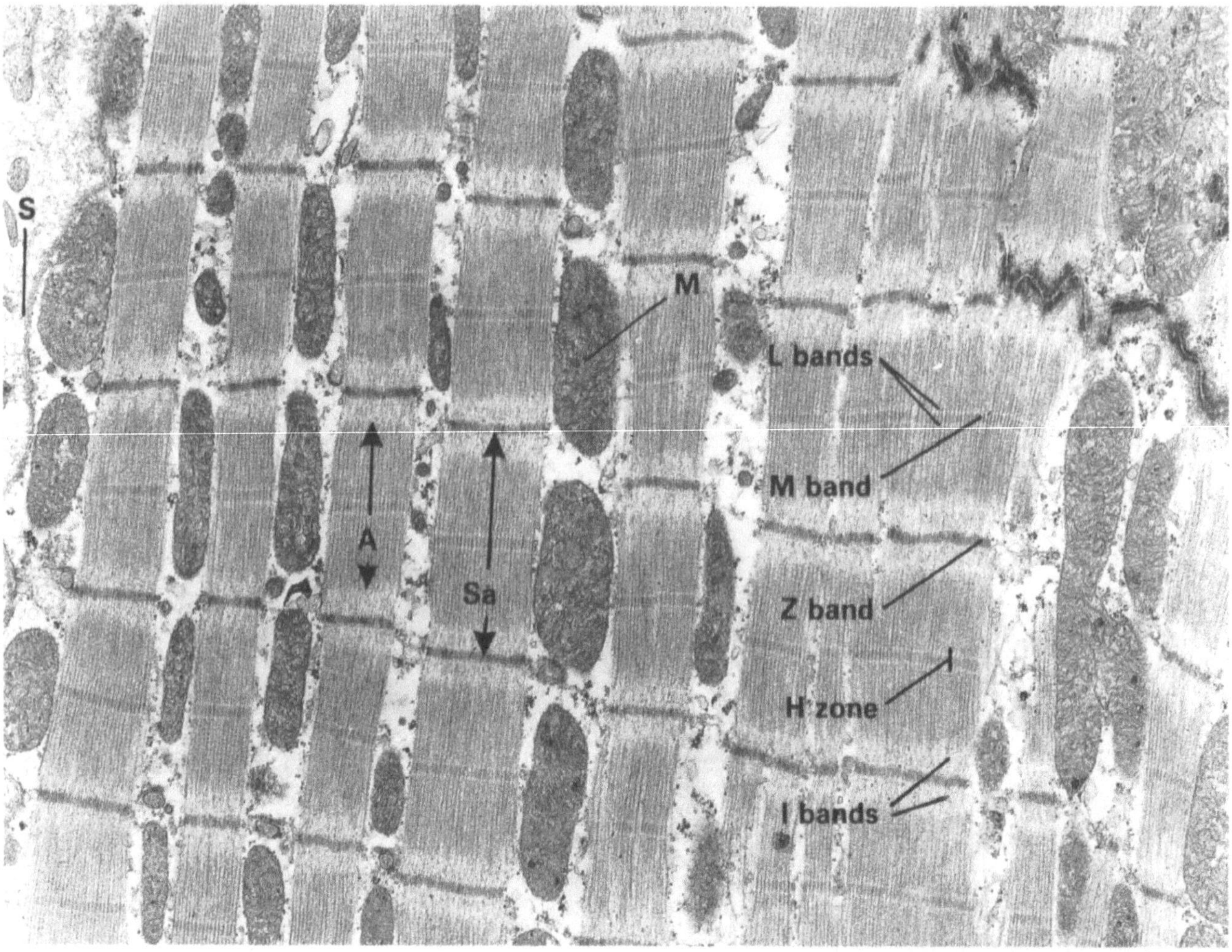

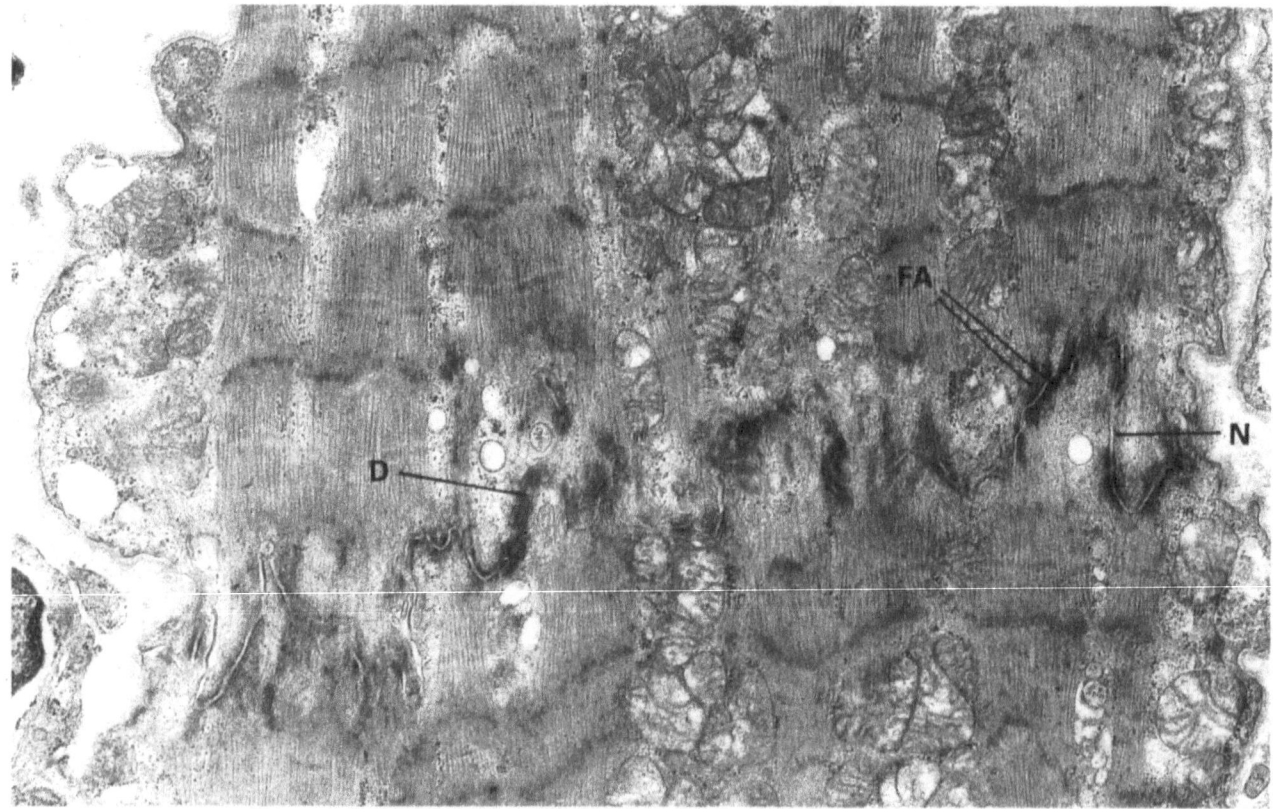

Figure 1.47 Electron micrograph showing the sarcolemma (S) at the left border of the illustration. The sarcomere (Sa) (the functional unit of a cardiac site) is delineated by two Z bands, on either side of which is a light band, the I band. Actin and myosin, alone or interdigitating give rise to the bands which characterise the sarcomeres. There is one mitochondrion (M) per two sarcomeres. (For a fuller description please see text.)   Lead citrate and uranyl acetate × 7500

Figure 1.48 The intercalated disc. Specialised regions can be recognised. FA = Fascia adhaerens; D = Desmosomes (macula adhaerens) N = Nexus (fascia occludens).   Lead citrate and uranyl acetate × 5900

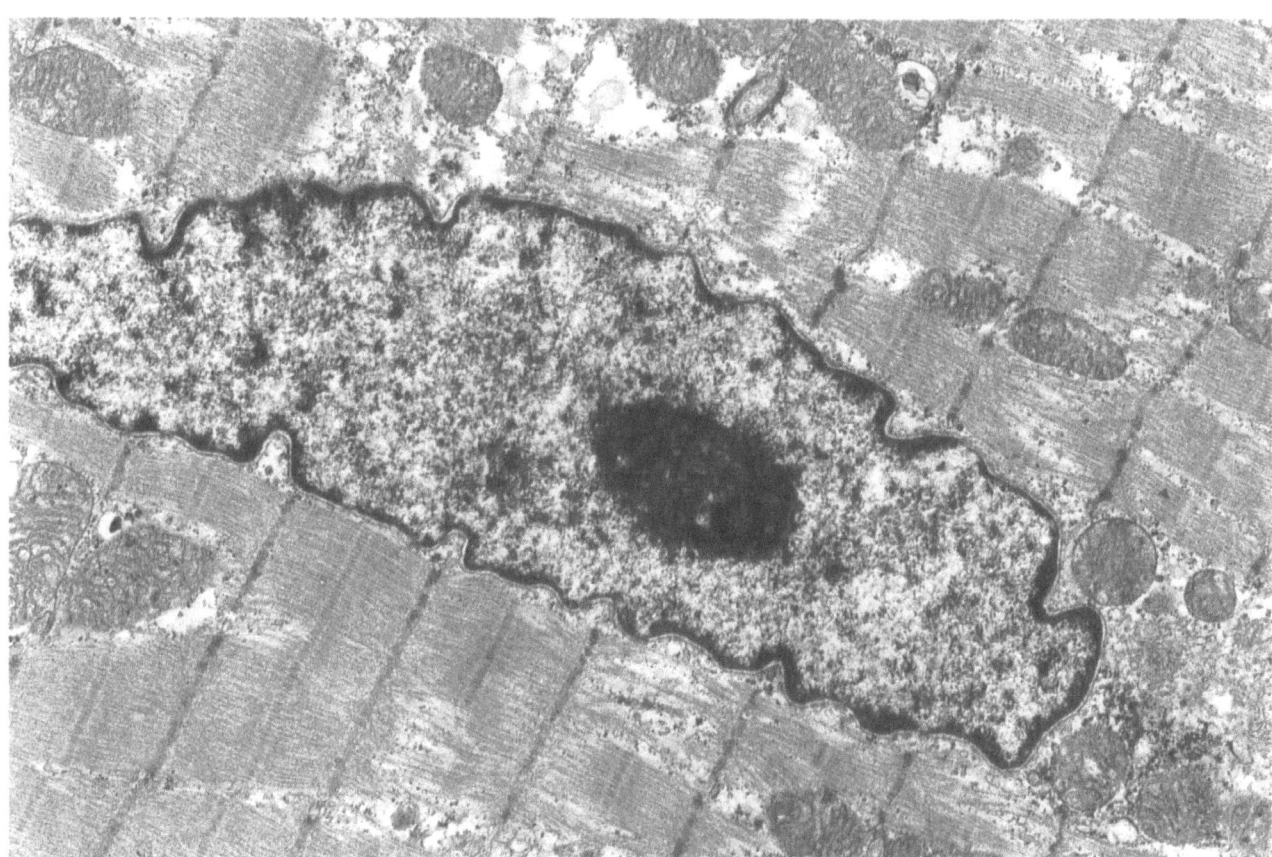

Figure 1.49   A nucleus showing a uniform distribution of chromatin and a nucleolus.   Lead citrate and uranyl acetate × 5900

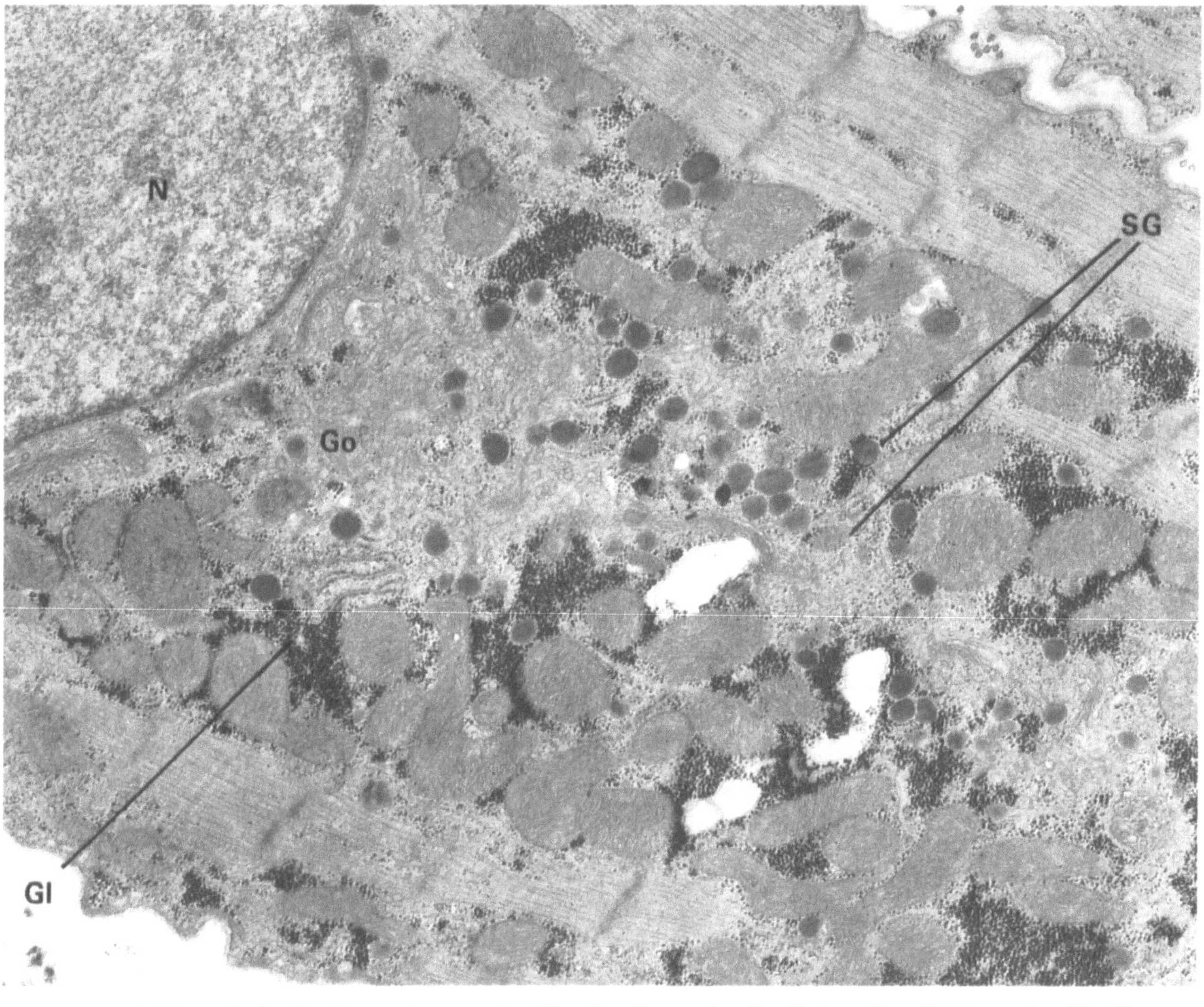

Figure 1.50   Atrial muscle showing characteristic granules. SG = Specific granules; N = Nucleus; Go = Golgi apparatus; Gl = Glycogen. Lead citrate and uranyl acetate × 9800 (By permission of The Macmillan Press, London and Basingstoke)

pores can be identified. The outer layer is continuous with sarcoplasmic vesicles (Figure 1.49).

The Golgi apparatus, close to the nucleus, consists of flattened sacs with paired membranes. Some vesicles are also identified in this area; see also Figure 2.13.

So far, ventricular muscle has been described.

Atrial Muscle

Atrial cardiocytes differ from ventricular cells in being shorter, thinner and with sparse or absent T tubules and couplings. Dense and surface vesicles are more numerous. Specific granules, of which four types are recognised are present, many of which are not found in ventricular myocytes (Figure 1.50).

Conduction system

The reader is referred to texts such as James et al., 1966[25] and Viragh and Challice, 1973[26]. The latter author also describes in great detail the ultrastructure of the mammalian heart.

References

1. Olsen, E. G. J. (1980). The normal heart. In The Pathology of the Heart. Second Edition, p. 3. (London and Basingstoke: The Macmillan Press Ltd.)

2. Silver, M. D., Lam, J. H. C., Ranganathan, N. and Wigle, E. D. (1971). Morphology of the human tricuspid valve. Circulation, 43, 333

3. Wenick, A. C. G. (1977). The medial papillary complex. Br. Heart J., 39, 1012

4. Grant, R. P., Downey, F. M. and MacMahon, H. (1961). The architecture of the right ventricular outflow tract in the normal heart and in the presence of ventricular septal defects. Circulation, 24, 223

5. Anderson, R. H., Becker, A. E. and van Mierop, L. H. S. (1977). What should we call the 'crista'. Br. Heart J., 39, 856

6. Ranganathan, N., Lam, J. H. C., Wigle, E. D. and Silver, M. D. (1970). Morphology of the human mitral valve. II. The valve leaflets. Circulation, 41, 459

7. Wartman, W. B. and Souders, J. C. (1950). Localisation of myocardial infarcts with respect to muscle bundles of the heart. Arch Pathol. 50, 329

8. Rodbard, S. (1973). Structure of the ventricular myocardium and conducting system. Am. J. Cardiol., 32, 877

9. Anderson, R. H. and Becker, A. E. (1980). Cardiac Anatomy. pp. 5 and 14. (Edinburgh, London and New York: Gower Medical Publications, Churchill Livingstone)

10. Anderson, K. R., Ho, S. Y. and Anderson, R. H. (1979). The cellular architecture of the human atrioventricular node, with a note on its morphology in the presence of a left superior vena cava. J. Anat., 109, 443

11. Kugel, M. A. (1928). Anatomical studies on the coronary arteries and their branches. I. Arteria anastomotica auricularis magna. Am. Heart J., 3, 260.

12. Bradham, R. R. and Parker, E. F. (1973). The cardiac lymphatics. Ann. Thorac. Surg., 15, 527

13. Zeek, P. M. (1942). Heart weight. I. The weight of the normal human heart. Arch Pathol, 34, 820

14. Roessle, R. and Roulet, F. (1932), Mass und Zahl in der Pathologie, p. 144. (Berlin and Vienna: J. Springer)

15. Coppoletta, J. M. and Wolbach, S. B. (1933). Body length and organ weights of infants and children. A study of the body length and normal weights of the more important vital organs between birth and twelve years of age. Am. J. Pathol., 9, 55

16. Hislop, A. and Reid, L. (1972). Weight of the left and right ventricle of the heart during fetal life. J. Clin. Pathol., 25, 534

17. Hutchins, G. M. and Anaya, O. A. (1973). Measurement of cardiac size, chamber volumes and valve orifices at autopsy. Johns Hopkins Med. J., 133, 96

18. Wissler, R. W., Lichtig, C., Hughes, R., Al-Sadir, J. and Glagov, S. (1975). A new method for determination of postmortem left ventricular volumes: clinicopathological correlations. Am. Heart J., 89, 625

19. Okada, R. (1961). Clinicopathological study on the thickening of parietal endocardium in the adult heart. Jpn. Heart J., 2, 220

20. Gross, L. and Kugel, M. A. (1931). Topographic anatomy and histology of the valves in the human heart. Am. J. Pathol., 7, 445

21. Wearn, J. T. and Moritz, A. R. (1937). The incidence and significance of blood vessels in normal and abnormal heart valves. Am. Heart J., 13, 7

22. Lautsch, E. V. (1971). Functional morphology of heart valves. Methods Achiev. Exp. Pathol., 5, 214

23. Lev, M. (1954). Aging changes in the human sinoatrial node. J. Gerontol., 9, 1

24. Rossi, L. (1978). Ageing changes in the atrio-ventricular and nervous system. In Histopathology of Cardiac Arrhythmias, Second Edition, p. 36. (Milano: Casa editrice ambrosiano)

25. James, T. N., Sherf, L., Fine, G. and Morales, A. R. (1966). Comparative ultrastructure of the sinus node in man and dog. Circulation, 34, 139

26. Viragh, S. and Challice, C. E. (1973). The impulse generation and conduction system of the heart. In Challice, C. E. and Viragh, S. (eds.) Ultrastructure of the Mammalian Heart, Vol. 6, p. 43. (New York, London: Academic Press)

Hypertrophy and Dilatation

2

Hypertrophy is an increase in the size of an organ due to an enlargement of its constituent cells[1].

The myocardium can react in a very limited way to a large variety of external stimuli. Whenever the stimulus results in extra work, which may be due to rhythm disturbance or overload due to intra- or extracardiac causes, it will result in hypertrophy. Hypertrophy is, therefore, encountered in most congenital and acquired heart diseases.

It can, however, also occur in normal individuals engaged in heavy manual labour or in athletes.

Several years ago distinction between physiological and pathological hypertrophy was made. An increase of the heart weight to 500 g was considered to be physiological hypertrophy and was termed the critical heart weight. Hypertrophy alone was considered to be responsible for this increase in the weight of the heart. Weights over 500 g were termed pathological hypertrophy and were considered to be due to hypertrophy as well as hyperplasia[2].

There is now ample evidence that hyperplasia contributes little or nothing towards the increase in heart weight except in the very young and in extreme degrees of hypertrophy where hyperplasia by longitudinal cleavage may occur[3].

Compensatory Hypertrophy

Hypertrophy can occur as a result of hyperfunction or damage[4,5].

Compensatory Hypertrophy Due to Hyperfunction

This has been subdivided into two groups:

the mainly isometric type where hypertrophy occurs as a result of an increased response to ventricular ejection such as systemic hypertension, aortic, or pulmonary stenoses;

the mainly isotonic type where an increased inflow of blood to a cardiac chamber occurs in conditions such as atrial or ventricular septal defects, patent ductus arteriosus or anaemia.

The greatest heart weights are recorded when isometric and isotonic hyperfunction coexist, such as in aortic stenosis and insufficiency. If the heart weight exceeds 1000 g the term 'cor bovinum' has been employed (Figure 2.1).

Compensatory Hypertrophy Due to Damage

Please see below.

Assessment of Hypertrophy

Weighing of the heart has already been described in Chapter 1 and emphasis was laid on the fact that this provides only a crude estimate, as does measurement of the wall thickness. A more accurate assessment of hypertrophy can be achieved by detaching the right ventricle and weighing it separately from the left ventricle and the septum. The results are then expressed as a ratio of left to right ventricular weights[6].

Macroscopy

'Concentric' hypertrophy (Figure 2.2) and 'eccentric' hypertrophy (Figure 2.3) may be recognized.

Histology

The fibre diameter is increased (above 12 µm). Nuclei show blunting of the nuclear poles, assuming rectangular shapes in longitudinal sections (Figure 2.4). Pyknosis is typical. Staghorn or horseshoe-shaped forms can be observed in severe hypertrophy as well as vesicular forms (Figure 2.5). Degenerative changes consisting of vacuoles, an increase in lipofuscin granules, basophilic change or coagulative necrosis may accompany hypertrophy (See Chapter 4).

Methods of assessment Measurement of the width of the muscle fibre can readily be undertaken with either eye-piece micrometry or by specialized instruments such as a Projectina instrument adapted for the purpose.

Measuring the length of sarcomeres can be undertaken or assessment by phase-contrast microscopy or diffraction spectrometry can be carried out.

Stereological techniques including planimetry, cutting and weighing of various components, linear integration or point counting can all be applied.

Another technique using a computer high resolution video image digitizing system has also more recently been applied[7].

Histochemistry

An increase, normal amounts or a decrease of succinic dehydrogenase (Figure 2.6), monoamine oxidase, acid phosphatase and non-specific esterases may be found depending on the stage of hypertrophy (see below). An increase in glycogen is usually found in the early stages of hypertrophy (Figure 2.7). Myosin ATPase (adenosine triphosphatase) is equally distributed (Figure 2.8).

Ultrastructural Examination

An increase of mitochondria to more than one per two sarcomeres provides a quick assessment of whether or

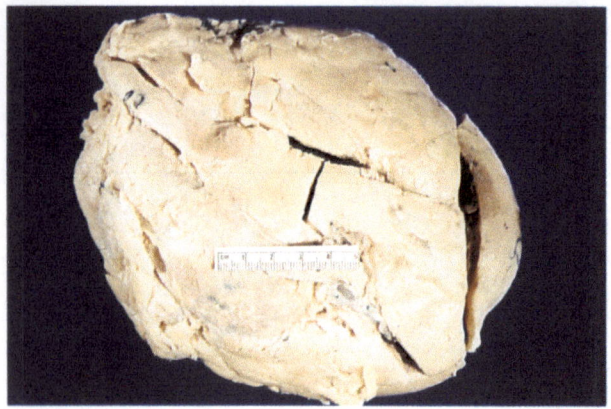

Figure 2.1 External view of a heart weighing 1250 g. The so-called 'cor bovinum'. From a patient with a combination of aortic stenosis and insufficiency

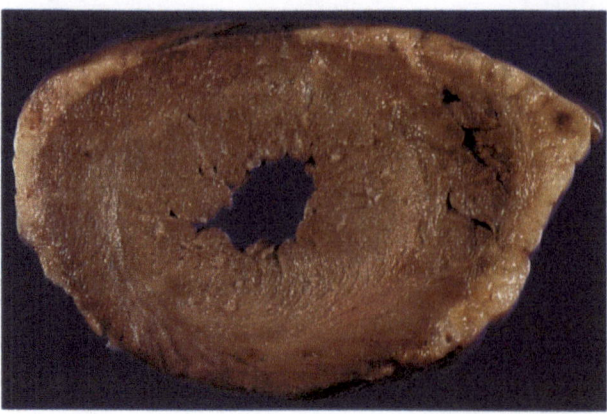

Figure 2.2 Cross-section of ventricles showing uniform hypertrophy of the left ventricle without dilatation of the ventricular cavity (concentric hypertrophy)

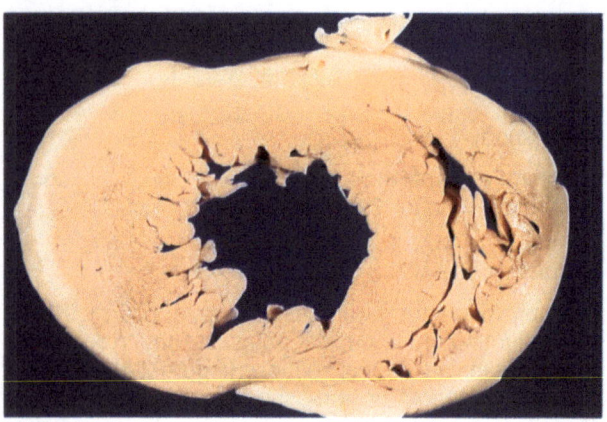

Figure 2.3 Eccentric hypertrophy, uniform hypertrophy with dilatation characterizes this form of hypertrophy

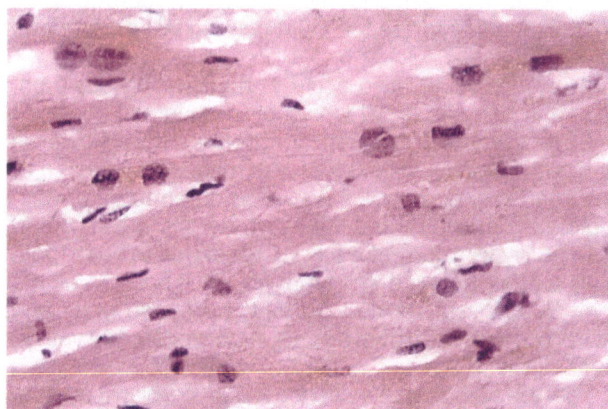

Figure 2.4 Photomicrograph of hypertrophied myocardial fibres showing nuclear changes of hypertrophy (hyperchromasia and blunting of nuclear poles as well as vesicular changes). H & E × 200

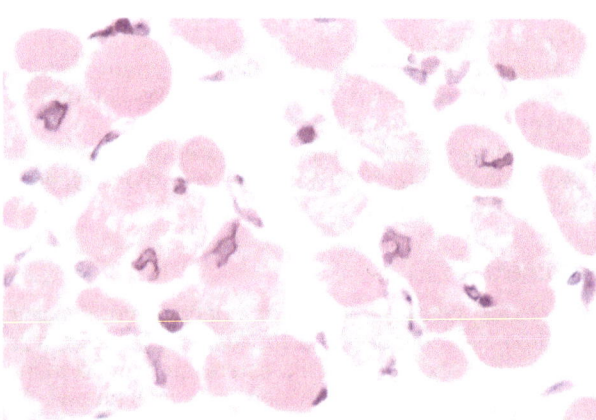

Figure 2.5 Severe hypertrophy showing great variation in nuclear shapes including staghorn or horseshoe-shaped outlines or severe vesicular changes. H & E × 400

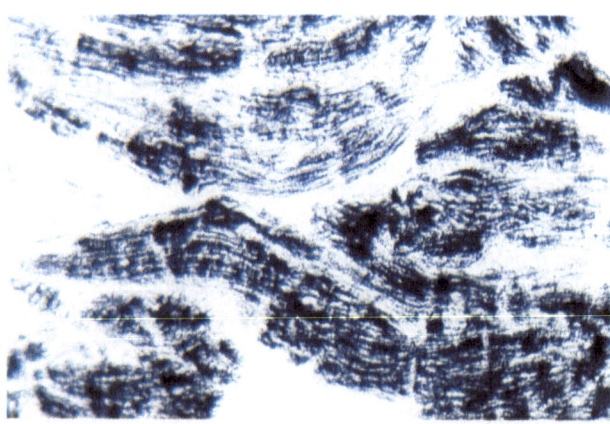

Figure 2.6 A patchy increase in succinic dehydrogenase is often seen in cases of hypertrophy (frozen section). MTT × 200

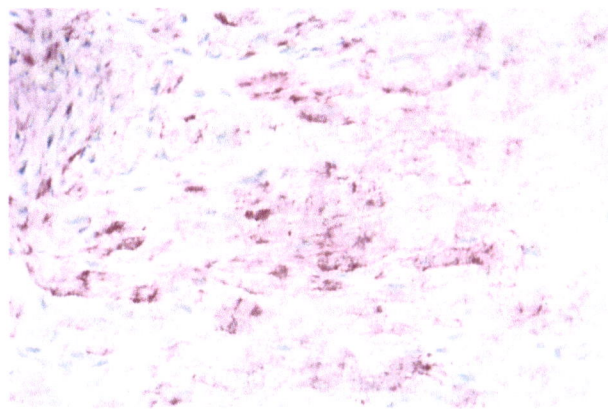

Figure 2.7 Focal increase of glycogen with accumulation, especially around nuclear poles (frozen section). PAS × 200

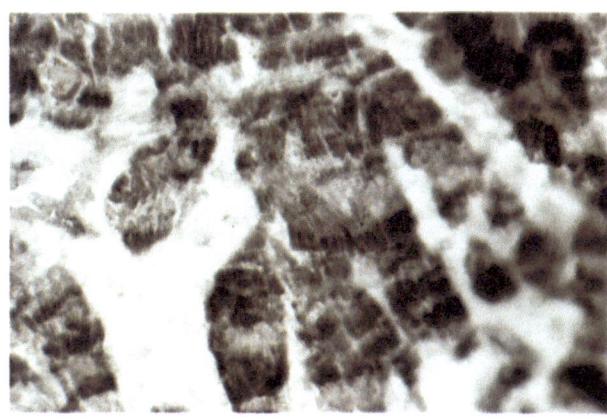

Figure 2.8 Myosin ATPase is not decreased and is evenly distributed (the ridging is due to contraction banding). Myosin ATPase × 250

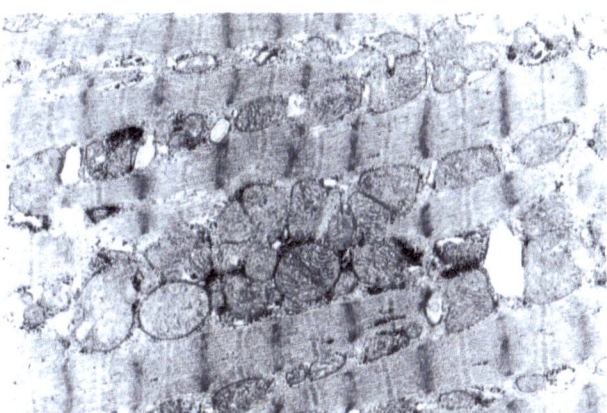

Figure 2.9 Electron micrograph showing an increase in the number (up to three) of mitochondria per two sarcomeres, providing a quick assessment of the severity of hypertrophy. Lead citrate and uranyl acetate × 7500

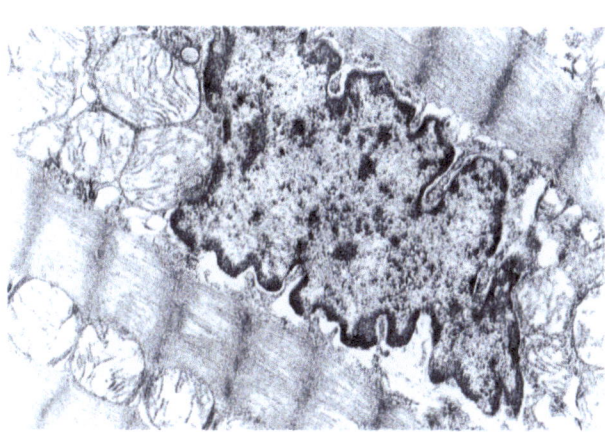

Figure 2.10 Crenellation of the nuclear membrane is typical of hypertrophy. Some chromatin clumping has occurred. Note also cristolysis in the mitochondria. In this section one mitochondrion per two sarcomeres is found but elsewhere evidence of hypertrophy existed. Lead citrate and uranyl acetate × 13000

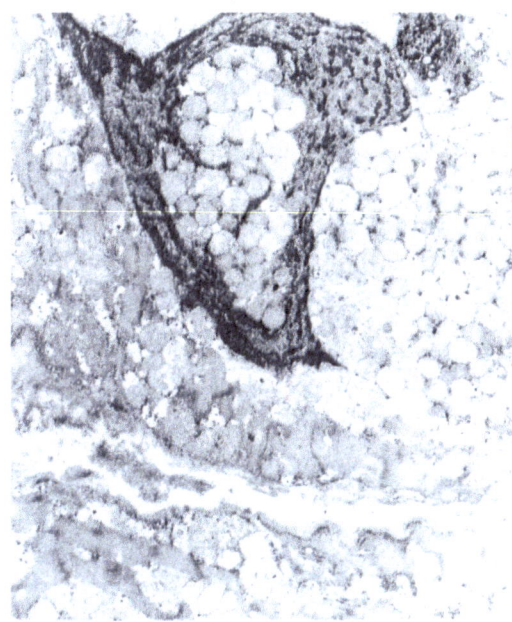

Figure 2.11 Electron micrograph showing pseudo-inclusion in the nucleus. Lead citrate and uranyl acetate × 5900

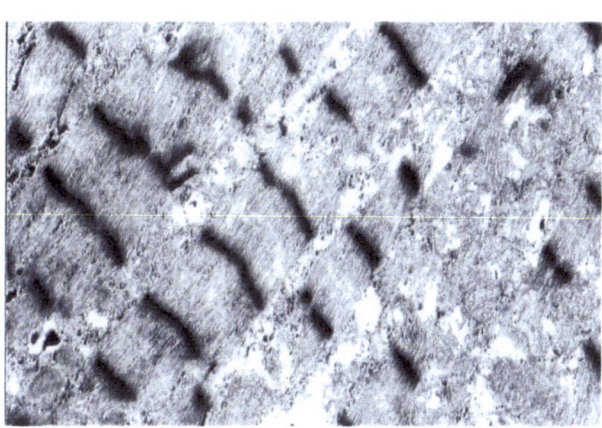

Figure 2.12 Diffusion of Z band material is often found in hypertrophy. Lead citrate and uranyl acetate × 9800

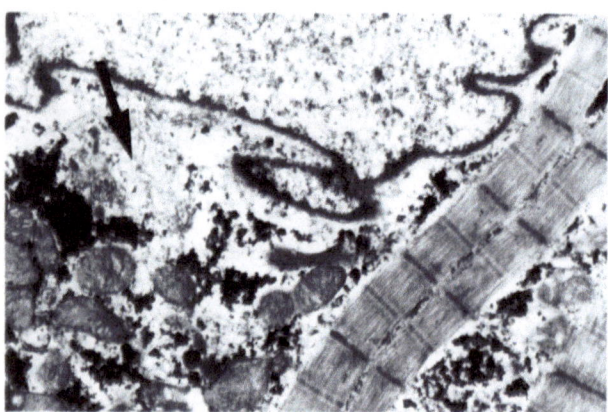

Figure 2.13 Illustrates a prominent Golgi apparatus (arrowed) and accumulation of glycogen, particularly in the perinuclear area.   Lead citrate and uranyl acetate × 7500

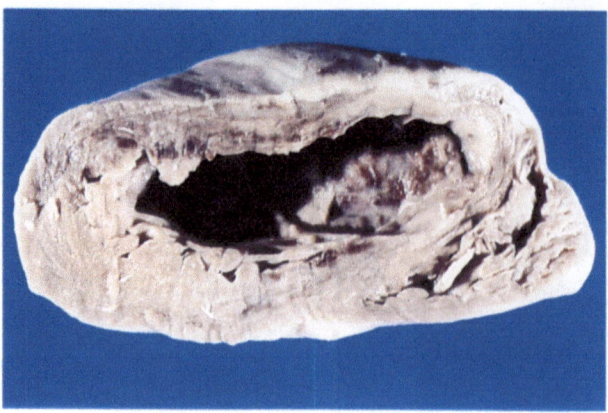

Figure 2.14 Cross-section of ventricles showing a myocardial infarct of approximately one week duration involving the interventricular septum and left anterior wall

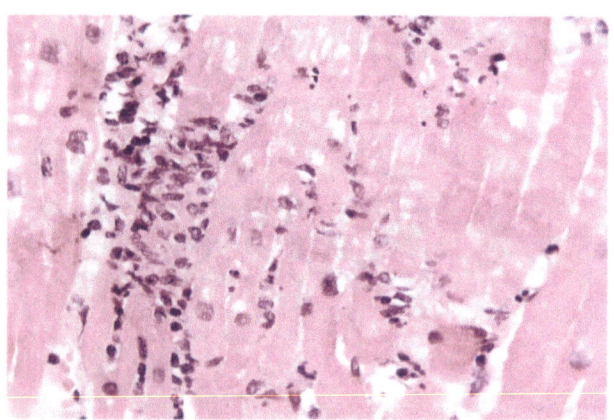

Figure 2.15 Photomicrograph of active myocarditis. H & E × 200

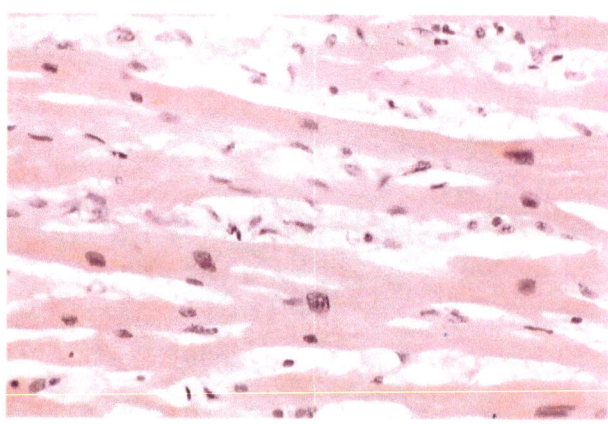

Figure 2.16 Hypertrophied, attenuated myocardial fibres in normal alignment together with a mild increase of interstitial collagen tissue. The changes are non-specific; from a patient with a clinical diagnosis of dilated cardiomyopathy. Damage of muscle due to infarction or inflammation or due to unknown causes (dilated cardiomyopathy) leads to compensatory hypertrophy due to damage. H & E × 200

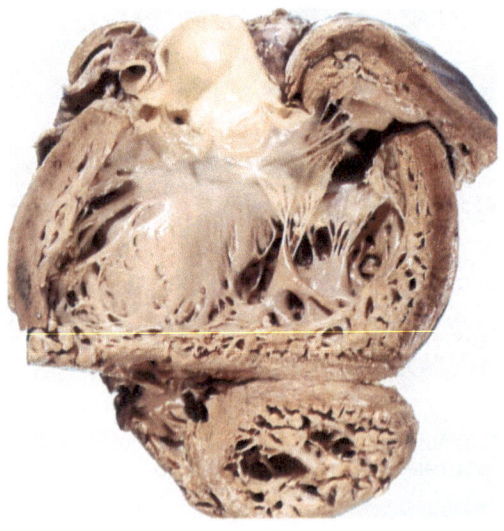

Figure 2.17 The left ventricle is displayed to show severe dilatation. Despite hypertrophy the left ventricular wall thickness is normal. Cross-section of the apex also shows right ventricular dilatation; from a patient in congestive heart failure

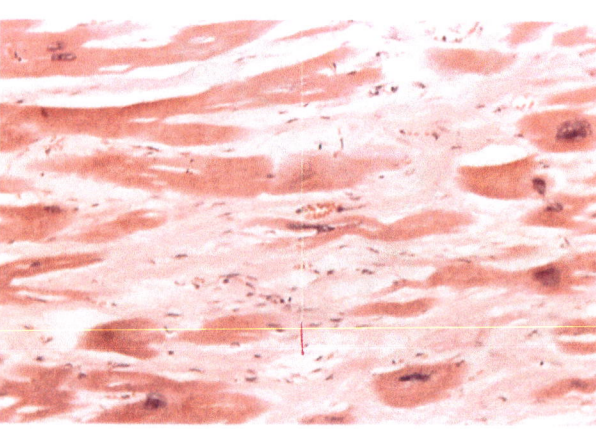

Figure 2.18 Photomicrograph from a patient in congestive heart failure of long duration. Interstitial fibrosis is severe.   H & E × 200

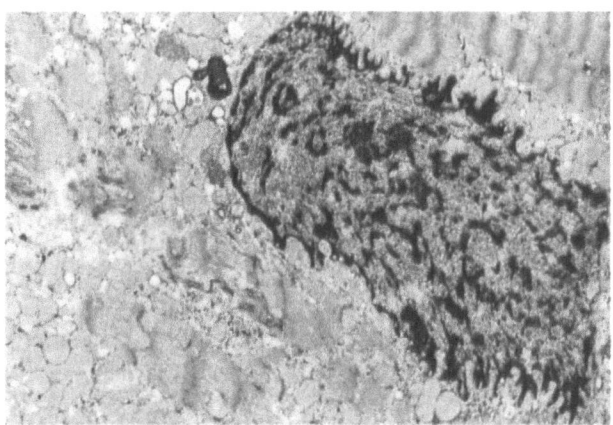

Figure 2.19 Electron micrograph showing extensive changes of degeneration. Note particularly the clumping of nuclear chromatin. Lead citrate and uranyl acetate × 4300

not hypertrophy is present[8]. Mitochondria may show swelling, irregularities in size and shape and cristolysis (Figure 2.9).

Enlarged nuclei may be prominent and varying degrees of convolutions of the nuclear membranes may be found (Figure 2.10). Pseudo-inclusions may be recognized (Figure 2.11).

The myofibrils may show disorganization, particularly in the region of the I and Z bands. Accumulation of Z band material is frequent (Figure 2.12). Prominence of the T tubular system and of the Golgi apparatus occurs and glycogen increase is usual[8] (Figure 2.13).

Methods of assessment Measurements of sarcomere length, histological techniques and autoradiography have all been undertaken. Photographing and cutting out and weighing of the various organelles have also been used in assessing hypertrophy at electron-microscopic level[7].

Experimental Studies

These have permitted insight into the process of hypertrophy. Sequential changes following induction of isometric hyperfunction have been described. Three stages are recognized.

(1) *First stage or stage of damage.* Cloudy swelling and a fatty change together with faintly eosinophilic staining of myocardial fibres can be observed. Trauma and rupture of the papillary muscle or chordae tendineae are encountered clinically in this stage of hypertrophy.

(2) *Second stage or the stage of relatively stable hyperfunction.* Morphological evidence of hypertrophy (increase in fibre diameter, etc.) is observed. The degenerative changes seen in the first stage have now disappeared. This stage is seen in all congenital and acquired heart diseases.

(3) *Third stage or stage of gradual exhaustion and progressive cardiosclerosis.* Dilatation becomes established. Hypertrophy, atrophy and vacuolar degeneration and breakdown of muscle fibres as well as hyalinization can all be observed. Fibrous replacement, an increase in interstitial fibrous tissue and fatty degeneration are also frequently seen[4,9].

Compensatory Hypertrophy Due to Damage

The stages leading to compensatory hypertrophy due to damage are similar to those described for overload of the isometric type of hypertrophy. Clinical examples include ischaemia, myocarditis or cardiomyopathies (Figures 2.14 – 2.16)[5].

Insufficiency – Dilatation

Cardiac insufficiency may be defined as a condition in which the load imposed on the heart exceeds the ability of the latter to perform its work of propelling the blood from the venous bed into the arterial bed[5].

It is the third stage (see above), i.e. the stage of gradual exhaustion and progressive cardiosclerosis. Heart failure supervenes.

Macroscopic Examination

Dilatation of cardiac chambers is typical (Figure 2.17). Depending on the underlying disease process the left side or the right side of the heart or both chambers may be affected. Hypertrophy is invariably present, yet this may be completely masked by the dilatation.

Histology

Myocardial fibres may be normal in diameter but the nuclear changes of hypertrophy (see above) are identified and this disproportion is due to stretching of the myocardial fibres. Degenerative changes may be widespread and evidence of fibrosis may be striking (Figure 2.18).

Histochemistry

Patchy or uniform depletion of the enzyme systems, already mentioned above, and of glycogen occurs.

Ultrastructural Changes

Extensive degeneration of mitochondria and myocardial fibrils (myosin and actin), severe enlargement of the sarcoplasmic tubules and dehiscence of the intercalated discs are usually present. Chromatin clumping in nuclei may be striking (Figure 2.19).

Mechanisms of Dilatation

Lengthening of the myocardial sarcomeres, more severe in the inner layers of the myocardial walls than in the sub-epicardial regions, is one important component of dilatation; the other is a decrease in muscle fibre layers[10]. When severe dilatation is present the heart operates under unfavourable geometric conditions.

Weakness and destruction of the connective tissue may also play a role in dilatation.

Sudden or acute overdistension of one ventricle is possible but overdistension of both ventricles is prevented by the pericardium. In 'chronic dilatation' concomitant 'growth' of the pericardium permits enormous dilatation to occur.

Hypoxia may play an important role in hypertrophy and dilatation (heart failure).

References

1. Olsen, E. G. J. (1980). Hypertrophy, hyperplasia and dilatation. In *The Pathology of the Heart*. Second Edition, p. 133. (London and Basingstoke: The Macmillan Press Ltd)

2. Linzbach, A. J. (1976). Hypertrophy, hyperplasia and structural dilatation of the human heart. *Adv. Cardiol.*, **18**, 1

3. Hatt, P. Y. (1977). Cellular changes in mechanically overloaded heart. *Basic Res. Cardiol.*, **72**, 198

4. Meerson, F. Z. (1965). A mechanism of hypertrophy and wear of the myocardium. *Am. J. Cardiol.*, **15**, 755

5. Meerson, F. Z. (1976). Insufficiency of hypertrophied heart. *Basic Res. Cardiol.*, **71**, 343

6. Fulton, R. M., Hutchinson, E. C. and Morgan Jones, A. (1952). Ventricular weight in cardiac hypertrophy. *Br. Heart J.*, **14**, 413

7. Olsen, E. G. J. (1980). In *The Pathology of the Heart*. Second Edition, p. 45. (London and Basingstoke: The Macmillan Press Ltd)

8. Olsen, E. G. J. (1976). Structural and ultrastructural basis of myocardial disease. *Proc. R. Soc. Med.*, **69**, 195

9. Meerson, F. Z. (1969). The myocardium in hyperfunction, hypertrophy and heart failure. *Circulation Res.*, **25**, Supplement II

10. Hort, W. (1960). Untersuchungen zur funktionellen Morphologie des Bindegewebesgerustes und der Blutgefasse der linken Herzkammerwand. *Virchows Arch. Pathol. Anat.*, **333**, 565

Changes in the Endocardium

3

Examination of the endocardium not only permits conclusions to be drawn about the haemodynamic situation that had existed in a cardiac chamber but also aids in establishing a diagnosis. Knowledge of the normal arrangement of the various components of the endocardium is mandatory (see Chapter 1).

Jet lesions can easily be recognized with the naked eye standing out as white fibrous plaques from the surrounding normal endocardium (Figure 3.1).

When the jet is at *right angles* to the surface, histological examination shows all components of the endocardium, collagen, elastic tissue and smooth muscle, haphazardly arranged (Figure 3.2).

When the *jet impaction is oblique* to the surface of the endocardium then heaping of normal endocardial components occurs which, however, is frequently overlain by fibrin[1]. This results in characteristic pocket-like lesions, the so-called Zahn–Schmincke pockets (Figure 3.3). These pockets resemble small semilunar leaflets. The direction of opening of these leaflet-like structures provides morphological evidence of significant valvar insufficiency or stenosis. For example, if the pockets are found in the outflow part of the left ventricle and the opening is directed towards the aortic valve, valvar insufficiency has been present; if on the other hand, the opening faces the apex, significant stenosis has then existed.

These pockets are also located in other sites, for example, the under surface of the anterior mitral valve leaflet and in ventricles or atria depending upon the involvement of the cardiac valves that have given rise to the abnormal haemodynamic situation.

Histology of the pockets shows all the components of the endocardium. Fibrin superimposition is frequently found (Figure 3.4).

Parallel streaming of blood over the endocardium results in some thickening with an increase of the elastic component, the elastic fibres being arranged in parallel bands (Figure 3.5).

One of the most impressive changes in the endocardium is that of *dilatation* which, if of long standing, can result in severe thickening by hypertrophy and hyperplasia of the smooth muscle component[2] (Figure 3.6). Smooth muscle is, of course, a normal constituent of the endocardium and can readily be identified in the normally thick endocardium of the left atrium (see Chapter 1). Though smooth muscle is also found in the endocardium of the ventricles, only a very occasional fibre can be identified after some searching. When dilatation supervenes, an increase in smooth muscle, which is focal at first but after some time becomes confluent, can be found (Figure 3.7a and b). The degree of smooth muscle increase also depends on the severity of the dilatation. Increase in the smooth muscle component

is a sensitive indicator of dilatation and can easily be observed in endomyocardial biopsies even though radiologically dilatation may not have been evident. An increase in smooth muscle is usually easily recognized three to five weeks after the onset of dilatation.

Friction and the effects of turbulence result in a spectrum of the lesions detailed above, especially when accompanied by dilatation (Figure 3.8).

Changes of *insufficiency of the valve leaflets* can also be readily identified. This consists of superimposition of collagen tissue occasionally admixed with some elastic fibres on the deformed face of the valve leaflet, clearly demarcated by the elastic layers of the deformed face (Figure 3.9).

Pathogenesis of Thickening

Thickening of the endocardium and valve leaflets is brought about by superimposition of fibrin and thrombus[3]. Mural endocardial thickening is most likely due to occlusion of the Thebesian veins and small arterioluminal vessels, resulting in degeneration of the superficial layers and thus in fibrin superimposition. Smooth muscle prominence is consequent to stretching.

Endocardial Thickening Consequent to Myocardial Infarction

When the infarct reaches the endocardial region, damage of the subendocardial muscle results in necrosis of the endocardium which may become detached and swept away in the bloodsteam leaving an exposed area. Thrombus becomes superimposed (Figure 3.10) and thick collagen overlying myocardial infarction is the result of the organization of this thrombus (Figure 3.11). The endocardium may survive and can be extremely thick and, here also, thrombus may be superimposed. Distinction from endocardial involvement by endomyocardial fibrosis is possible. In the last mentioned condition zonal layering is characteristic, indeed diagnostic. Beneath the layer of thrombus or fibrin a layer of collagen tissue is found beneath which the so-called granulation tissue layer is identified. This layer consists of loosely arranged connective tissue in which dilated vascular channels and inflammatory cells can be identified. Eosinophils, frequently abnormal, can also be found. It is from this layer that the septae extend into the underlying myocardium (see Chapter 9).

This zonal layering is not observed in the thickened endocardium over an infarcted area, although for both conditions organizing thrombus or fibrin is held responsible for the immense thickening of the endocardium.

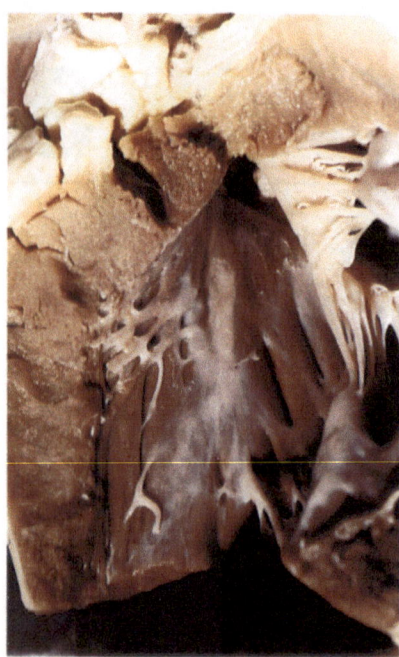

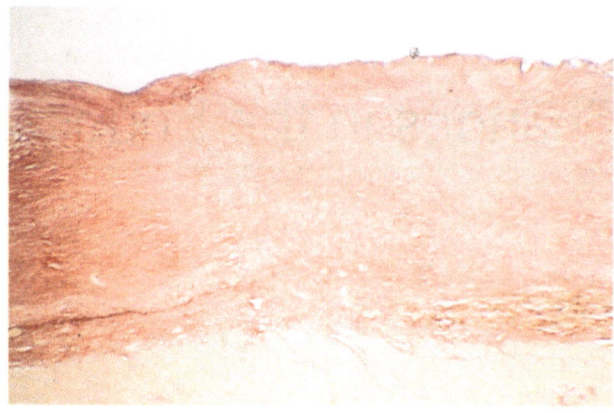

Figure 3.1 Endocardial thickening of the outflow part of the left ventricle due to an insufficent aortic valve

Figure 3.2 Severe endocardial thickening due to a jet of blood at right angles to the surface of the endocardium. All components of the endocardium are haphazardly arranged. Elastic van Gieson × 25

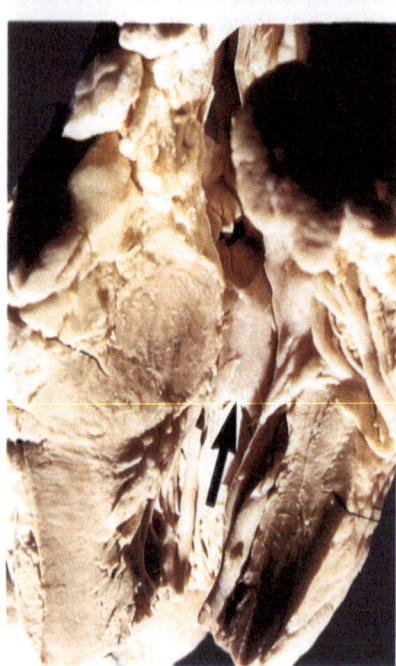

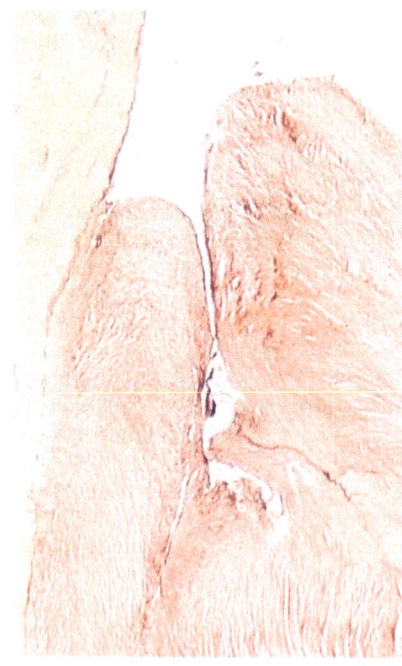

Figure 3.3 Zahn–Schmincke pocket (arrow) due to an oblique jet in a patient with aortic stenosis

Figure 3.4 Photomicrograph of a Zahn–Schmincke pocket (systolic pocket). Elastic van Gieson × 25

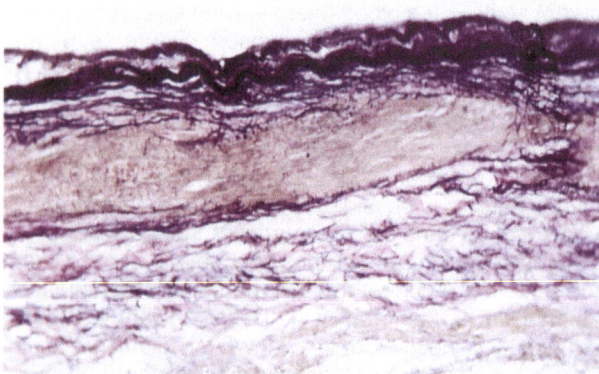

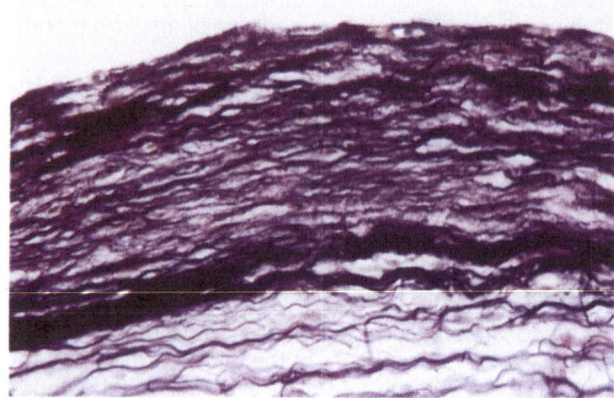

Figure 3.5 Streaming of blood parallel to the surface of the endocardium results in thickening; an increase in elastic tissue is typically arranged in parallel bands. Elastic van Gieson × 200

Figure 3.6 Long-standing severe dilatation resulting in striking prominence of the smooth muscle component of the endocardium. The sample illustrated has been obtained from the left atrium. Elastic van Gieson × 50

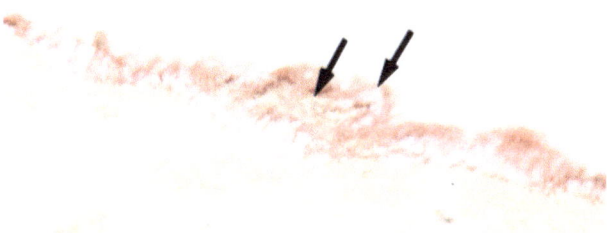

Figure 3.7a Focal prominence of the smooth muscle (arrowed) of the endocardium is found in this left ventricular sample.   Elastic van Gieson × 250

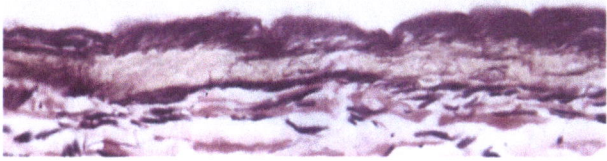

Figure 3.7b In another case of long duration a uniform increase of the smooth muscle can be seen.   Elastic van Gieson × 100

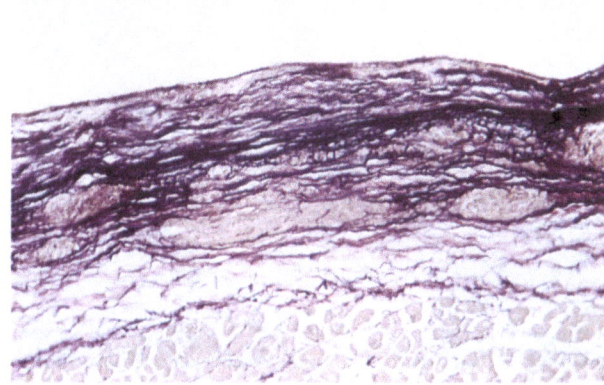

Figure 3.8 Illustration of predominantly parallel streaming and dilatation.   Elastic van Gieson × 100

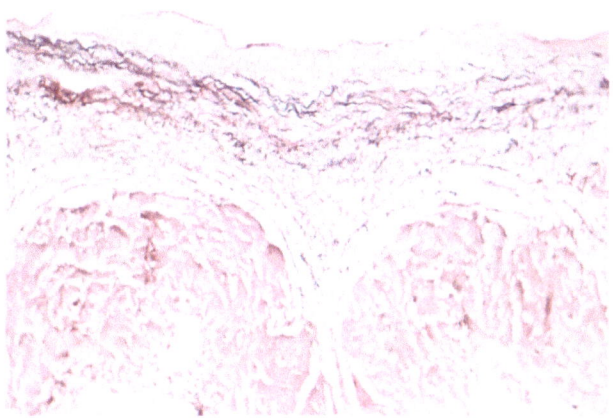

Figure 3.9 Superimposition of collagen tissue on the 'deformed face' of the valve (mitral) which indicates valvar insufficiency. Note also the prominent zona spongiosa.   Elastic van Giesen × 50

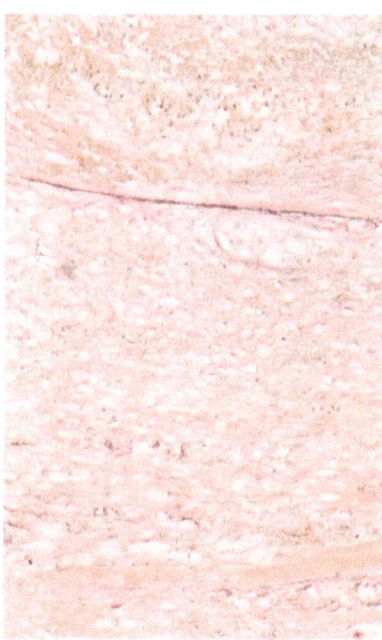

Figure 3.10 Superimposition of recent thrombus has occurred above the external elastic lamina of the endocardium (which is otherwise missing), in a case with subendocardial infarction. Elastic van Gieson × 50

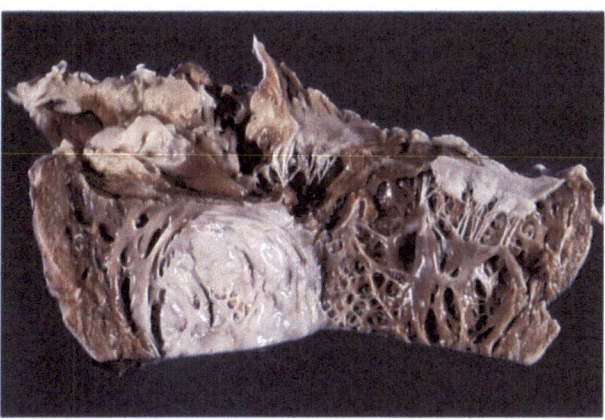

Figure 3.11a Thick endocardium over an old infarcted area

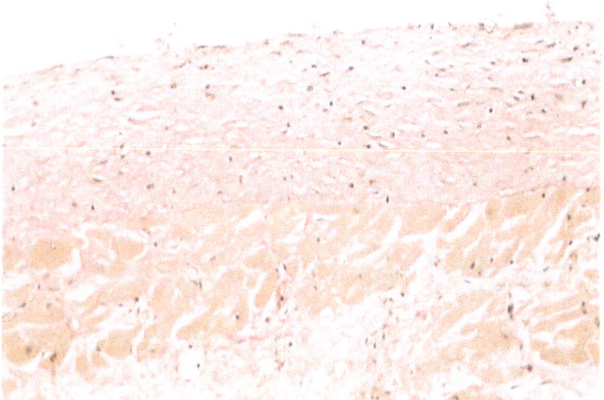

Figure 3.11b A thick layer of collagen tissue resulting from organized thrombus covering an area of old infarction. Some superficial myocardial fibres have survived ischaemic damage. Elastic van Giesen × 50

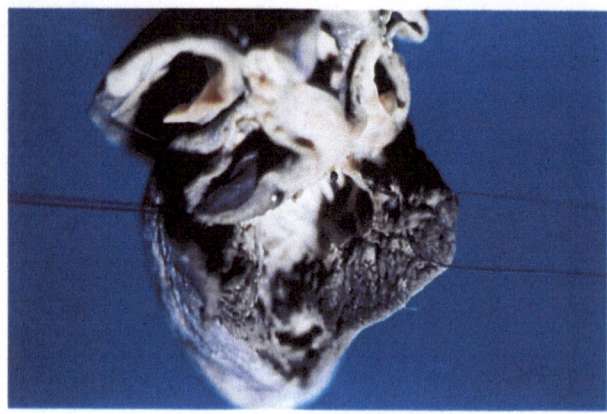

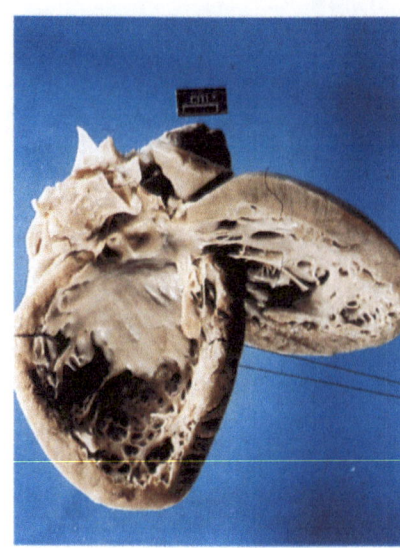

Figure 3.12 Isolated endocardial fibroelastosis of the newborn involving the left ventricle. The chamber is small. The changes must be distinguished from premature closure of the foramen ovale which results in non-specific endocardial thickening

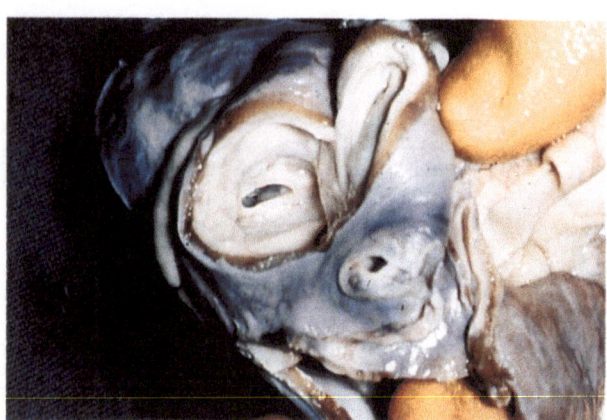

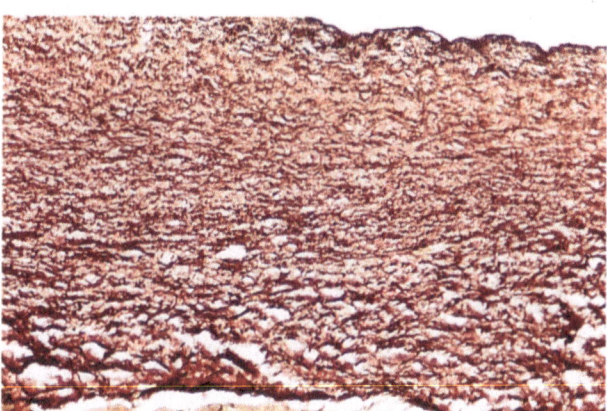

Figure 3.14 Isolated endocardial fibroelastosis having involved the mitral and aortic valves (By courtesy of Professor M. J. Davies)

Figure 3.15 Photomicrograph of the extremely thick endocardium from a patient with isolated endocardial fibroelastosis. The irregular arrangement of the elastic tissue is highly characteristic. Elastic van Gieson × 100

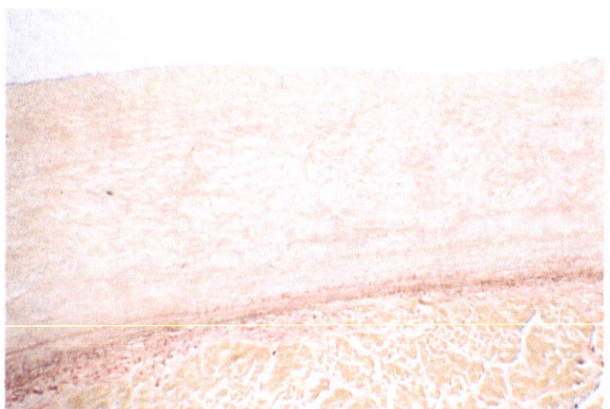

Figure 3.16 Carcinoid heart disease; the thickening is due to superimposition of abnormal material typically devoid of elastic tissue on the otherwise near normal endocardium. Elastic van Gieson × 25

Isolated Endocardial Fibroelastosis of the Newborn

This terminology actually includes two clinical forms of the disease. One occurs in the newborn and is associated with a small cardiac chamber (Figure 3.12). The other, the so-called adolescent form, is found in older children and is associated with a dilated chamber (Figure 3.13). In both instances characteristic features can be observed permitting distinction from other forms of endocardial thickening. In endocardial thickening from any other cause the trabecular pattern is obscured and covered by the thickened endocardium, whereas in fibroelastosis every trabeculum is clearly picked out, giving great emphasis to the trabecular pattern. In cases of left ventricular involvement, the area beneath the aortic valve is characteristically involved; this area is only rarely involved in endomyocardial fibrosis. Valves may also be involved by the disease process (Figure 3.14).

Some doubt has been raised as to whether this condition can be diagnosed histologically. A severe increase in elastic tissue is highly characteristic[4]. The elastic tissue is arranged in regular bands almost resembling the aortic media (Figure 3.15). If, however, samples from an area not severely affected are obtained, for example, by the bioptome, difficulty in distinguishing this endocardial thickening from that due to parallel streaming may be experienced.

The pathogenesis of the condition remains obscure but intra-uterine viral infection has been suggested[5].

Carcinoid Heart Disease

The changes of the endocardium found in carcinoid heart disease are characteristic.

Fibrous plaques affecting particularly the right ventricular outflow tract, are located just beneath the pulmonary valve. The pulmonary valve leaflets may also become thickened and may contract. Commissural fusion may occasionally be observed. The tricuspid valve may also be involved as well as the chordae tendineae.

The fibrous thickening may be focal or more diffuse and may have a blueish appearance.

The lesions may also be encountered on the left side of the heart.

Histological appearances consist of superimposition of the abnormal material on the original endocardium, which is usually intact. The superimposed tissue consists of some spindle-shaped cells as well as a few collagen fibres enmeshed in an acellular metachromatic ground substance, typically devoid of elastic fibres (Figure 3.16). Some lymphocytes, plasma cells and mast cells can also often be identified.

Diagnosis, therefore, is easily achieved by the presence of metachromasia and the absence of elastic tissue. The latter is found in all other types of endocardial thickening.

Pathogenesis of the endocardial lesion

Three factors in the production of the heart lesions have been proposed although their pathogenesis is still debated:

(1) dilatation of the right side of the heart during an attack of flushing;

(2) local serotonin action resulting in deposition of fibrin and platelets;

(3) altered tryptophan metabolism, together with hypoproteinaemia and hypovitaminosis, which leads to lowering of tissue resistance to trauma[6].

References

1. Still, W. J. S. (1961). Endocardial thickening associated with diseased valves. *Br. Heart J.*, **23,** 155

2. Fisher, E. and Davis, E. R. (1958). Observations concerning the pathogenesis of endocardial thickening in the adult heart. *Am. Heart J.*, **56**, 553

3. Still, W. J. S. (1961). Endocardial fibroelastosis. *Am. Heart J.*, **61**, 579

4. Davies, J. N. P. (1963). Pathology and pathogenesis of endocardial disease. *Cardiologia*, **42**, 161

5. Olsen, E. G. J. (1980). In *The Pathology of the Heart*. Second Edition, p. 329. (London and Basingstoke: The Macmillan Press Ltd)

6. Thorson, A. and Nordenfelt, O. (1959). Development of valvular lesions in metastatic carcinoid disease. *Br. Heart J.*, **21**, 243

Degeneration, Deposition and Diseases of Connective Tissue

4

Various degenerative changes can be found in the myocardium among which are so-called cloudy swelling, basophilic (mucinous) degeneration, and hyaline change.

Cloudy Swelling, Hydropic and Vacuolar Degeneration

It is believed that each of these changes belongs to the same process, reflecting an increase in water content of the cell and a decline of the efficiency of the sodium pump.

Macroscopically no changes can be found but the myocardium may be flabby and greyish-brown in appearance. In cloudy swelling the myocardial cell diameter is increased and the cytoplasm is granular (Figure 4.1). The changes may also be seen in autolysis and as an artefact in tissue obtained by bioptome.

The changes of 'cloudy swelling' merge with hydropic change when individual fibrils become separated by ill-defined light areas (Figure 4.2).

Vacuolar degeneration is present when clear spaces can be seen with a well-defined edge (Figure 4.3). These spaces may surround nuclei and must be distinguished from the perinuclear halos seen in hypertrophic cardiomyopathy which are by contrast ill-defined and also show fibrillar degeneration.

Basophilic (Mucinous) Degeneration

Basophilic degeneration may be found in normal hearts and in hypertrophied myocardium irrespective of the cause of the hypertrophy and is usually most frequently found with increasing age[1]. It has been shown to be a glycoprotein and stains positively with PAS stains, Best's Carmine and Langhan's Iodine and Alcian Blue[2].

Basophilic change can only be identified microscopically and takes the form of a blueish-purple granular change affecting the entire myocardial fibre or part of it when examined on haematoxylin and eosin staining, occasionally small groups of adjacent fibres are affected (Figure 4.4). On transverse sections the material is located in the outer rim of the fibres and in partly affected fibres nuclei and cytoplasm are normal.

Basophilic change can readily be observed in the ventricular myocardium, particularly the posterior aspect of the left ventricle. It has also been identified in the left atrial appendage.

Hyaline Change

Myocardial fibres affected by this change show a homogeneous refractile cytoplasm and stain deeply eosinophilic. The nuclei may be pale or absent (Figure 4.5).

The changes are most readily identified in myocardial infarction but can also be found in any part of hypertrophied myocardium or in patients treated with chemotherapy[3]. The cause remains obscure.

Electron microscopy shows indistinct myofibrils and lamellae in the mitochondria.

Amyloid

According to the WHO/ISFC definition and classification of cardiomyopathies and specific heart muscle diseases[4], amyloid belongs to the second group and is classified into the following types:

primary;
secondary;
familial, hereditary cardiac amyloidosis;
familial Mediterranean fever; and
senile.

Other classifications have been proposed such as subdivision into peri-reticulin and peri-collagen types, or according to the chemical structure[5,6].

Amyloid resembles interfibrillary glycoproteins of the ground substance of connective tissue and by means of peptide mapping similar, but not identical, chemical compositions between different individuals have been found. Amyloid proteins of immunological origin and non-immunoglobulin proteins have also been demonstrated. Theories of deposition include abnormal protein synthesis of plasma cells or secretion of histiocytes/mesenchymal cells.

The heart is involved in all types and in the primary form cardiac involvement may be as high as 90%[7]. Macroscopically, the heart is overweight and the walls are rigid having a glass-like appearance (Figure 4.6). Not only is the myocardium involved but endocardium and valves as well as the epicardium may all be affected. The areas of deposition can readily be identified by soaking slices of tissue in aqueous iodine solution (Figure 4.7).

Microscopically, amyloid consists of laminated deposits which are occasionally related to blood vessels. Alternatively amyloid may be diffusely distributed between myocardial fibres. Adjacent myocardial fibres may show evidence of degeneration. A chronic inflammatory cell infiltrate may also be found making distinction from viral myocarditis difficult unless care is taken to identify amyloid. Vessels are frequently involved. A form where amyloid is confined to the left atrium is also recognized.

Amyloid has a flaky appearance and may be laminated. On haematoxylin and eosin staining it has a hyaline pink appearance (Figure 4.8). Staining with Methyl Violet shows a rose-violet discoloration (Figure 4.9). The time-honoured staining with Congo Red viewed under cross-polaroid light shows an apple-green change (Figure 4.10 a and b). Staining with thioflavine T shows yellow-green fluorescence when viewed under ultraviolet light (Figure 4.11). Highly reliable recognition has been reported by using sodium sulphate–Alcian Blue stains which result in a green colour[8] (Figure 4.12).

Electron microscopy allows definitive diagnosis. Amyloid has a fibrillar structure; often up to eight lateral aggregates of filaments each 7.5 nm wide with a periodicity of 10 nm can be recognized. Thicker fibrils (14–45 nm) which occasionally show beading can also be identified (Figure 4.13).

Familial Amyloidosis

The symptomatology of genetically determined amyloidosis has been well defined. Polyneuropathy is a constant manifestation.

Familial Mediterranean Fever

The fibrillar protein has an amino acid sequence distinct from any known human protein. Morphologically it is typical of 'secondary' amyloid.

Senile Amyloidosis

An incidence of between 3 and 90% in individuals over the age of 60 years has been noted. Nodules can be found in the atrial endocardium, more commonly in the left than in the right. Deposits around myocardial cells can also be seen[9].

Amyloid may also occur in association with myelomatosis but the heart is rarely affected; when it is, it is only to a mild degree.

Disturbances of Fat Metabolism

Characteristically in anaemia the so-called 'thrush breast' changes are found. More frequently the diffuse form is present which is not recognizable with the naked eye.

Microscopically, fat globules of varying size accumulate and may coalesce to form small cysts within myocardial fibres (Figure 4.14). It has already been noted in myocardial infarction but has also been described in toxaemia of pregnancy, alcohol abuse, carbon monoxide poisoning and in nutritional deficiency[10].

Fat change of myocardial fibres must be distinguished from infiltration of fat when fat cells extend from the epicardium into the myocardium between myocardial fibres (Figure 4.15). It is a frequent accompaniment of obesity, but in the right ventricle and atrium it can occur in individuals of normal weight. Fatty replacement is also found in muscular dystrophy and Friedreich's ataxia.

Disturbances of Carbohydrate Metabolism

Carbohydrate disturbances are well-recognized in conditions such as Pompe's disease (Figure 4.16) when severe glycogen accumulation is found. Glycogen also increases in hypertrophy from known causes but decreases in heart failure. (See Chapter 2).

Calcification

Three forms are recognized: dystrophic, metastatic and idiopathic[11].

Dystrophic Calcification

This is the most frequently found form of calcification and accompanies degeneration. It may affect valves, for example in rheumatic heart disease and in the aortic valve in calcific aortic disease (Figure 4.17), but it may also be found in advancing age. Areas of infarction in the myocardium may also be affected (Figure 4.18).

Metastatic Calcification

This occurs in previously normal tissue and may take place when ionized serum calcium is increased, a local rise in the pH value occurs, or when serum phosphorus is elevated. Diseases which may lead to this form of calcification include hyperparathyroid disease, renal failure, hypervitaminosis D, or widespread bone disease due to neoplasm (Figure 4.19).

Idiopathic Calcification

This occurs in normal tissue but without any recognizable underlying cause.

Calcification in infants and in the newborn is well recognized. Coronary arteries are usually affected but calcium may not always be found[12] (See Chapter 11).

Calcification is recognized in the tissue by staining with Alizarin red (red colour) (Figure 4.20) and by the Von Kossa silver method (Figure 4.21) (black colour).

Wherever calcification is seen ossification may occur (Figure 4.22); it is rarely found in the heart.

Pigmentation

The most commonly encountered pigmentation in the heart is deposition of iron in the myocardium which may be endogenous or exogenous.

Endogenous Iron Deposition

Haemochromatosis, an inborn error of metabolism, frequently involves the heart. Macroscopically, the myocardium may show a brownish tinge together with fibrosis (Figure 4.23). Histologically, iron deposition usually occurs at the nuclear poles and extends throughout the myocardial fibre with the greatest concentration in the centre of the cell (Figure 4.24 a and b). If they are severely affected, degeneration of the myocardial fibres is found which may result in necrosis and subsequently in varying degrees of fibrosis. The conduction tissue may be involved, but valves and coronary arteries are spared[13].

Other endogenous forms of pigmentation include lipofuscin, particularly in the elderly (Figure 4.25 a and b); lipochrome, seen in brown atrophy of the heart; haemofuscin and bile pigments.

Exogenous Iron Deposition

Exogenous iron deposition is most frequently due to transfusion and is morphologically indistinguishable from endogenous iron deposition[14]. The distribution of iron within the myocardium is, however, uneven. Degenerative changes and fibrosis are rare.

Electron microscopy reveals siderin granules containing iron particles approximately 6 nm in diameter scattered between fibrils (Figure 4.26). Degenerative changes may, however, be found.

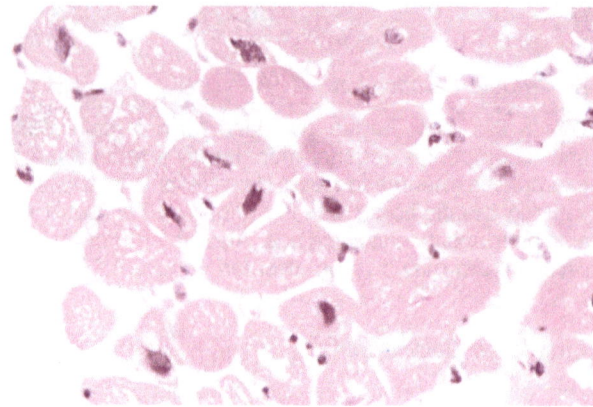

Figure 4.1 So-called cloudy swelling can be identified by the granular change of the myocardial fibres due to focal separation of myofibrils by oedema.   H & E × 400

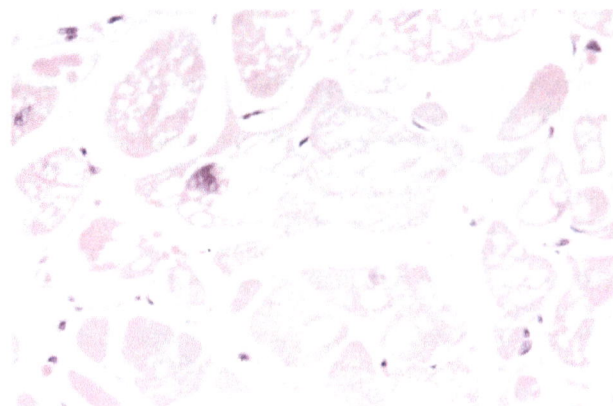

Figure 4.2 Hydropic change is characterized by more severe separation of myofibrils.   H & E × 400

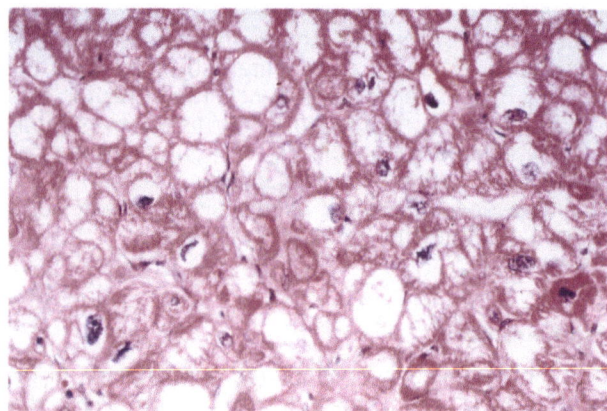

Figure 4.3 Vacuolar degeneration is present when clear, well demarcated central zones in the myocardial fibres predominate giving a lace-like appearance. Not infrequently a thin rim of myofibrils is all that remains.   H & E × 400

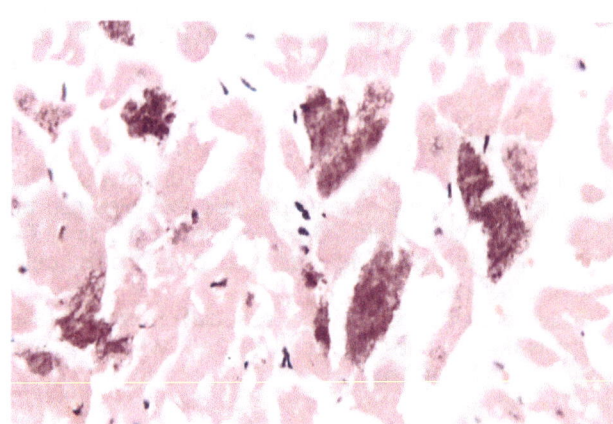

Figure 4.4 Photomicrograph illustrating basophilic change.   H & E × 200

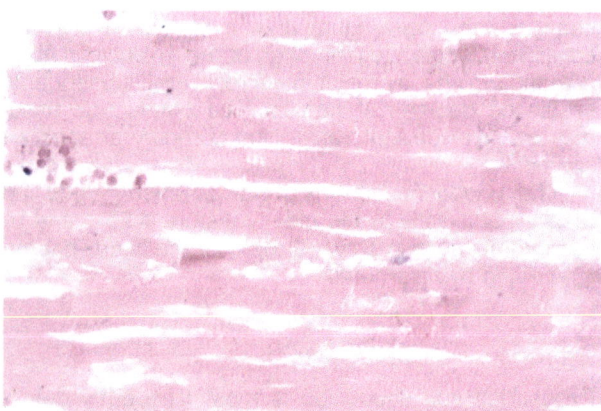

Figure 4.5 Hyaline change of the myocardial fibres is characterized by eosinophilic staining of the fibres and usually absent nuclei. Note that there is no inflammatory cell infiltrate.   H & E × 200

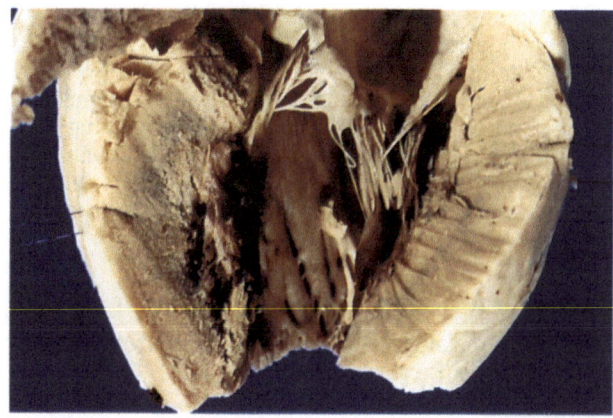

Figure 4.6 Amyloid heart disease. The left ventricle has been opened to illustrate the thick (and rigid) walls and the 'glass-like' appearance

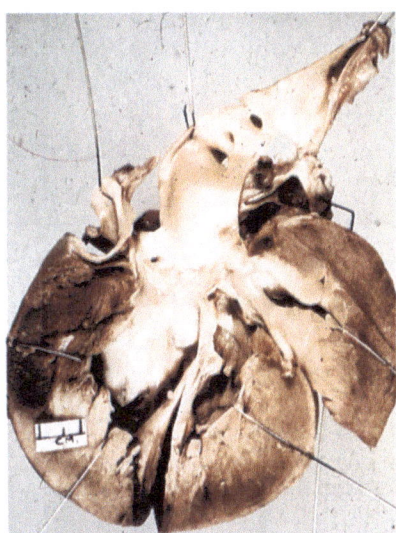

Figure 4.7 Part of the left ventricular wall has been immersed in aqueous iodine solution permitting identification of amyloid by the naked eye (brown colour)

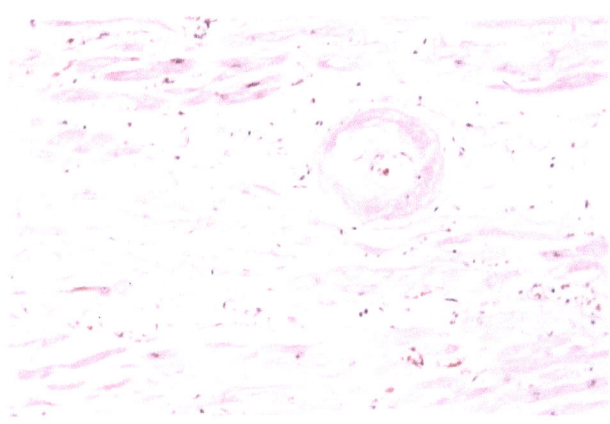

Figure 4.8 Amyloid deposition staining pink on haematoxylin and eosin preparation. The arteriole in the illustration also shows involvement of the wall characterized by uniform pink staining. H & E × 100

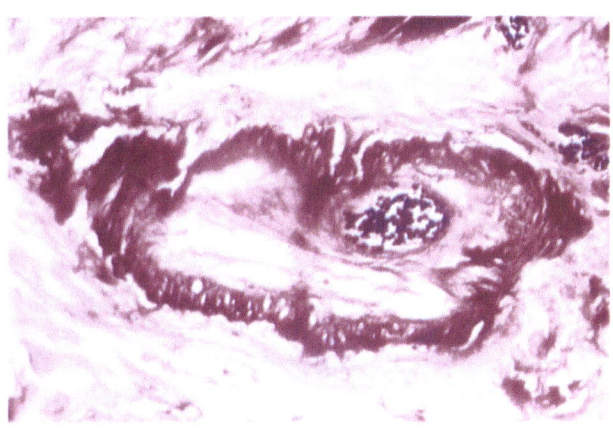

Figure 4.9 Amyloid deposition shown in an arteriolar wall and surrounding connective tissue demonstrating a rose-violet discolouration. Methyl Violet × 200

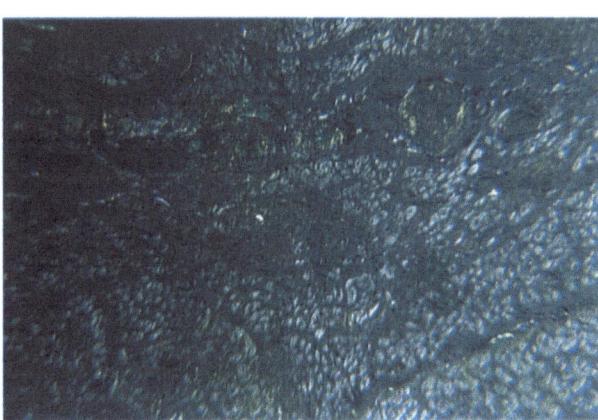

Figure 4.10a Illustration of staining for amyloid with Congo Red viewed under crossed polaroids resulting in apple-green fluorescence. Congo Red × 50

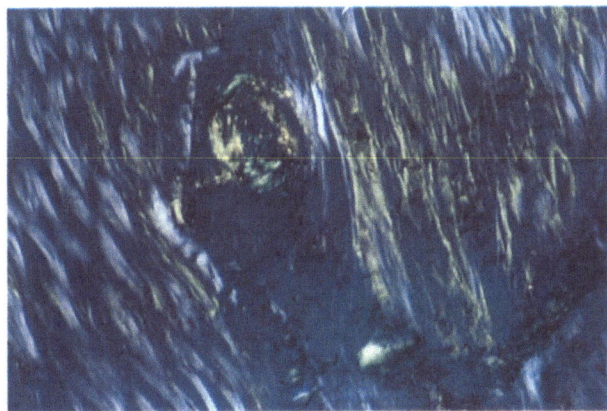

Figure 4.10b As in Figure 4.10a. Congo Red × 100

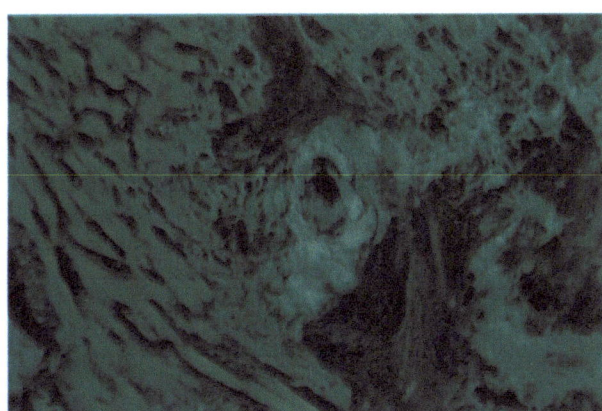

Figure 4.11 Amyloid giving a yellow-green fluorescence stained with Thioflavine T viewed under ultraviolet light × 100

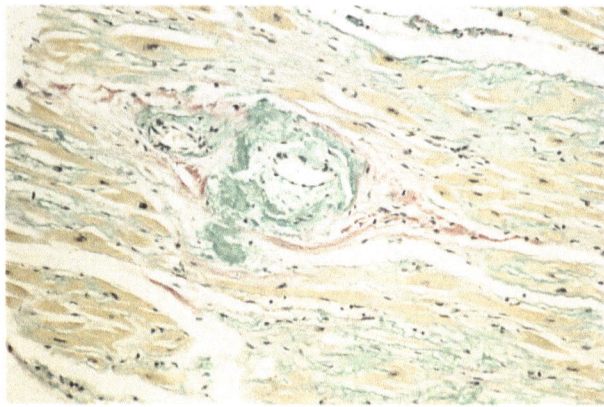

Figure 4.12 Staining for amyloid by sodium sulphate–Alcian Blue, a most reliable stain for demonstrating amyloid × 100

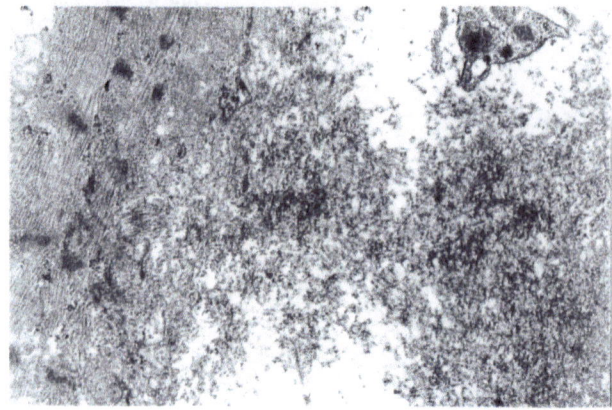

Figure 4.13 Electron micrograph illustrating the characteristic, finely fibrillar structure of amyloid. Lead citrate and uranyl acetate × 13000

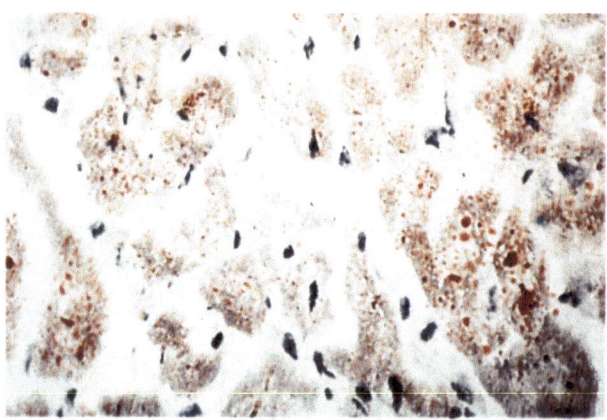

Figure 4.14 Focal accumulation of fat globules from the myocardium of a severely anaemic patient. Fat globules can be found in many conditions including early myocardial infarction. Oil Red O × 200

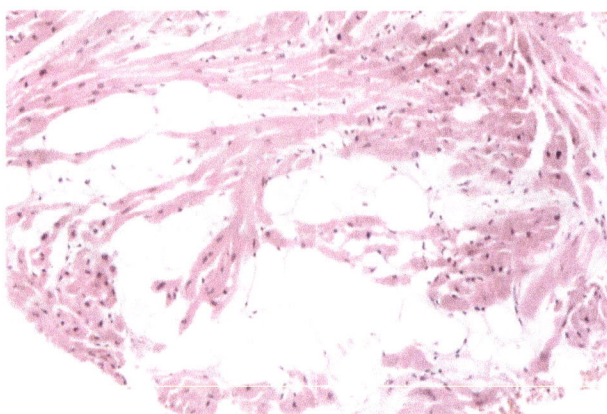

Figure 4.15 Fatty infiltration. Fat globules between myocardial fibres can be readily seen. The tissue illustrated comes from a right ventricular endomyocardial biopsy. H & E × 100

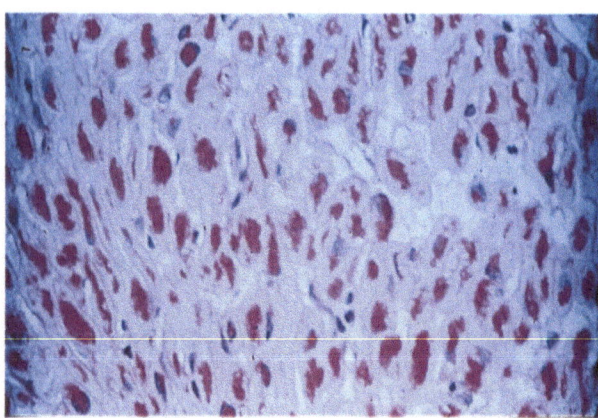

Figure 4.16 Photomicrograph from a child with Pompe's disease showing severe accumulation of glycogen. On haematoxylin and eosin staining the myocardial fibres exhibit a lace-like pattern. (See Figure 4.3). PAS × 160. (By courtesy of Dr L Becu)

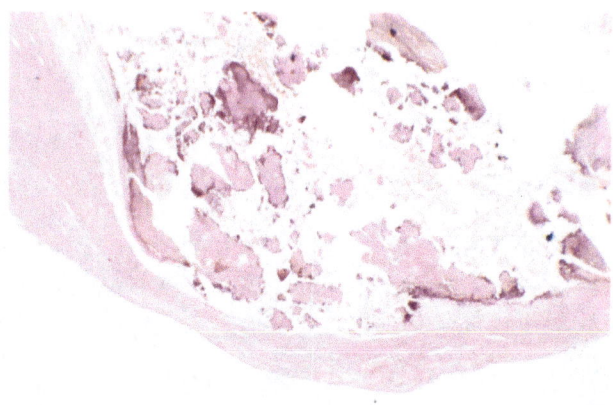

Figure 4.17 Calcific aortic valve disease showing distortion of the normal valvar architecture and large foci of calcification. H & E × 25

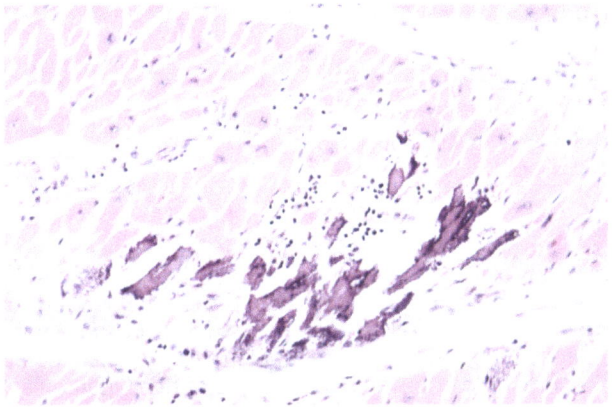

Figure 4.18 Dystrophic calcification of myocardial fibres in an area of necrosis in a patient with myocardial infarction. H & E × 100

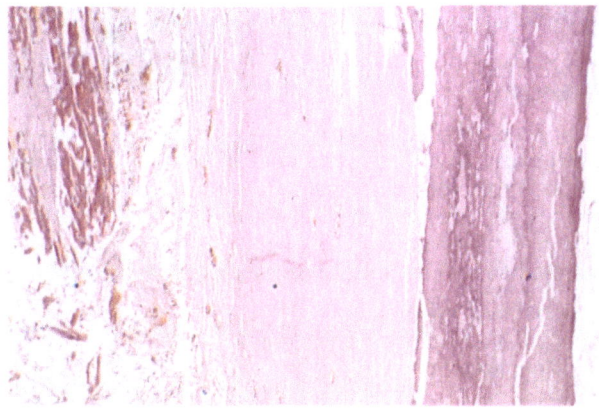

Figure 4.19 Metastatic calcification. A band of calcification in myocardium is seen from a patient with hyperparathyroidism. H & E × 25

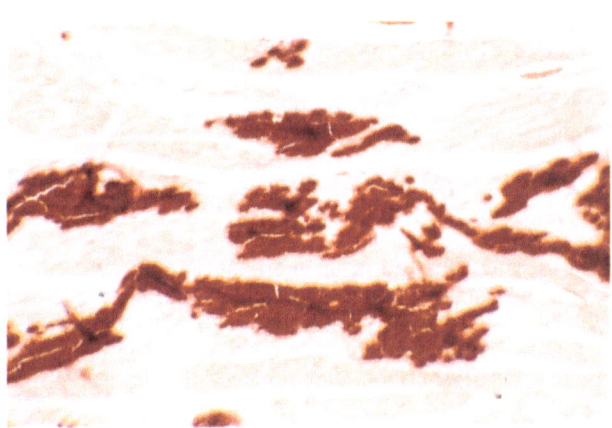

Figure 4.20 Calcification in tissue is characterized by Alizarin red staining giving a red discoloration. Alizarin Red × 200

Figure 4.21 Calcification characterized by Von Kossa staining (phosphate) resulting in black staining. Von Kossa × 100

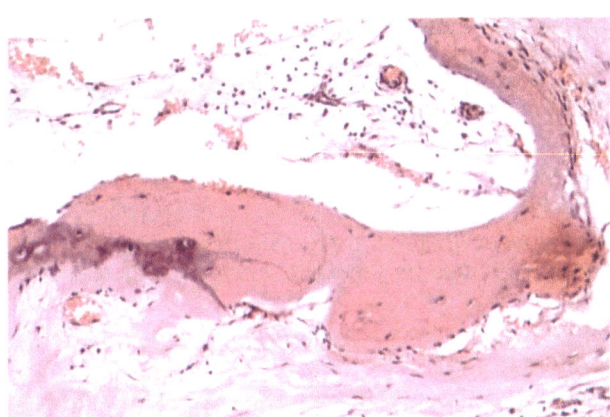

Figure 4.22 Illustration of ossification in the myocardium in a case with widespread dystrophic calcification. H & E × 100

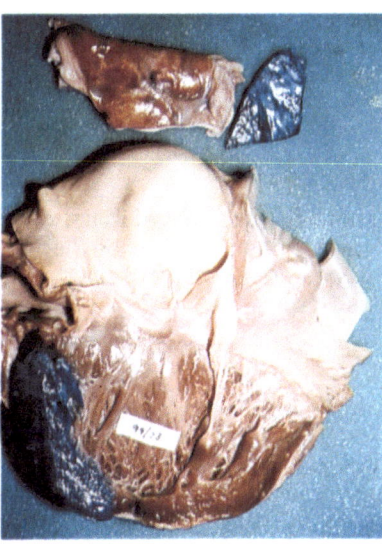

Figure 4.23 The left ventricle has been opened to show extensive iron deposition (Perl's Prussian Blue reaction)

Necrosis

Necrosis is defined as an irreversible cellular change or death of a cell or groups of cells in contact with living tissue. It may follow severe degenerative changes such as vacuolar change or if hypertrophy is particularly severe. It is of course frequently seen in myocardial infarction. Three types of necrosis are recognized[15]:

coagulation necrosis;
coagulative myocytolysis; and
colliquative myocytolysis

Coagulation Necrosis

Changes include early myocardial cell acidophilia, nuclear changes (pyknosis), karyolysis or karyorrhexis and a polymorphonuclear cell infiltrate (Figure 4.27).

Coagulative Myocytolysis

This form of necrosis may be found in normal myocardium either close to coagulation necrosis or in the region of the wall affected by myocardial infarction. Changes in this type of necrosis include hypercontraction of the fibre or a segment of the fibre (Figure 4.28), stretching and breakdown of myofibrils in other segments or adjacent cells, and an increase in affinity for acidophilic stains.

In the later stages the contractile part of the fibre is removed by macrophages and the sarcolemmal tube is all that remains (Figure 4.29). Later still a fibrous scar results.

Colliquative Myocytolysis

Changes include dissolution of myofibrils following intracellular fluid accumulation otherwise this form has similar appearances to coagulative myocytolysis.

Atrophy

Myocardial fibres are smaller than normal. Atrophy occurs as an accompaniment to myocardial infarction, in areas of severe fibrosis or in acromegaly. Brown atrophy of the heart implies a distinctive atrophy with a reduction in size such that adult hearts resemble those of infants. The myocardium is deep brown in colour and coronary arteries pursue a tortuous course.

The myocardial fibres are severely reduced in size and accumulation of lipid-containing granules (indistinguishable from haemofuscin) are found.

Mitral Valve Prolapse

Although the pathogenetic mechanisms of mitral valve prolapse are not fully established, in view of the fact that degenerative changes are usually observed, this topic is included in this Chapter.

Definition

Mitral valve prolapse may be defined as a recognizable condition with characteristic clinical and pathological changes. The entity has become increasingly recognized in recent years and an incidence of up to 6% has been reported on echocardiographic screening of normal females[16]. All ages can be affected but most frequently those between 30 to 50 yrs suffer from this syndrome. In younger age groups females predominate, but with advancing years the sex incidence tends to be equal.

Clinically, chest pain, a non-ejection mid-to-late systolic click followed by a late systolic murmur characterize the condition[17].

Pathology

Not infrequently both valve leaflets are affected but the changes are usually much more pronounced in the posterior mitral valve leaflet, particulary in the middle third. Varying degrees of redundant tissue, which results in doming, can be recognized postmortem, particularly when water under pressure is introduced into the left ventricle (Figure 4.30). In Chapter 1 the normal mitral valve was discussed and this showed a large surface area of the anterior mitral valve leaflet. In mitral valve prolapse it is the posterior mitral valve leaflet which in surface area often exceeds the anterior mitral valve leaflet[18] (Figure 4.31).

The leaflets are transparent, gelatinous in appearance with a bluish tinge. These changes extend into the chordae tendineae which are elongated and may show beading along their course (Figure 4.32). Rupture is not infrequent and may be the reason for surgical removal of affected valves. Secondary changes due to mitral valve insufficiency may result in some thickening of the leaflets giving rise to some opaqueness.

Histology

The striking change is an increase in the layer of the zona spongiosa which may occupy over 90% of the total thickness of the valve leaflet (Figure 4.33). Degenerative changes in the zona fibrosa are typical and consist of eosinophilic smudges with loss of the fibrillar nature characteristic of collagen tissue. Vascularity is not increased. A layer of collagen tissue on the deformed face results in macroscopic opaqueness and a uniform thickening. This is found when insufficiency has been present for some time.

Histochemistry

The mucinous material consists of uronic acid mucopolysaccharides and stains positive with Alcian Blue at pH 2.5 (Figure 4.34) and also positive with the PAS stain. The material is metachromatic with Toluidine Blue at low pH, strongest between pH 3 and 5. Positive reactions with Congo Red (green fluorescence on crossed polaroid examination) have also been found.

Electron Microscopy

Amorphous material surrounded by irregular collagen fibrils with loss of periodicity is typical (Figure 4.35).

Nature of Mitral Valve Prolapse

The nature and pathogenesis of mitral valve prolapse is controversial but myxomatous degeneration of the zona spongiosa, which may be prominent from birth resulting in doming, is the likely cause particularly if myocardial abnormalities which interfere with normal mitral valve function are present[19]. Abnormal or decreased chordal insertion has also been suggested. A biochemical fault may be a causal factor in promoting degeneration of collagen. Familial occurrence has been described.

Complications

The more common complications include chordal rupture, infective endocarditis and calcification. The aortic valve may be involved showing identical features.

The relationship with Marfan's disease is also controversial. Although mitral valve prolapse is found in patients with overt Marfan's disease and, conversely, Marfan's disease in patients with mitral valve prolapse, it is unlikely to represent a *forme fruste* of Marfan's disease[20]. (See Chapter 11).

Other Degenerative Changes

Other degenerative changes include Ehlers–Danlos syndrome, osteogenesis imperfecta, Holt–Oram syndrome and pseudoxanthoma elasticum (Figures 4.36 and 4.37). For a fuller account of this topic the reader is referred to Olsen, 1980[20].

References

1. Rosai, J. and Lascano, E. F. (1970). Basophilic (mucoid) degeneration of the myocardium. A disorder of glycogen metabolism. *Am. J. Pathol.*, **61**, 99

2. Scotti, T. M. (1955). Basophilic (mucinous) degeneration of the myocardium. *Am. J. Clin. Pathol.*, **25**, 994

3. Buja, L. M. and Ferrans, V. J. (1975). Myocardial injury produced by antineoplastic drugs. In Fleckenstein, A. and Rona, G. (eds). *Recent Advances in Studies on Cardiac Structure and Metabolism.* Vol. 6. *Pathophysiology and Morphology of Myocardial Cell Alterations.* p. 487. (Baltimore: University Park Press)

4. Report of the WHO/ISFC Task Force on the Definition and Classification of Cardiomyopathies (1980). *Br. Heart J.*, **44**, 672

5. Heller, H., Missmahl, H. P., Sohar, E. and Gafnı, J. (1964). Amyloidosis: Its differentation into peri-reticulin and peri-collagen types. *J. Pathol. Bacteriol.*, **88**, 15

6. Stirling, G. A. (1975). Amyloidosis. In Harrison, C. V and Weinbren, K. (eds). *Recent Advances in Pathology.* p. 249. (Edinburgh, London and New York: Churchill Livingstone)

7. Symmers, W. St. C. (1956). Primary amyloidosis: a review. *J. Clin. Pathol.*, **9**, 187

8. Lendrum, A. C., Slidders, W. and Fraser, D. S. (1972). Renal hyalin. A study of amyloidosis and diabetic fibrinous vasculosis with new staining methods. *J. Clin. Pathol.*, **25**, 373

9. Wright, J. R. and Calkins, E. (1975). Amyloid in the aged heart: Frequency and clinical significance. *J. Am. Geriatr. Soc.*, **23**, 97

10. Alavaikko, M., Hirvonen, J. and Rasanen, O. (1970). Fatty change in papillary heart muscle and in its arterioles. Analysis of a material of 262 autopsies. *Acta Pathol. Microbiol. Scand.*, **78**, 458

11. Olsen, E. G. J. (1980). In *The Pathology of the Heart.* Second Edition, p. 71. (London and Basingstoke: The Macmillan Press Ltd)

12. Witzleben, L. (1970). Idiopathic infantile arterial calcification – a misnomer? *Am. J. Cardiol*, **26**, 305

13. Keschener, H. W. (1951). The heart in haemochromatosis. *South Med. J.*, **44**, 927

14. Cappel, D. F., Hutchinson, H. E. and Jowett, M. (1957). Transfusional siderosis: the effects of excessive iron deposits on the tissues. *J. Pathol. Bacteriol.*, **74**, 245

15. Baroldi, G. (1975). Different types of myocardial necrosis in coronary heart disease: a pathophysiologic review of their functional significance. *Am. Heart J.*, **89**, 742

16. Brown, O. R., Kloster, F. E. and DeMots, H. (1975). Incidence of mitral valve prolapse in asymptomatic normal. *Circulation*, **52**, Supplement II, 77

17. Barlow, J. B. and Pocock, W. A. (1979). Mitral valve prolapse, the specific billowing mitral leaflet syndrome, or an insignificant non-ejection systolic click. *Am. Heart J.*, **97**, 277

18. Ranganathan, N., Silver, M. D., Robinson, T. I., Kostuk, W., Felderhof, C. H., Patt, N. L., Wilson, J. K. and Wigle, E. D. (1973). Angiographic–morphologic correlation in patients with severe mitral regurgitation due to prolapse of the posterior mitral valve leaflet. *Circulation*, **48**, 514

19. Olsen, E. G. J. and Al-Rufaie, H. K. (1980). The floppy mitral valve. Study on pathogenesis. *Br. Heart J.*, **44**, 674

20. Olsen, E. G. J. (1980). Degenerative and connective-tissue disorders of the cardiovascular system. In *The Pathology of the Heart.* Second Edition, p. 81. (London and Basingstoke: The Macmillan Press Ltd)

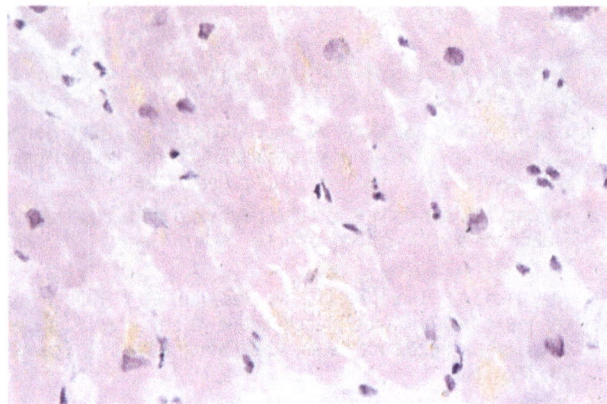

Figure 4.24a Endogenous iron deposition in haemochromatosis, showing brown staining granules in myocardial fibres. H & E × 400

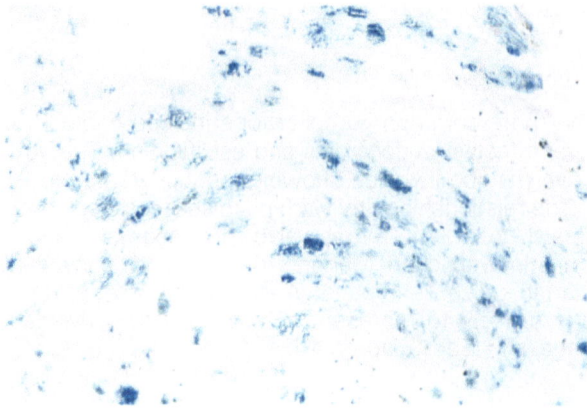

Figure 4.24b The same case as Figure 4.24a giving a positive result with Perl's Prussian Blue reaction × 200

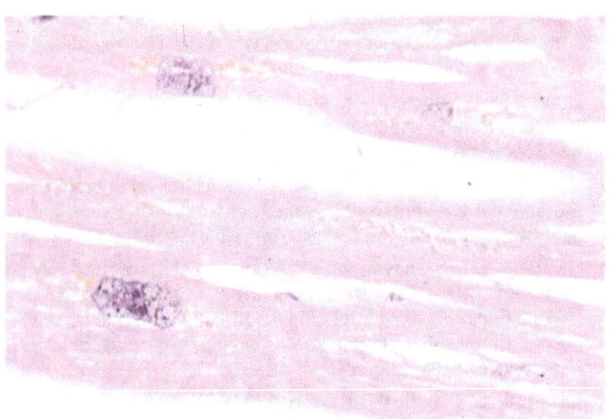

Figure 4.25a Lipofuscin deposition, particularly near the nuclear poles. H & E × 600

Figure 4.25b The same case as Figure 4.25a with Schmorl's reaction resulting in dark blue staining × 600

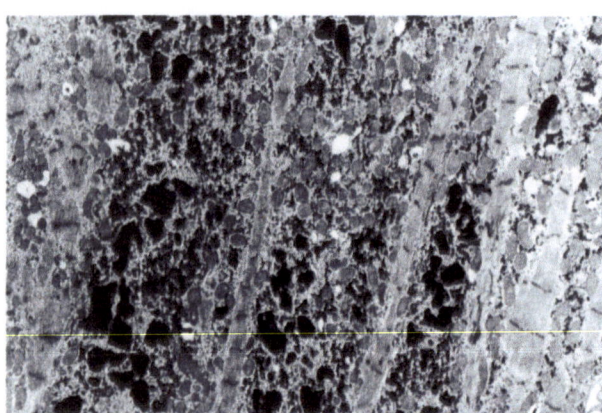

Figure 4.26 Electron micrograph showing exogenous iron deposition (electron-dense areas) between myocardial fibrils. Lead citrate and uranyl acetate × 4300

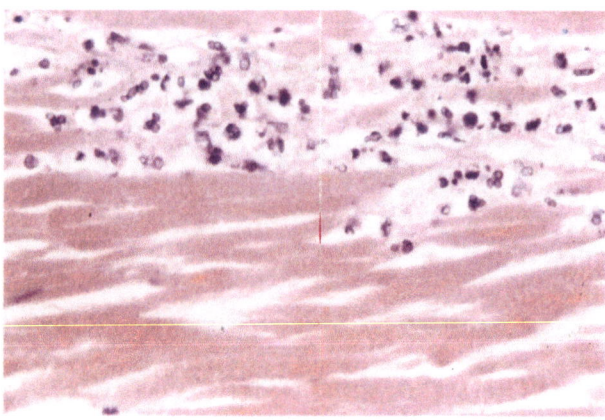

Figure 4.27 Photomicrograph of coagulation necrosis. The myocardial fibres show acidophilia (hyaline change). The nuclei have disappeared. A predominantly neutrophilic infiltrate can clearly be seen. From a patient with acute myocardial infarction. H & E × 200

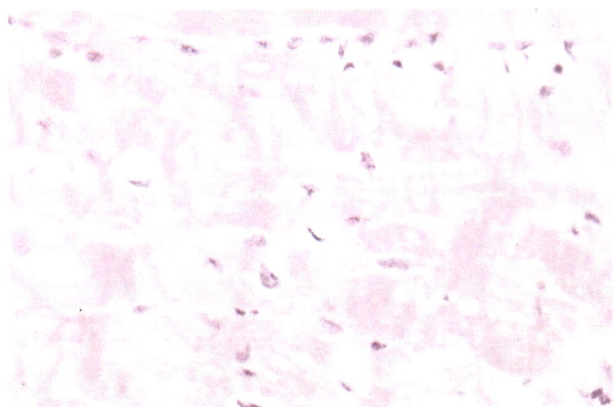

Figure 4.28 Coagulative necrosis. Note the extensive, severe contraction bands (hypercontraction).   H & E × 400

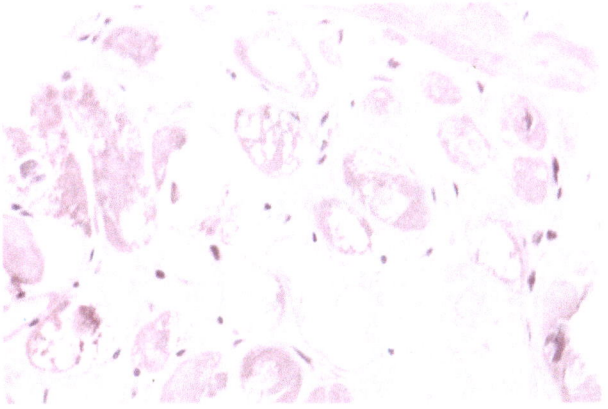

Figure 4.29 Coagulative necrosis. In some areas the sarcolemma is all that remains whilst in other fibres various stages of this form of necrosis can be identified.   H & E × 400

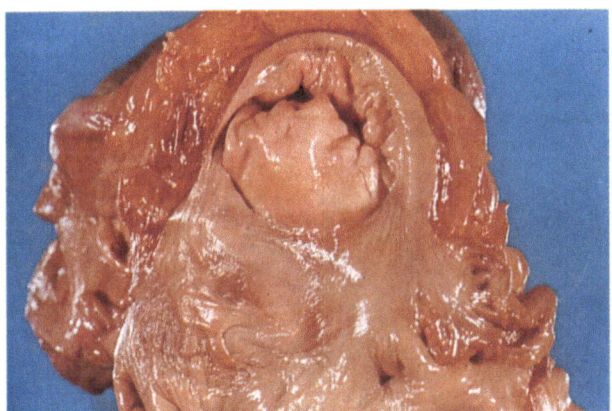

Figure 4.30 Mitral valve prolapse (atrial view). The prolapsing mitral valve bulges into the left atrium. The larger leaflet is the posterior mitral valve leaflet

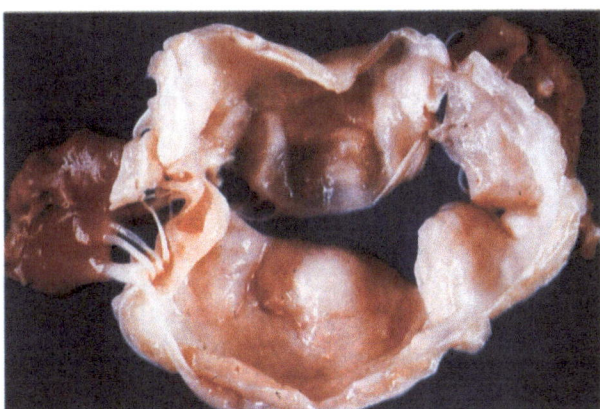

Figure 4.31 Surgical specimen of a prolapsing mitral valve. Note the larger surface area of the posterior leaflet compared to the anterior leaflet (top of the photograph)

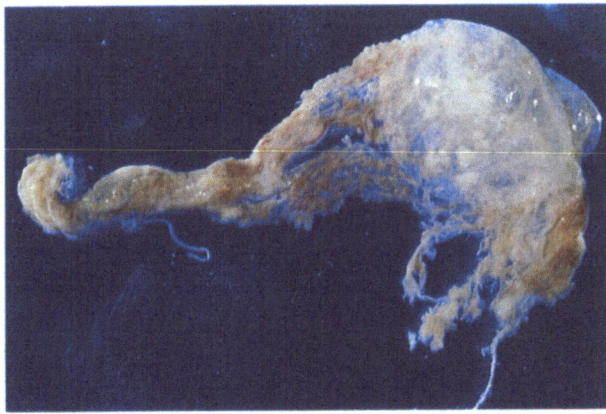

Figure 4.32 Posterior mitral valve leaflet from a patient with mitral valve prolapse. The valve leaflet is, in some areas, abnormally transparent. The chordae tendineae are also affected by the disease process and also have a gelatinous appearance. Beading can be seen

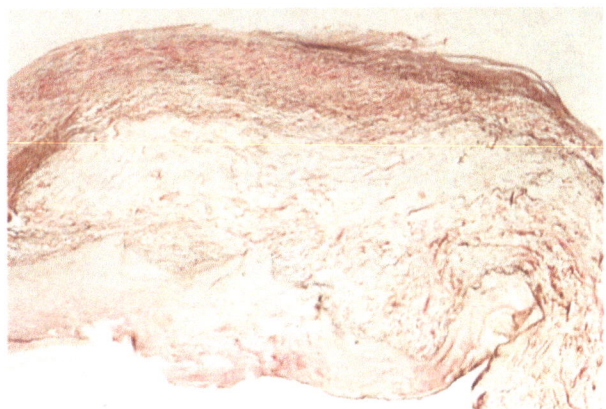

Figure 4.33 Mitral valve prolapse. The photomicrograph shows an extensive zona spongiosa involving especially the fibrosa (holding face) of the leaflet. The deformed face can clearly be seen on the upper aspect of the leaflet.   Elastic van Gieson × 25

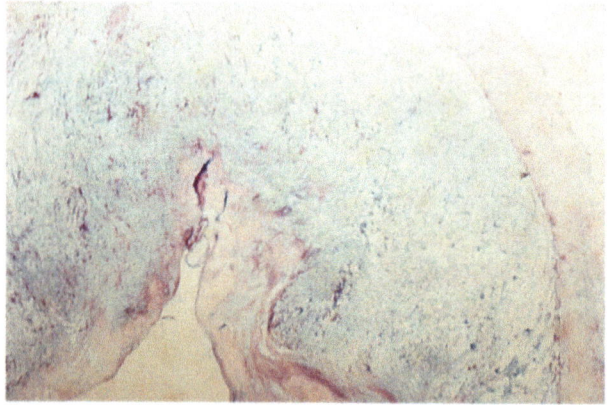

Figure 4.34 Alcian Blue-positive material is present in the severely widened zona spongiosa. Alcian Blue (pH 2.5) × 25

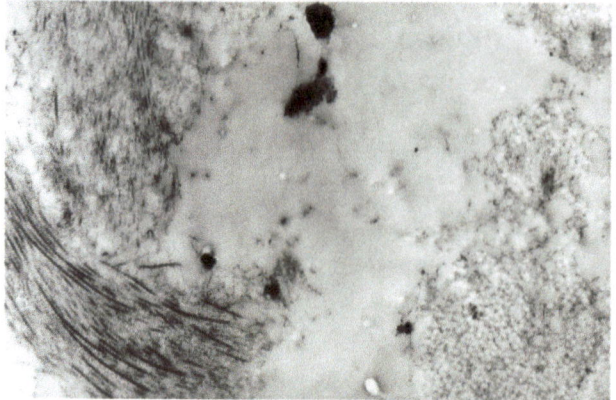

Figure 4.35 Electron micrograph showing loss of periodicity of the collagen bundles in the 'floppy valve'. Lead citrate and uranyl acetate × 9800

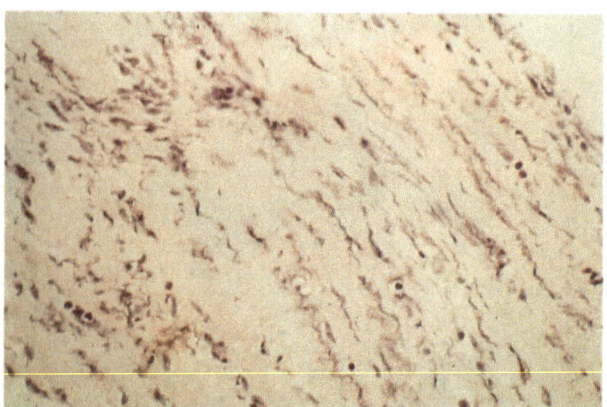

Figure 4.36 Pseudoxanthoma elasticum. Photomicrograph of the mitral valve showing calcification of collagen tissue which characterizes this condition histologically. H & E × 100

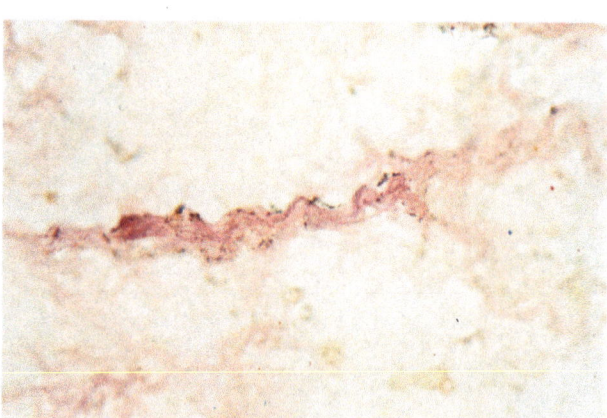

Figure 4.37 From the same case as Figure 4.36 showing calcium phosphate deposition on collagen tissue. Von Kossa × 400

Ischaemic Heart Disease and Myocardial Infarction

5

Ischaemia of the heart implies structural and functional abnormalities of the myocardium, resulting from inadequate blood supply. Many diseases may affect the coronary vessels including polyarteritis nodosa, giant cell or temporal arteritis, Takayasu's disease, systemic lupus erythematosus and thromboangiitis obliterans (Buerger's disease). (For description of these abnormalities please see Chapter 11.) Other causes include coronary embolism and stasis following ostial stenosis. Syphilis had been thought to be a major cause for such stenosis but it has more recently been shown that atherosclerosis is by far the most common abnormality[1].

Trauma, abnormalities of the blood favouring thrombosis, congenital abnormalities especially coronary arteries arising from the pulmonary trunk, viral infection and iatrogenic causes have all been described. As far as oral contraception is concerned, those patients that had suffered myocardial infarction also had at least one additional 'accepted' risk factor and therefore the influence of that type of contraception on myocardial infarction is unresolved.

By far the most common lesions are, however, those of atherosclerosis. Many risk factors have been documented over the years and an immense literature exists. Claims and counter-claims for such risks have been published. Amongst the more common risk factors are: cigarette smoking, diet, obesity, hypertension, level of physical activity, stress and drinking of soft water or coffee, as well as familial predisposition, sex of the patient and hyperlipidaemia[2].

Diabetes mellitus is also considered an 'accepted' risk factor. It has been shown that patients with diabetic capillaropathy are at greater risk of sustaining myocardial infarction compared to diabetic patients without such vascular involvement. Reports of the relationship between diabetes mellitus and subsequent development of cardiovascular disease are, however, not uniform[3].

Cigarette smoking results in catecholamine excretion and is related to high adrenergic activity and significant arrhythmia. Carbon monoxide, aryl hydrocarbon, nicotine and cadmium, have been implicated as active principles.

None of these risk factors should be considered in isolation but should be related to the countries where such studies have been undertaken. This is illustrated by the work of Dolder and Oliver[4] who carried out such studies in industrial and non-industrial countries.

Though some evidence of a decrease in the incidence of ischaemic heart disease and myocardial infarction exists in the USA following widespread publicity concerning the involvement of smoking, dietary habits and exercise, identification of patients likely to develop atherosclerosis and myocardial infarction is not, to date, possible. 'High risk' patients may not develop heart disease[5] whereas large numbers of 'low risk' patients have developed myocardial infarction[6].

The incidence of recorded death following ischaemic heart disease and myocardial infarction (Registrar General's figures) is high and some 160 000 patients are recorded annually as having died of this disease in England and Wales.

Definition and Classification of Terms

Those suggested by Haust, 1983[7] will be followed (see Table 5.1)

Table 5.1 Definitions and terminology of atherosclerotic lesions

I.	Early lesions	1. Fatty dots and streaks (Figure 5.1a and b)
		2. Gelatinous elevations
		3. Microthrombi
II.	Advanced lesions	1. White or pearly-white fibrous plaques (free of basocentral atheroma) consisting entirely of fibrous tissue or partly organized mural thrombi (Figure 5.2a and b)
		2. Atheromatous plaques consisting of a basocentral atheroma and fibrous cap (Figure 5.3)
III.	Complicated lesions (atherosclerotic plaques)	Advanced lesions with ulceration, thrombosis, haemorrhage, and marked calcification (Figure 5.4a and b)
IV.	Atheroma	The basocentral 'pool' of homogeneous proteinaceous and fatty substances in atheromatous plaques (II–2)
V.	Atheromatous lesions	Atheroma-containing lesions (II–2, any form of III)
VI.	Atherosclerotic lesions	A generic term referring to all or any form and stage of lesions

Atherogenesis

A number of major theories have been advanced to explain atherogenesis.

(1) *Encrustation Theory*: platelets and fibrin are deposited from the blood stream.

(2) *Haemodynamic Stress*: This theory suggests mural strain resulting from stress of pulsatile blood flow.

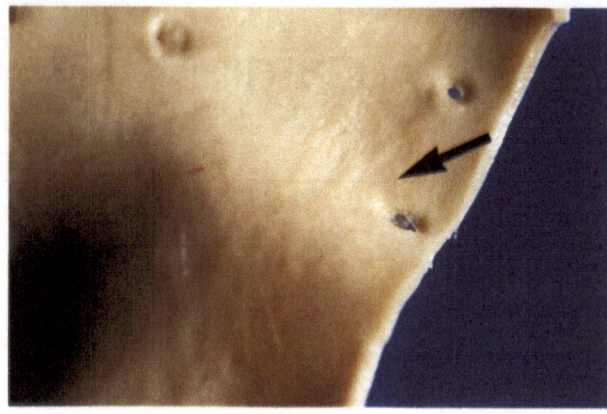

Figure 5.1a Fatty streaks (arrowed)

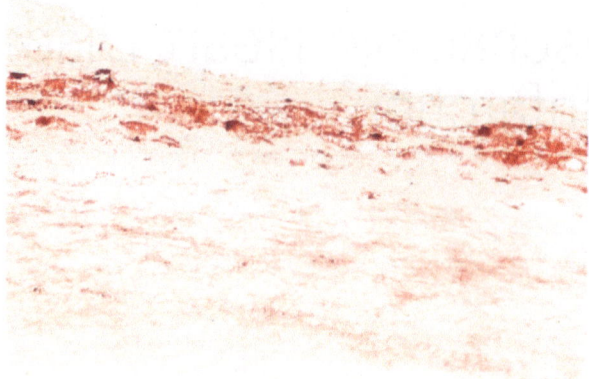

Figure 5.1b Fatty streak showing lipid deposition and lipid droplets in macrophages. Oil red O × 200

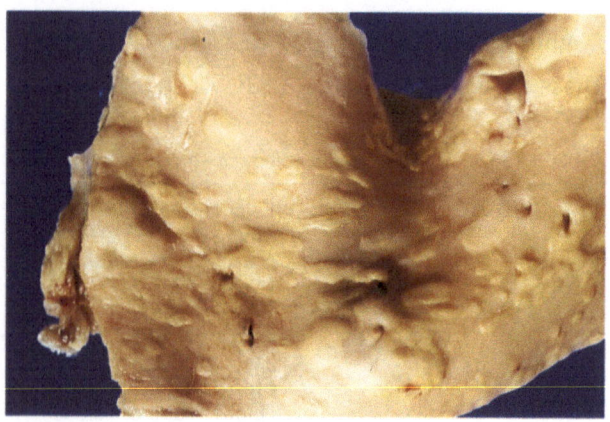

Figure 5.2a Fibrous plaques

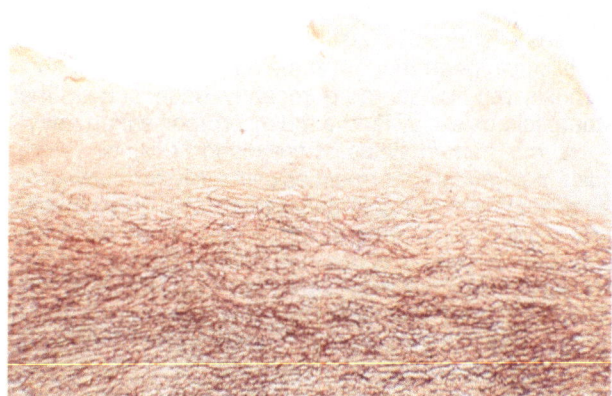

Figure 5.2b Advanced lesion showing a patchy organized thrombus which will result in a fibrous plaque (see Figure 5.2a). Elastic van Gieson × 50

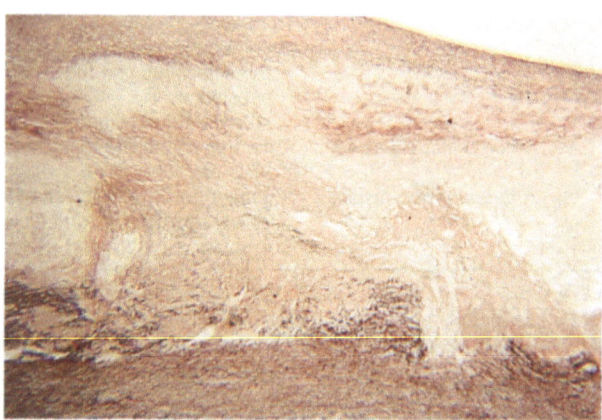

Figure 5.3 Atheromatous plaque showing basocentral atheroma and a fibrous cap. Elastic van Gieson × 50

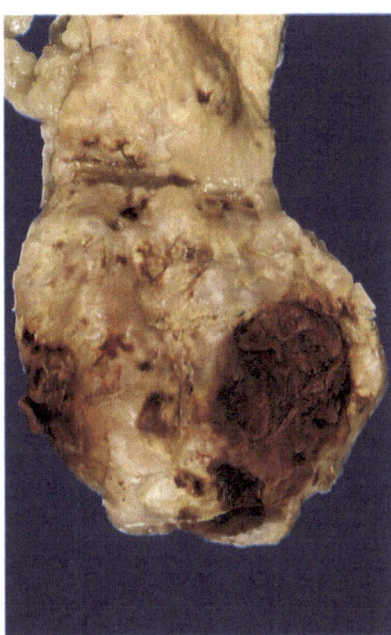

Figure 5.4a Complicated lesion with thrombus superimposition

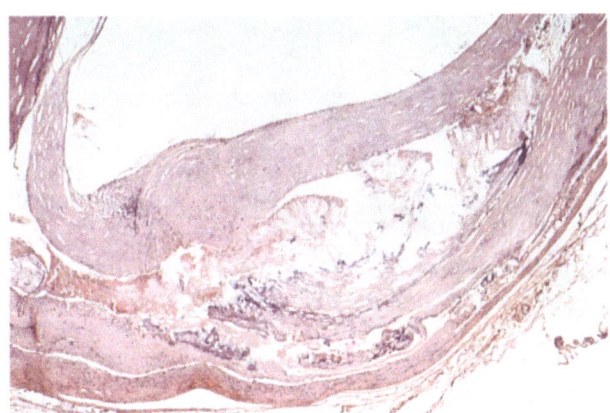

Figure 5.4b Complicated lesion showing a fibrous cap, atheroma and calcification. Ulceration is not evident. Elastic van Gieson × 25

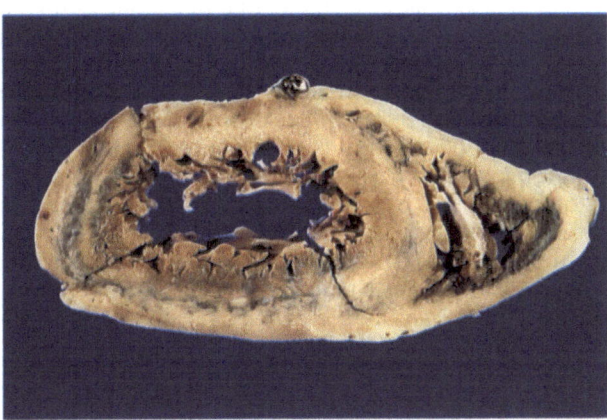

Figure 5.5 Postero-lateral ventricular and lateral right ventricular myocardial infarction of approximately one week's duration, showing extensive damage of the wall but the inner third of the left ventricular wall has been spared

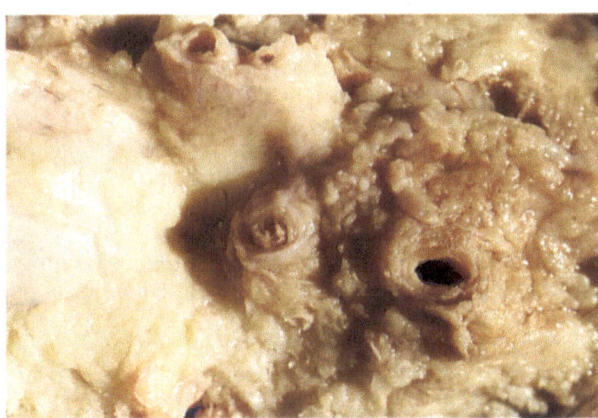

Figure 5.6a Total occlusion by thrombus of a coronary artery in a patient with recent myocardial infarction

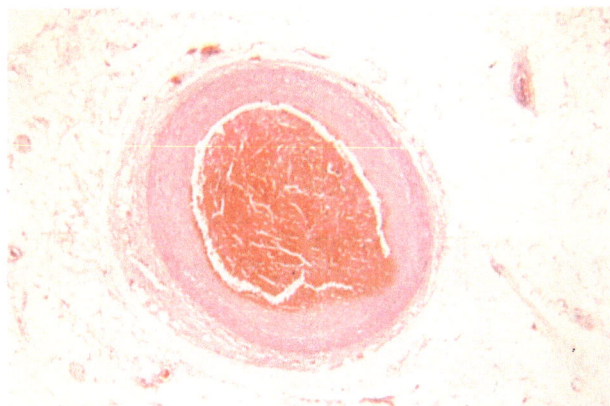

Figure 5.6b Total occlusion by a recent thrombus of a coronary artery superimposed on an area of mural erosion. The clear space surrounding the thrombus is fixation artefact. H & E × 25

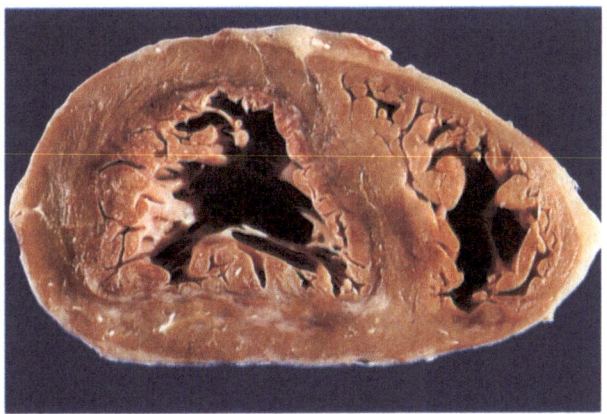

Figure 5.7 Cross-section of the ventricles midway between the apex and the atrio-ventricular junction. A recent subendocardial infarct can clearly be seen. In addition, focal areas of fibrosis in the posterior left ventricular wall are present

(3) *Filtration Theory*: low density lipoproteins enter the vascular wall.

(4) *Mural Hypoxia*: this is linked with the filtration theory in that hypoxia permits accumulation of lipoproteins (cholesterol)[2].

(5) *Monoclonal Theory*: this theory was promulgated by Benditt and Benditt[8] and suggested that genetically transformed smooth muscle cells give rise to atherosclerotic lesions. It has been suggested that the plaque arises from a single type of genetically transformed smooth muscle cells and hence the term 'monoclonal'.

Protagonistic and antagonistic views on each of these theories have been expressed and at our state of knowledge it is likely that all of these mechanisms may in some way be involved in atherogenesis.

Pathology

There are no consistent morphological changes for ischaemic heart disease which manifests itself as angina pectoris. Pathophysiologically, angina pectoris may result from temporary deficiency of oxygen supply to meet myocardial requirements.

In a more recent study comparison of patients with angina pectoris, suffering between 1 and 12 years and who died suddenly, with patients who also died suddenly but had no history of angina pectoris (except terminally), has shown slightly more extensive atherosclerosis and calcification in the group with angina pectoris[9].

It must be remembered that angina pectoris can also occur with normal arteries in conditions such as dilated or hypertrophic cardiomyopathies. No strict correlation between symptoms and damage of the myocardium, particularly in the form of fibrosis exist (see Chapter 9). Angina could be related to necrosis following inflammation or lack of oxygen supply resulting from the need to meet the requirements of the immense hypertrophy encountered in hypertrophic cardiomyopathy. In the syndrome 'angina pectoris, normal coronary arteries' endomyocardial biopsies have shown no morphological abnormalities of vessels at the histological or the electron-microscopic level of investigation. Possible metabolic causes have been suggested.

Types of Myocardial Infarction

Regional Infarction

This type of infarction is usually accompanied by occlusion of a vessel resulting in damage of the myocardium in the area of distribution of that artery. The damage may or may not be full thickness (Figure 5.5). Not infrequently, there is total arterial occlusion by thrombus (Figure 5.6a and b) but the problem of whether or not thrombus precedes myocardial infarction or is a secondary event, has so far not been fully solved. Table 5.2 indicates the localization of the infarct according to the vessel involved.

Great variation does, however, exist being dependent on the dominance of the arterial supply. Dominance is determined by that vessel which forms the posterior descending artery which, in the majority of cases studied, is formed by the right coronary artery. In addition, the absence or presence of collateral circulation determines the size of the infarct[2].

Table 5.2 Localization of infarcts in relation to arteries

Artery	Location of infarct
Anterior descending (left)	Anterior wall left ventricle or antero-septal. Involvement of bundle and right bundle branch
Circumflex (left)	Posterior or lateral aspect of left ventricle. Atrioventricular node and sinu-atrial node rarely involved (if left artery dominant)
Right coronary	Posterior or posteroseptal of left ventricle. Posterior wall right ventricle. Sinu-atrial node, atrioventricular node and bundle of His involved

Sub-Endocardial Infarction

If all three major coronary arteries are affected by severe atherosclerosis, an increase in the small vessels supplying the myocardial wall will occur, as well as an increase in the sub-endocardial plexus[10]. If the patient now suffers a period of hypotension, either due to fainting or rhythm disturbances, it is the area furthest away from the blood supply that will be affected, which is the sub-endocardial area (Figure 5.7). An infarct of this type may result in rupture of the papillary muscle or of the apex and because the endocardium is being denuded, may lead to thrombus superimposition. Due to the fact that severe atheroscleroses of all three vessels are present, an infarct of this type may be too small to evoke a change in the patient's symptoms. The small damage to the myocardium may also not result in elevation of enzymes in the blood.

Pathology of Myocardial Infarction

Irrespective of the type of infarct present the earliest changes visible to the naked eye consist of oedema resulting in pallor of the muscle. By 36h, the centre of the infarcted area becomes opaque and yellowish, surrounded by a haemorrhagic border which is clearly visible 3 to 4 days after infarction. The sequential events are shown in Table 5.3.

Table 5.3 Sequential changes observed in myocardial infarction

Time after the event	Observed changes
1. 15h	Muscle pale and oedematous
2. 36h	Infarct centre opaque or yellowish, border haemorrhagic
3. 3–4 days	Rubbery centre, distinct haemorrhagic border
4. 1 week	Rubbery centre, slight shrinkage of infarct (Figure 5.8)
5. 3 weeks	Thinning of myocardium
6. 6–8 weeks	Scarring; there may be a brownish tinge preceding this (Figure 5.9a and b)
7. 3 months	White and firm scar
8. Eventually	Tough white scar[11]

Histology

Sequential changes take place and the earliest change occurs at around 5h when the myocardial fibres become eosinophilic (Figure 5.10) on haematoxylin and eosin staining, and nuclear changes in the form of karyolysis and pyknosis make their appearance. At 6h, neutrophils begin to invade the infarcted area (Figure 5.11) and lymphocytes make their appearance around the fourth day. On that day, fibroblasts can also be identified and by the ninth day collagen fibres can be recognized (Figure

Table 5.4 Sequential histological changes in myocardial infarction (from reference 11, by courtesy of the Author and Publishers)

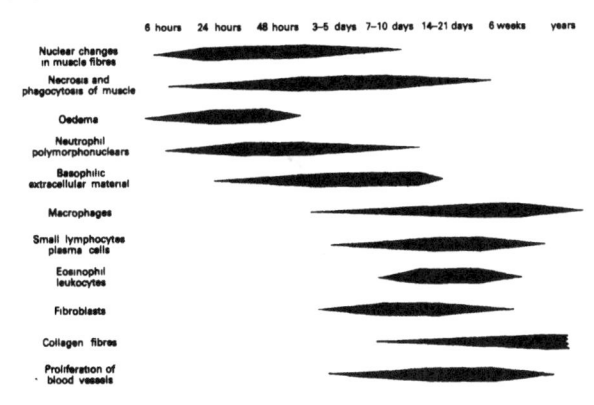

5.12a and b). The changes are summarized in Table 5.4. Fairly accurate dating up to approximately 3 weeks is possible but this can only be achieved if, apart from haematoxylin and eosin staining, an elastic van Gieson stain is also carried out.

It is, of course, important to know the changes that occur prior to those recognizable by routine histological techniques. In addition to the eosinophilic change already referred to, waviness of underperfused muscle, which will result in myocardial infarction, may be found[12] (Figure 5.13) but this is not a reliable guide.

Histochemical and electron-microscopic examination are more reliable for delineating early myocardial infarction but, for conventional techniques, fresh myocardial tissue is essential.

Early Recognition of Myocardial Infarction

Macroscopic Evaluation

This can be achieved by either perfusing the coronary arteries (Figure 5.14) and/or cutting transverse sections of the ventricles and soaking the slices in substances such as Nitro-Blue Tetrazolium (BT) (Figure 5.15)[13]. The ensuing reactions are dependent on enzymes present in the myocardium. In areas not previously damaged, endogenous substrate coenzymes and dehydrogenases are present which reduce Nitro-BT to a dark blue formazan. In the infarcted areas where leakage of enzymes has occurred reduction of Nitro-BT does not occur and the area remains pale. This reaction is not specific for any particular enzyme system, but is a general dehydrogenase reaction. Positive results are observed 6–8 h after infarction has occurred[13].

Microscopy

At microscopic level, stains for glycogen (Figure 5.16), fat globules (Figure 5.17), succinic dehydrogenase (Figure 5.18a) or cytochrome oxidase (Figure 5.18b) can be undertaken. Glycogen begins to disappear almost immediately (within a few minutes after cessation of blood supply to the area), and has completely disappeared from the damaged myocardium, 6 to 8 h after the event. Fat globules become clearly visible 2 to 3 h after shut-off of the blood supply and become increasingly bigger up to about 7 h, when they begin to disappear. They are completely absent from the myocardial fibres in the centre of the infarct at 24 h.

At the interface between infarcted and viable muscle,

fat globules are recognizable for longer periods and thus provide an accurate assessment of infarct size.

As far as succinic dehydrogenase and cytochrome oxidase are concerned, after approximately 2 to 3 h, a rapid increase takes place up to about 6 h, followed by a gradual increase. After 24 h, these substances begin to disappear rapidly from the damaged myocardial fibres[2].

In man it is frequently difficult to obtain fresh myocardial tissue. Histochemical staining is particularly valuable in experimental work, especially when the influence of a drug on the size of an infarct is being investigated.

Two other methods deserve special mention. The haematoxylin–basic fuchsin–picric acid (HBFP) stain is a valuable way of investigating early myocardial infarction[14]. Underperfused muscle will retain basic fuchsin 30 min after cessation of blood supply (Figure 5.19). If the muscle is normally perfused basic fuchsin is not retained (Figure 5.20). This stain is also independent of autolysis and can be undertaken on paraffin-embedded sections. Differentiation with picric acid can result in false positive or negative findings and it is for this reason that this stain has fallen into disrepute with some workers. If, however, complete transverse sections of the ventricular walls are available positive areas can usually be defined conforming with electrocardiograms (Figure 5.21). Complete transverse sections have, therefore, a built-in control and if the staining procedures are properly carried out this stain is an invaluable adjunct to diagnosing the earliest form of myocardial damage at microscopic level.

The other technique is that of eosinophilic fluorescence on haematoxylin and eosin preparations viewed under ultraviolet light. Characteristic fluorescence can be observed. Comparison of this technique with the HBFP stain has shown yellow fluorescence in the same position where the HBFP stain has been found positive[15] (Figure 5.22).

Biochemical techniques are also available but these are beyond the scope of this atlas.

Electron Microscopic Changes

These, like the conventional histochemical changes are dependent on autolysis and therefore fresh tissue is essential. The earliest changes consist of swelling of the mitochondria together with extensive cristolysis. These changes are potentially reversible (Figure 5.23).

Sequential changes also take place at this level of investigation[16] and these are summarized in Table 5.5. The subject has been reviewed by Olsen, 1975[17].

Examination of myocardial tissue at electron-microscopic level has contributed to making prolonged open heart surgery possible. The sequence of events that have just been mentioned are those that occur at body temperature. If, however, the body is cooled the sequence of events are slowed up and the potential reversible mitochondrial changes, instead of becoming evident at 20 min, are seen at 45 min. This permits more extensive corrective surgery to be carried out with safety.

Rarer Types of Myocardial Infarction

Infarction of the Atria

This is a not infrequent accompaniment to ventricular infarction but it may be extremely difficult to recognize early changes as inflammatory cellular elements are not infrequently found in atrial walls. The only reliable diagnostic feature is superimposition of thrombus or examination by Nitro-BT.

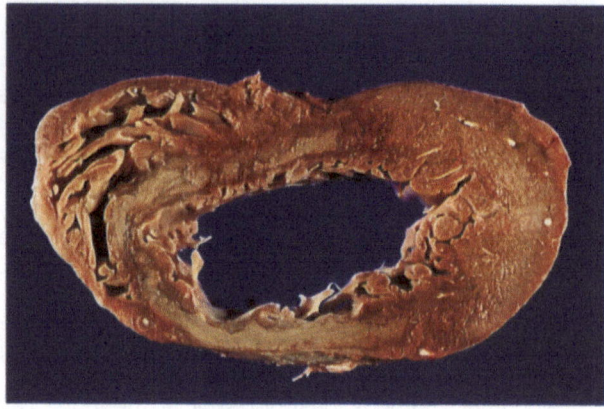

Figure 5.8 Myocardial infarct of one week's duration involving the anterior wall, the interventricular septum and part of the posterior left venticular wall. Shrinkage has occurred. The centre of the infarct has a 'rubbery' appearance and is surrounded by a haemorrhagic border

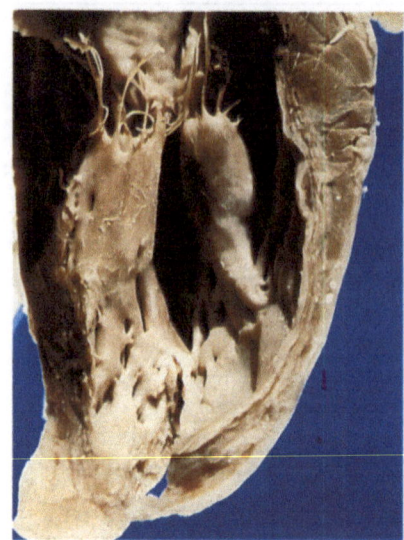

Figure 5.9a Extensive thinning of the left ventricular wall has occurred following infarction of approximately six weeks' duration

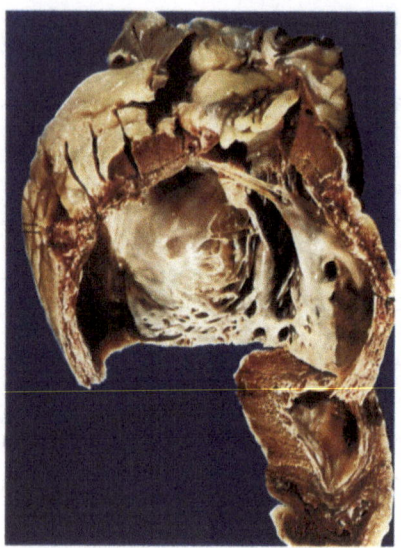

Figure 5.9b Myocardial infarction of approximately 8 weeks duration

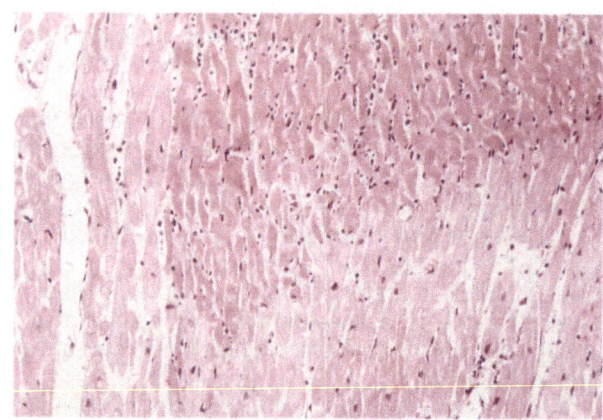

Figure 5.10 Photomicrograph of a recent myocardial infarction showing eosinophilia of the top half of the area chosen for illustration. A sparse cellular infiltrate can already be noted. H & E × 50

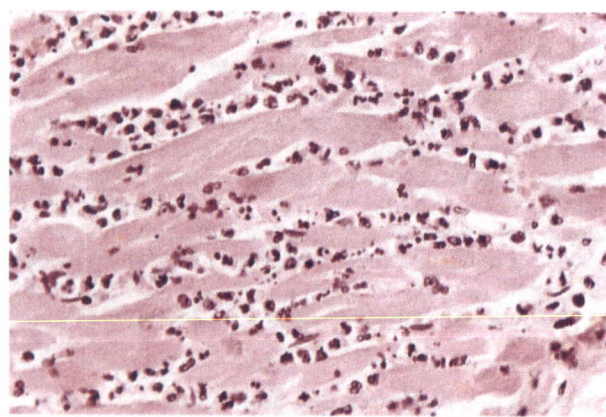

Figure 5.11 Recent myocardial infarction showing a predominantly neutrophilic inflammatory infiltrate. Nuclei cannot be identified in this area of eosinophilia of the myocardial cells. H & E × 200

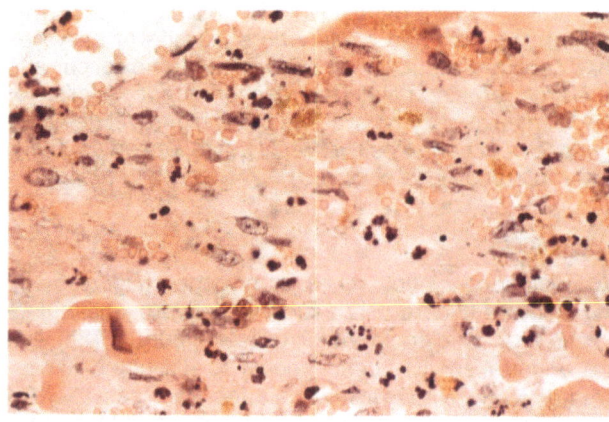

Figure 5.12a Area of infarction showing a central zone of amorphous material, a few inflammatory cells, many of which are disintegrating, fibroblasts (large vesicular nuclei) and damaged myocardial fibres with nuclear karyolysis. H & E × 200

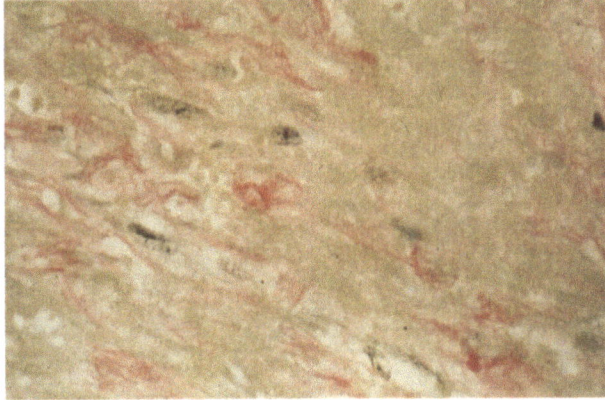

Figure 5.12b The same area as Figure 5.12a, showing collagen fibres staining with Elastic van Gieson × 250

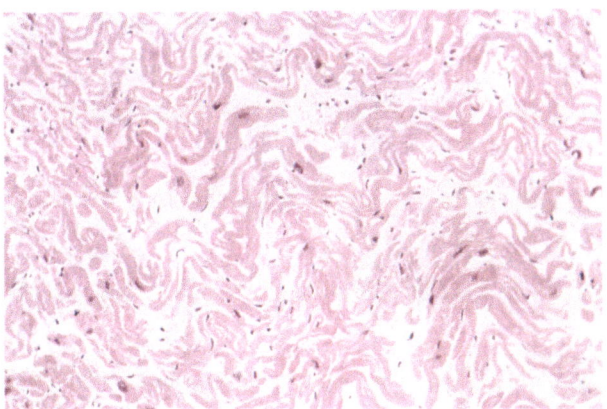

Figure 5.13 Waviness of ventricular muscle fibres may indicate underperfusion which results in infarction. H & E × 50

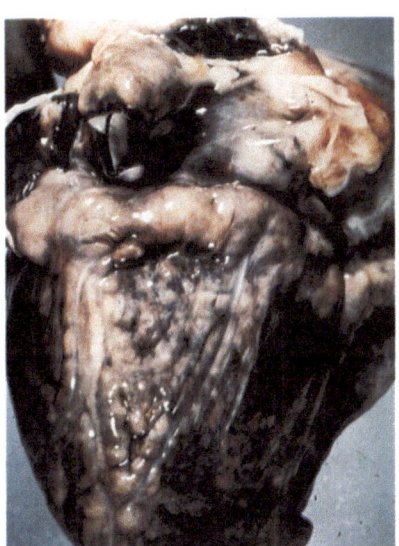

Figure 5.14 Posterior aspect of the heart with recent myocardial infarction of approximately 8 h duration. The coronary arteries have been perfused with Nitro-BT. The pale areas indicate abnormal perfusion or infarction

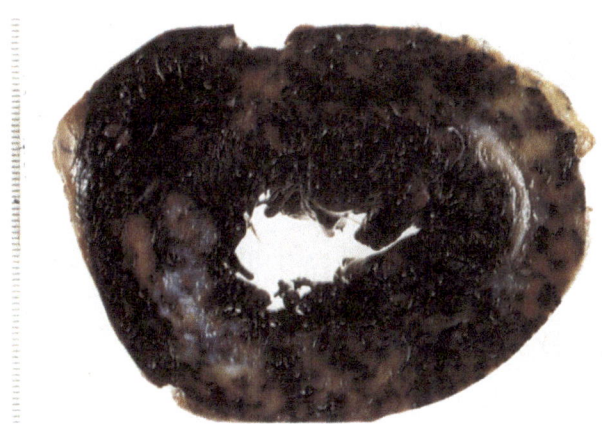

Figure 5.15 Cross-section of the left ventricle. The slice had been soaked in Nitro-BT. Muscle damage, especially of the posterior and lateral regions, can clearly be identified (pale areas). In addition, previous damage of the wall had occurred (fibrotic areas)

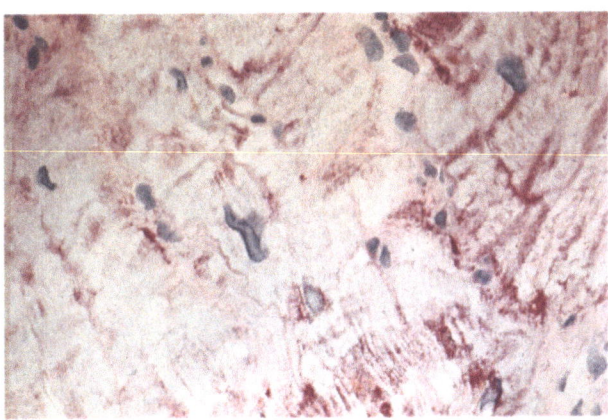

Figure 5.16 Patchy depletion of glycogen 2 h after infarction. PAS × 400

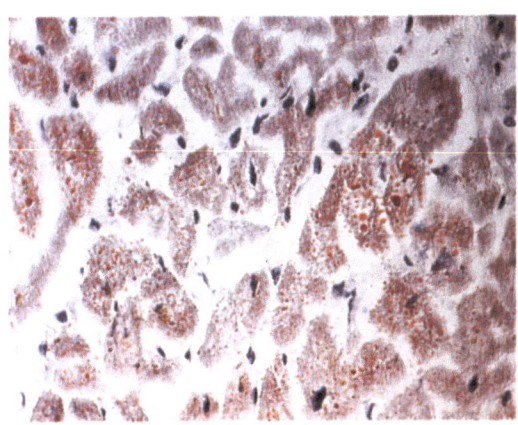

Figure 5.17 Fat globules in the centre of a recently infarcted area (3 h duration). Oil Red O × 200

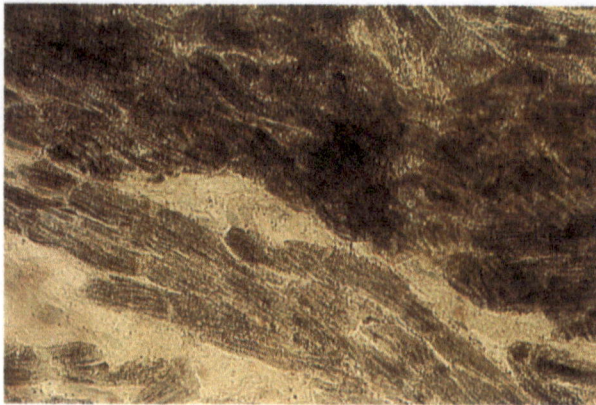

Figure 5.18a Succinic dehydrogenase. The apparent increase in the upper two-thirds of the photomicrograph indicates damage following infarction × 250

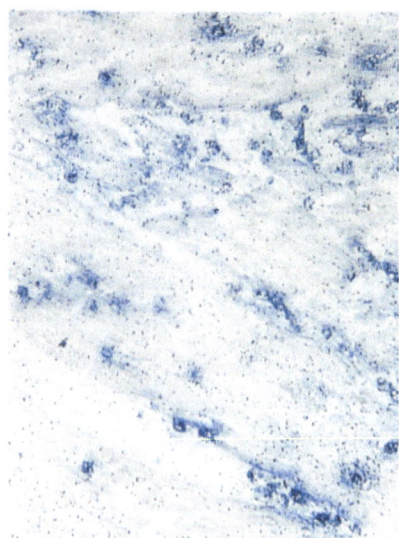

Figure 5.18b The same area stained for cytochrome oxidase × 250

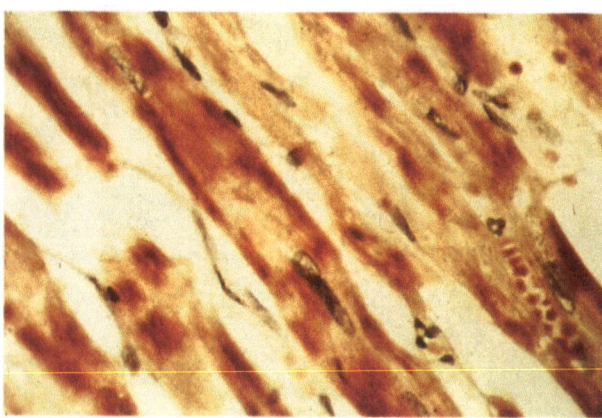

Figure 5.19 Area of underperfusion (myocardial infarction) 45 min after the event. Retention of basic fuchsin is striking. HBFP × 400

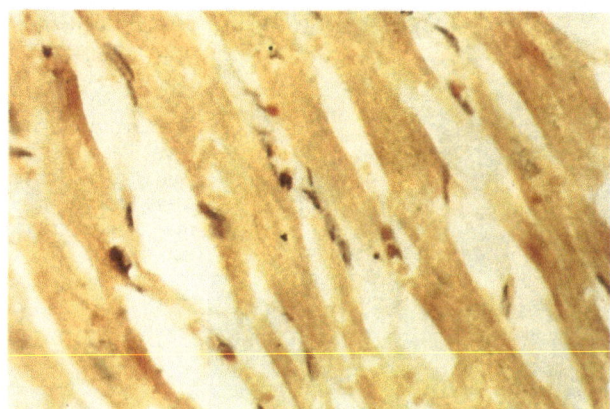

Figure 5.20 For comparison with Figure 5.19, basic fuchsin is not retained in normally perfused myocardial fibres. HBFP × 400

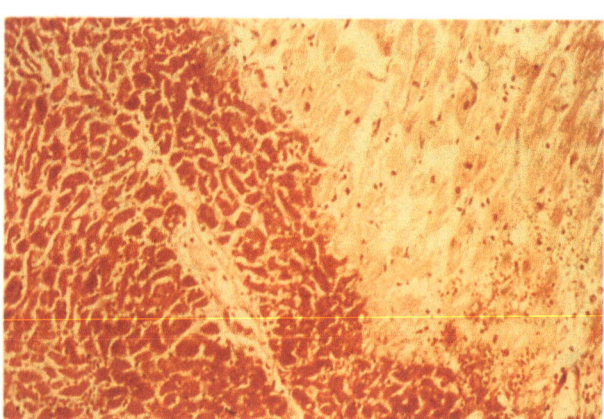

Figure 5.21 Junction of underperfused and normally perfused myocardial fibres. HBFP × 50

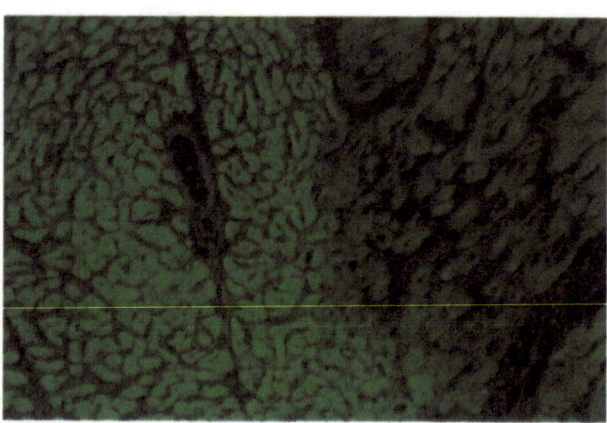

Figure 5.22 Eosinophilic fluorescence viewed under ultraviolet light from the identical area illustrated in Figure 5.21 × 50

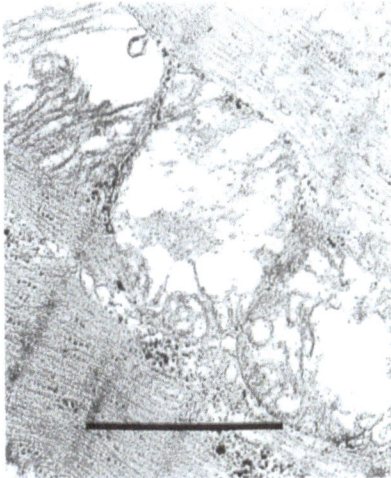

Figure 5.23 Electron micrograph showing swelling of mitochondria and cristolysis, 20 min of cessation of blood flow. The remaining cristae are apparently more prominent. Lead citrate and uranyl acetate. Scale bar = 1 μm

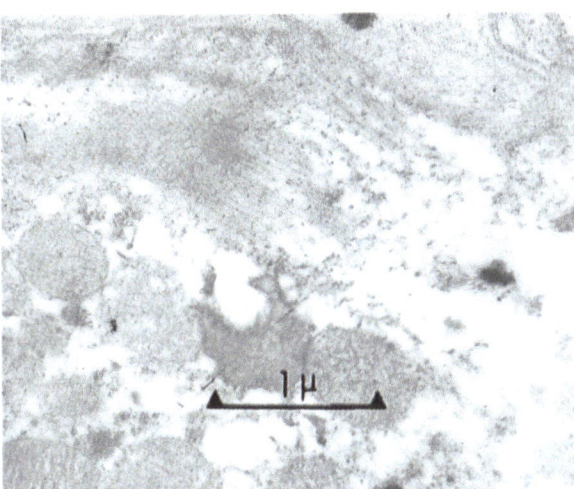

Figure 5.24 Transverse tearing of myocardial fibrils in infarction of approximately 4 h duration. Despite this extensive damage some mitochondria are normal indicating that death is not necessarily uniform within a cell. Lead citrate and uranyl acetate. Scale bar = 1 μm

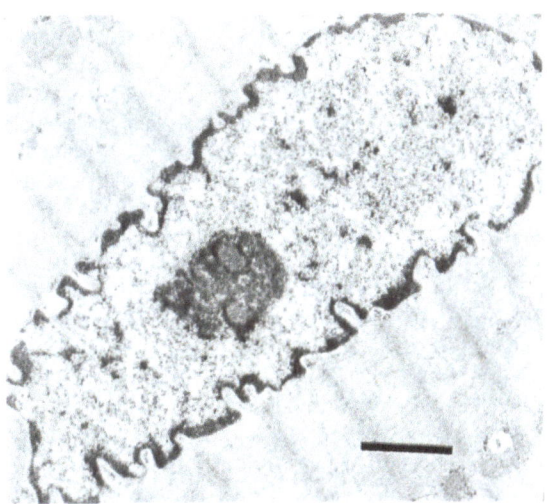

Figure 5.25 Clumping of nuclear chromatin has begun. From an area of infarction 30 min after the event. Lead citrate and uranyl acetate. Scale bar = 1 μm

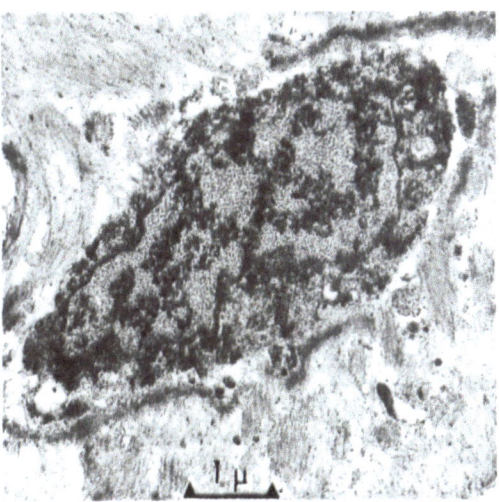

Figure 5.26 A nucleus in an infarcted area of 4 h duration. Lead citrate and uranyl acetate. Scale bar = 1 μm

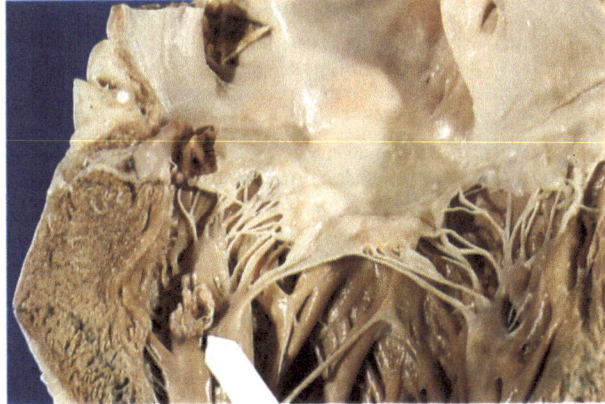

Figure 5.27 Rupture of the papillary muscle. The site of the rupture is indicated by the white arrow. The tip of the papillary muscle can be seen on the atrial side of the mitral valve

Table 5.5 Ultrastructural sequential changes observed in myocardial infarction

Time after the event	Observed changes
A. *Glycogen and myocardial cells*	
1. 5 min	After total ischaemia glycogen begins to diminish and the space between myofibrils increases
2. 10–15 min	Separation of cells is clearly evident
3. 1 h	Increase in the I disc is clearly established
4. 4 h	Transverse tearing of myofibrils is seen (Figure 5.24)
5. 5 h	Rupture of the sarcolemma occurs
B. *Mitochondria*	
1. Up to 20 min	No change detected
2. Thereafter	Swelling noted and cristae more distinct (as a result of decrease in matrix density) (Figure 5.23)
3. 4 h	Cristae disrupt and disappear
4. 5 h	Rupture of mitochondria occurs
C. *Endoplasmic reticulum and nuclear changes*	
1. 35 min	Tubules begin to swell; the Golgi apparatus is prominent
2. 5 min	Nucleoplasm begins to show clumping (Figure 5.25) with drifting towards nuclear membrane after 2–3 h
3. About 4 h	Rupture of nuclear membranes (Figure 5.26)

Right Ventricular Infarction

This is also rare. Not infrequently it accompanies extensive left ventricular infarction (see Figure 5.5). One of the reasons why the right ventricular myocardium escapes is most likely to be the lower metabolic requirements of the right ventricular muscle and the presence of sufficient collateral blood supply to meet these requirements. There are also anatomical differences in the deep branches of the right coronary artery; the branches continue in the same plane as the parent trunk and are thus less liable to bending, whereas branches of the left coronary artery arise at right angles. Protection by the nutritive Thebesian venous system may also contribute to the relatively rare occurrence of right ventricular myocardial infarction. The incidence of isolated right ventricular infarction is approximately 2%[18].

Complications

These include cardiogenic shock, disturbances of conduction, including the Wolff–Parkinson–White syndrome, syncope and thrombo-embolism. Cardiac rupture may occur which can be external (at ventricular or atrial level) or internal (of the inter-ventricular septum, the papillary muscle (Figure 5.27) or chordae tendineae). It may be slow or rapid.

Ventricular aneurysms, pericarditis, abscess formation of the myocardium, calcification, hypertension and deep vein thrombosis complete the morphologically recognizable complications[2].

Percutaneous Coronary Transluminal Angioplasty

This method of relieving severe narrowing of a coronary artery by introducing and inflating a non-deformable, plastic, balloon-tipped arterial catheter into the affected artery is used with increasing frequency in special units. Histopathological features have only rarely been documented. A case is illustrated in Figures 5.28–5.32. For detailed information the reader is referred to Raphael and Donaldson[19].

References

1. Rissanen, V. (1975). Occurrence of coronary ostial stenosis in a necropsy series of myocardial infarction, sudden death and violent death. *Br. Heart J.*, **37**, 182

2. Olsen, E. G. J. (1980). Myocardial infarction. In *The Pathology of the Heart.* Second Edition, p. 99. (London and Basingstoke: The Macmillan Press Ltd.)

3. Kannel, W. B. and McGee, D. L. (1979). Diabetes and cardiovascular risk factors: The Framingham study. *Circulation*, **59**, 8

4. Dolder, M. A. and Oliver, M. F. (1975). Myocardial infarction in young men. Study of risk factors in 9 countries. *Br. Heart J.*, **37**, 493

5. Oliver, M. F. (1977). Predictions of acute heart attacks. *Scot. Med. J.*, **22**, 42

6. Elmfeldt, D., Wilhelmsen, L., Wedel, H., Vedin, A., Wihlmsson, C. and Tibblin, G. (1976). Primary risk factors in patients with myocardial infarction. *Am. Heart J.*, **91**, 412

7. Haust, M. D. (1983). Atherosclerosis – lesions and sequelae. In Silver, D. M. (ed.) *Cardiovascular Pathology.* Volume 1, p. 191. (New York, Edinburgh, London, Melbourne: Churchill Livingstone)

8. Benditt, E. P. and Benditt, J. M. (1973). Evidence for a monoclonal origin of human atherosclerotic plaques. *Proc. Natl. Acad. Sci. USA*, **70**, 1753

9. Crawford, T. (1977). *Pathology of Ischaemic Heart Disease.* p. 12. (London-Boston: Butterworth)

10. Fulton, W. M. F. (1956). Chronic generalized myocardial ischaemia with advanced coronary disease. *Br. Heart J.*, **18**, 341

11. Lodge-Patch, I. (1951). The aging of cardiac infarcts and its influence on cardiac rupture. *Br. Heart J.*, **13**, 37

12. Bouchardy, B. and Majno, G. (1974). Histopathology of early myocardial infarcts. *Am. J. Pathol.*, **74**, 301

13. Ramkissoon, R. A. (1966). Macroscopic identification of early myocardial infarction by dehydrogenase alterations. *J. Clin. Pathol.*, **19**, 479

14. Lie, J. T., Holley, K. E., Kampa, W. R. and Titus, J. L. (1971). New histochemical method for morphologic diagnosis or early stages of myocardial ischaemia. *Mayo Clin. Proc.*, **46**, 319

15. Al-Rufaie, H. K., Florio, R. A. and Olsen, E. G. J. (1983). Comparison of the haematoxylin basic fuchsin acid method and the fluorescence of haematoxylin and eosin stained sections for the identification of early myocardial infarction. *J. Clin. Pathol.*, **36**, 646

16. Caulfield, J. and Klionsky, B. (1959). Myocardial ischaemia and early infarction: an electron microscopic study. *Am. J. Pathol.* **35**, 489

17. Olsen, E. G. J. (1975). Pathological aspects of ischaemic heart disease. In Longmore, D. R. (ed.), *The Current Status of Cardiac Surgery.* Chapter 61, p. 401. (Lancaster: MTP Press)

18. Kherdekar, A. and Nevins, M. A. (1973). Right ventricular infarction. *J. Med. Soc. NJ.*, **70**, 374

19. Raphael, M. J. and Donaldson, R. M. (1985). Coronary transluminal angioplasty. *Br. J. Hosp. Med.*, **33**, 18

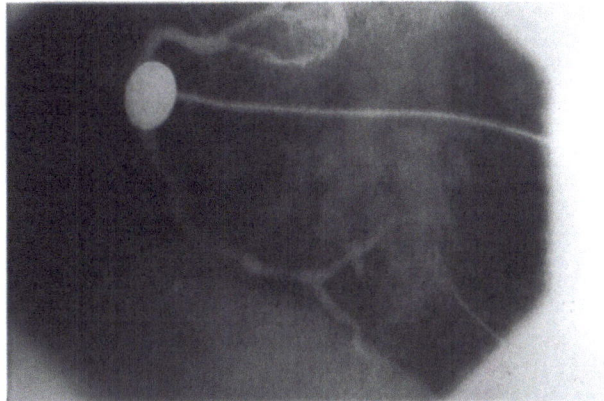

Figure 5.28a Angiogram illustrating the right coronary artery before the procedure showing severe narrowing of the lumen below the ECG electrode

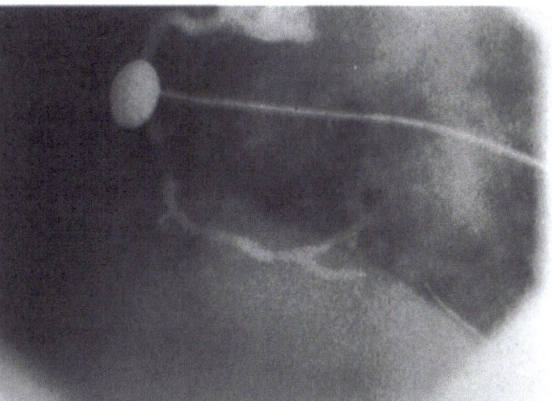

Figure 5.28b Angiogram after the intervention showing great improvement of the patency of the right coronary arterial lumen

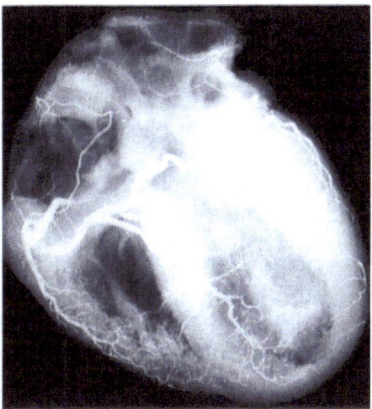

Figure 5.29 Postmorten angiogram illustrating a good-sized lumen of the right coronary artery, but some filling defect just below the origin of the marginal artery can be seen

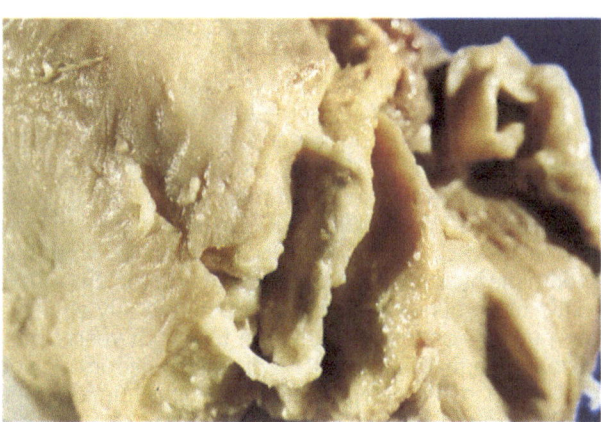

Figure 5.30 Dissection of the right coronary artery displaying the segment showing irregular filling with contrast medium in Figure 5.29

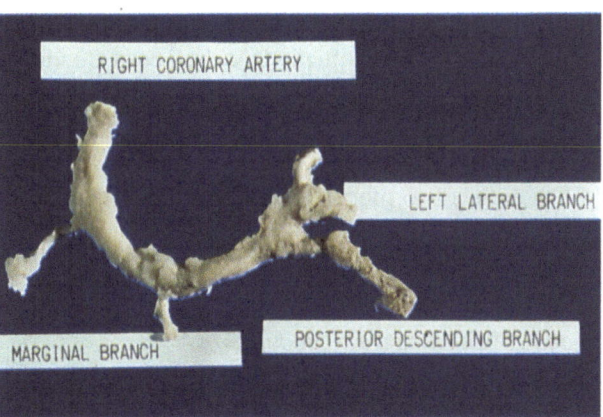

Figure 5.31 The dissected right coronary artery. The first branch is the artery of the sinus node

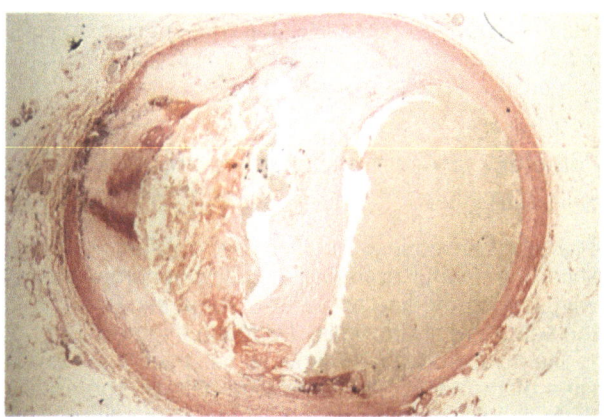

Figure 5.32 Photomicrograph showing rupture of the fibrous cup of the atheromatous plaque. The functional lumen is filled with contrast medium. Elastic van Gieson × 10

Rheumatic Heart Disease

6

Rheumatic fever is an inflammatory non-suppurative systemic disease affecting predominantly the heart and the joints and has a tendency to recur.

Though many reports from various parts of the world testify to a decrease in rheumatic fever, particularly in the developing countries, rheumatic fever, developing into chronic involvement of the heart, is still widespread and can even today be found in some industrialized countries. It has therefore a world-wide distribution but is particularly prevalent in the tropical zones, so much so that it is considered by some to be a tropical disease[1].

The incidence in England and Wales has remarkably declined. In the year 1901 67 per million patients were recorded as having died from rheumatic fever, this had declined to 23 per million in 1939 and two patients per million in 1965. In countries such as India, however, rheumatic heart disease remains a great problem. Rheumatic heart disease affects any race and any age, but the peak incidence lies between 5 and 15 years; both sexes are equally affected. Predisposing factors include climate, particularly where there is high humidity and overcrowding[2].

Aetiology

The aetiology has been well established in relationship to an upper respiratory infection by β-haemolytic streptococci, Lancefield group A. The actual mechanism of how damage is brought about is still not clear. It has been shown that the bacteria have varying rheumatogenic potentials, the most potent of which is type A5. The M protein attached to the fimbria on the surface of the bacterial wall is responsible for type-specific acquired antibodies and forms the basis of type-specific immunity in man[3].

Pathology of Acute Rheumatic Heart Disease

Macroscopy

The valves are oedematous and have a glistening appearance and careful examination will show small whitish wisps along the line of closure. Some early erosion of the valve leaflets may also be found (Figure 6.1).

The myocardium may show some speckling in certain sites of the ventricular walls (see below). The pericardium shows evidence of a fibrinous pericarditis.

Histology

The valve leaflets show thickening due to oedema which can readily be recognized by separation of the collagen bundles. On the line of closure vegetations consisting entirely of fibrin are evident (the wisps seen macroscopically). The cellular reaction of the valve leaflets varies in intensity but usually shows Aschoff cells, Anitschkow cells and chronic inflammatory cells (Figure 6.2). Aschoff nodules are usually not observed in valvar tissue.

In the myocardium Aschoff nodules can be identified. Three stages of formation are recognized.

(1) The first stage (the alternative stage), after approximately 2 to 3 weeks following infection with streptococci, results in a basophilic change of the ground substance and an occasional focus of fibrinoid necrosis as well as a few plasma cells and lymphocytes[4] (Figure 6.3).

(2) The second stage, evident approximately one month after infection, shows typical Aschoff nodules (Figure 6.4) which measure approximately $800 \times 80\,\mu m$. They are usually oval in shape and can just be recognized with the naked eye. A typical Aschoff nodule consists of: *Aschoff cells* which are large mononuclear or multinucleated cells with two or three nuclei, with the nuclear chromatin arranged as in Anitschkow cells, these cells have an irregular outline and the cytoplasm is basophilic; several *Anitschkow cells*, the nucleus of which consists of a central chromatin bar and radiating hair-like chromatin condensation (the owl-eyed nuclei on the cross-section) (Figure 6.5); *lymphocytes* and *plasma cells*. The cellular elements are arranged in a variety of ways and they have, from a descriptive point of view, names such as coronal type or syncytial type[5] (Figures 6.6 and 6.7).

(3) The third stage, the healing phase, is reached 3 to 6 months after infection. Aschoff cells are the first cells to disappear, followed by Anitschkow cells, which in turn are followed by the majority of the cellular elements that form the Aschoff nodule. The disappearance of cells follows in reverse the order of formation. Finally, all that is identifiable are some onion-shaped scars in which some reticulum and chronic inflammatory cells can be found (Figure 6.8).

Localization of Aschoff Nodules

These are haphazard in distribution but are found particularly in the posterior left ventricular wall, the pulmonary conus, the posterior wall of the left atrium and the myocardial wedge between the aorta and the left atrium[6].

Although in the acute phase valvar lesions may not be prominent, myocardial hypertrophy is usually evident, together with some of the endocardial changes of dilatation (see Chapter 3).

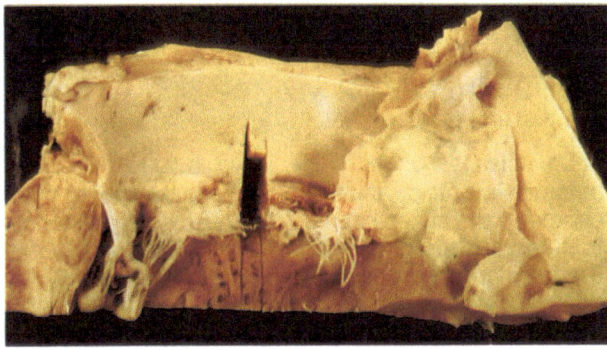

Figure 6.1 Tiny wisps of fibrin can be identified along the line of closure (one is clearly seen against the haemorrhagic background to the right of the cut made for selection of tissue for histological examination). Erosion of the atrial surface of the mitral valve is also seen in this case of acute rheumatic heart disease

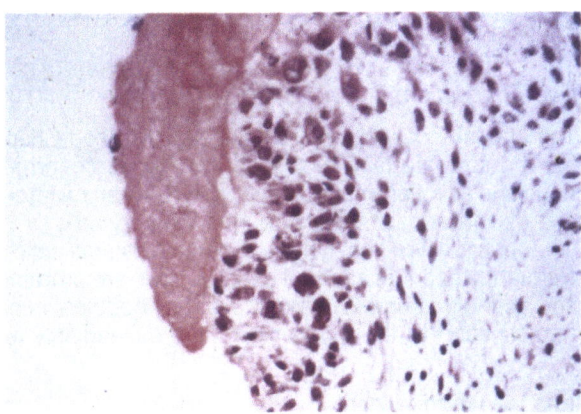

Figure 6.2 Acute rheumatic heart disease. Beneath the fibrin 'cap' a mixed cellular infiltrate is found in which Anitschkow cells and Aschoff cells abound in this section of the mitral valve leaflet. H & E × 400

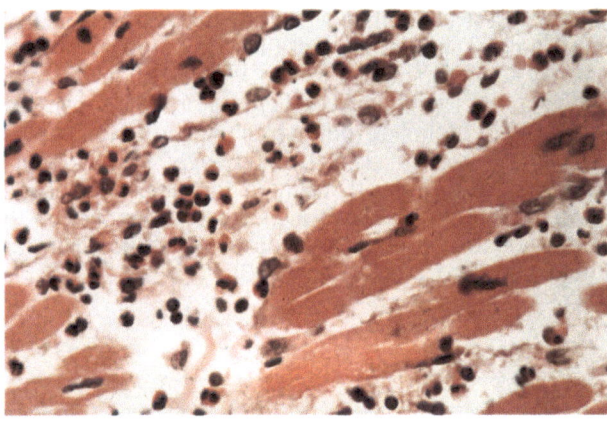

Figure 6.3 The first stage of the development of an Aschoff nodule consisting of a mixed cellular infiltrate rich in lymphocytes and plasma cells in connective tissue having a bluish tinge.   H & E × 250

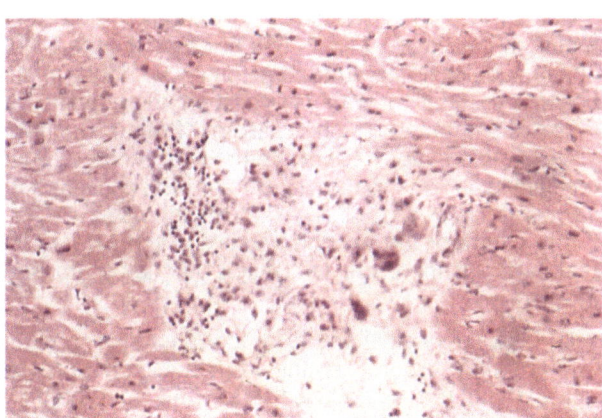

Figure 6.4 An Aschoff nodule showing all the characteristic features (see text).   H & E × 50

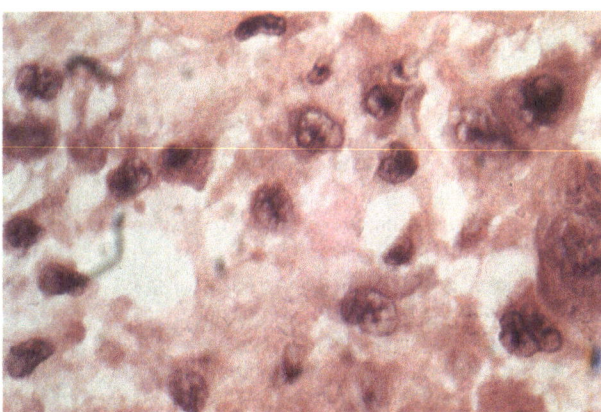

Figure 6.5 High power view of Aschoff and Anitschkow cells showing characteristic arrangement of chromatin (owl-eyed nuclei).   H & E × 800

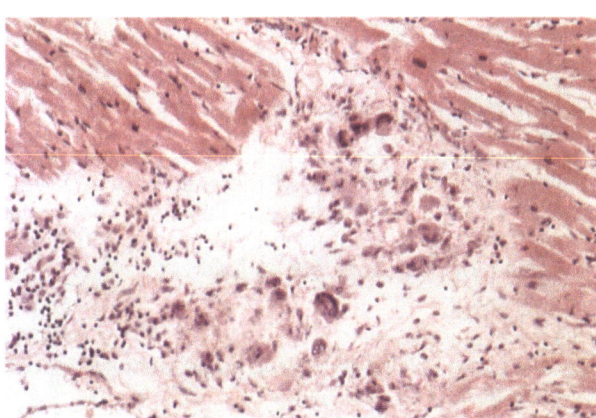

Figure 6.6 Aschoff nodule. According to the way in which the cellular elements are arranged a variety of terms have been used. The description 'coronal type' has been applied to the type illustrated in this figure.   H & E × 50

The Pericardium

The appearances are entirely non-specific (see Chapter 8). The inner surface of the pericardium is covered by fibrin and an inflammatory infiltrate which can be intense and usually consists of acute inflammatory cells. In the sub-pericardial region, lymphocytes and plasma cells are frequently seen. In addition small vessels are prominent and fibrinoid necrosis is found. Aschoff nodules, in contradistinction to the myocardium, are exceedingly rare.

Changes in the Heart

As mentioned above, hypertrophy and dilatation of the myocardium takes place often in the absence of any marked valvar changes, but the most striking feature is dilatation of the left atrium. In the posterior wall roughening of the surface is found, to which the name McCallum's patch is applied. This persists into the chronic stage (Figures 6.9 and 6.11).

Examination of the endocardial changes in the atrial appendages, which have been routinely examined since the onset of intracardiac surgery, have shown the presence of Aschoff nodules or constituent cellular elements in between 37 and 75% of cases (Figure 6.10). These nodules in the atrial appendages do not have any positive correlation with clinical symptomatology but reflect the pathogenetic mechanism of rheumatic heart disease; this suggests that the process is one of ever-continuing damage to the myocardium and endocardium with only occasional clinical manifestations.

The nature of the Aschoff nodules is somewhat controversial but there are two major theories as to how they arise.

(1) The connective tissue theory suggests that the primary lesion, i.e. the immunological process, affects the connective tissue of the heart or joints and is followed by the sequential cellular infiltrates described above[5].

(2) The other theory is the myogenic theory which suggests that the brunt of the pathogenetic process falls on the myocardial and smooth muscle fibres and that the cells observed in Aschoff's nodules represents fragments of damaged muscle fibres. Fibrinoid necrosis represents non-nucleated sarcoplasmic remnants of myocardial tissue[7].

Recent studies suggest that the connective tissue theory is the more likely process.

Chronic Rheumatic Heart Disease

The valves involved are most frequently the mitral valve followed by a combination of mitral and aortic valves. Lone aortic valve involvement is exceedingly rare. Valvar involvement has been studied by Lannigan, 1966[8], and the results of 298 cases are as follows:

Mitral alone	48.3%
Mitral and aortic	42.3%
Aortic alone (excluding calcific aortic stenosis)	2.0%
Mitral, aortic and tricuspid	4.4%
Mitral, aortic, tricuspid and pulmonary	0.6%
Mitral and pulmonary	0.3%
Mitral and tricuspid	2.0%

Valvar changes of the mitral valve include thickening, commissural fusion and shortening and thickening of the chordae tendineae (Figure 6.11). These characteristic features are found in approximately 45% of patients. Predominantly cuspal (Figure 6.12) or chordal involvement has also been recognized[9].

Involvement of the aortic valve leaflets consists of commissural fusion and thickening of the valve leaflets. In chronic valvar disease calcification may be superimposed (Figure 6.13). Similar changes are found in the tricuspid and pulmonary valves.

Histological examination of the valves consists of deformation or destruction of the normal architecture. The thickening is predominently due to collagen tissue and frequently also due to foci of calcification (Figure 6.14). Vascularity is increased. Normally some thin-walled vascular channels can reach the tip of the valve leaflets (see Chapter 1) but following inflammation thick-walled capillary sized vessels become numerous and may extend to the tip of the valve leaflets (Figure 6.15).

This stage in the myocardium consists of non-specific changes in the form of focal interstitial fibrosis or onion-skin-like lesions found in the vicinity of small blood vessels. A few chronic inflammatory cells can also usually be identified but typical Aschoff nodules are usually not present. They can, however, be observed in the endocardium, particularly in the atrial appendages (see above). Numerous adhesions are identified in the pericardium and both surfaces of the pericardium are thick and fibrous (see Chapter 8).

References

1. Louis-Gustave, A. (1977). Concerning rheumatic fever and rheumatic heart disease. (Letter). Am. Heart J., 93, 536

2. Olsen, E. G. J. (1980). Rheumatic heart disease. In The Pathology of the Heart. Second Edition, p. 133. (London and Basingstoke: The Macmillan Press Ltd)

3. Olsen, E. G. J. (1983). Rheumatic heart disease, aetiology, pathology, epidemiology and prevention. In Sleight, P. and Vann Jones, J. (eds). Scientific Foundations of Cardiology, p. 297. (London: William Heinemann Medical Books Ltd)

4. Klinge, F. (1933). Der Rheumatismus. Ergeb. Allg. Pathol. Anat., 27, 1

5. Gross, L. and Ehrlich, J. C. (1934). Studies on the myocardial Aschoff body. I. Descriptive classification of lesions. Am. J. Pathol., 10, 467

6. Gross, L., Antopol, W. and Sacks, B. (1930). A standardized procedure suggested for microscopic studies of the heart, with observations on rheumatic hearts. Arch. Pathol., 10, 841

7. Murphy, G. E. (1963). The characteristic rheumatic lesions of striated and non-striated or smooth muscle cells of the heart. Medicine (Baltimore), 42, 73

8. Lannigan, R. (1966). In Cardiac Pathology, p. 116. (London: Butterworth)

9. Rusted, I. E., Scheifley, C. H. and Edwards, J. E. (1956). Studies of the mitral valve. II. Certain anatomic features of the mitral valve and associated structures in mitral stenosis. Circulation, 14, 398

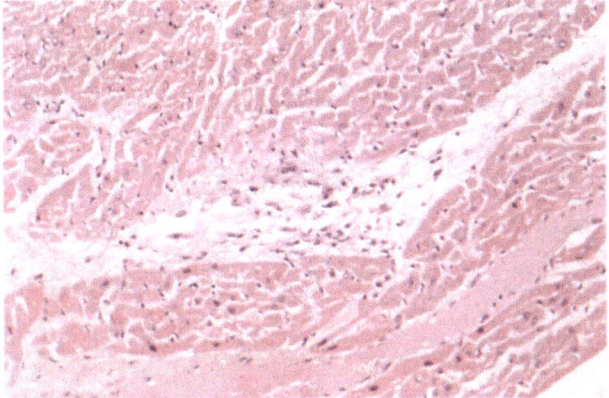

Figure 6.7 Illustrates the so-called 'syncytial type'. H & E × 50

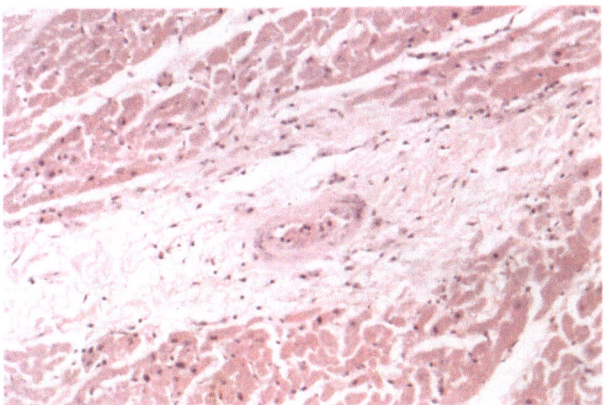

Figure 6.8 The late healing/healed phase is non-specific consisting of 'onion skin-like' arrangement of collagen in the peri-arteriolar region and a few chronic inflammatory cells. H & E × 50

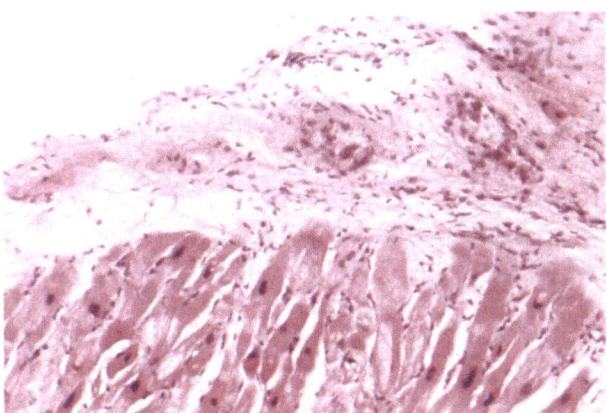

Figure 6.9 Photomicrograph of the posterior wall of the left atrium (McCallum's patch). An interendocardial band of hyalin tissue in which two Aschoff nodules can be seen. Chronic inflammatory cells can also be identified. H & E × 100

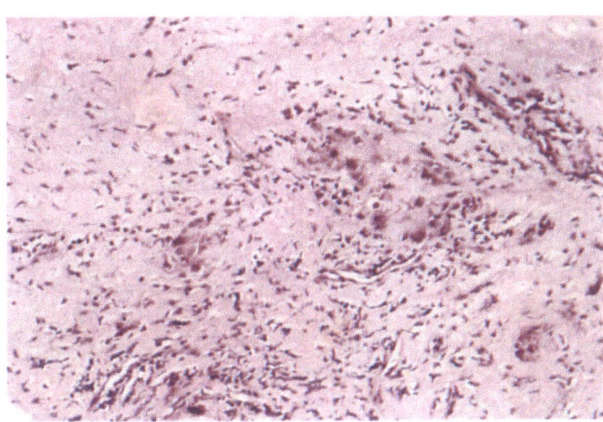

Figure 6.10 Aschoff nodules in the endocardium of the left atrial appendage removed during valve replacement for chronic rheumatic heart disease. H & E × 75

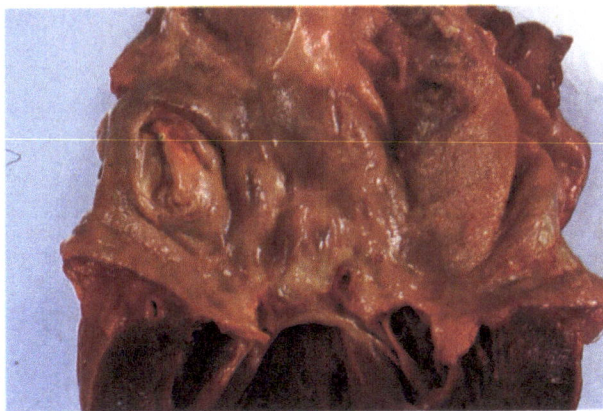

Figure 6.11 Chronic rheumatic heart disease. The mitral valve apparatus shows the characteristic triad: valvar thickening, commissural fusion and chordal thickening. Note the severe enlargement of the left atrium on the posterior wall of which a McCallum's patch can clearly be seen (above the posterior mitral valve leaflet)

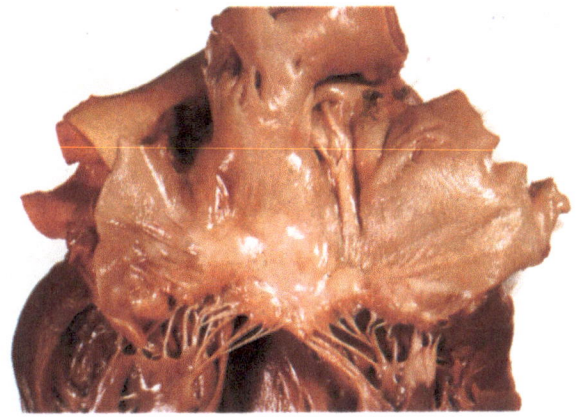

Figure 6.12 Chronic rheumatic heart disease showing predominantly cuspal thickening of the mitral valve. The chordae tendineae are largely unaffected

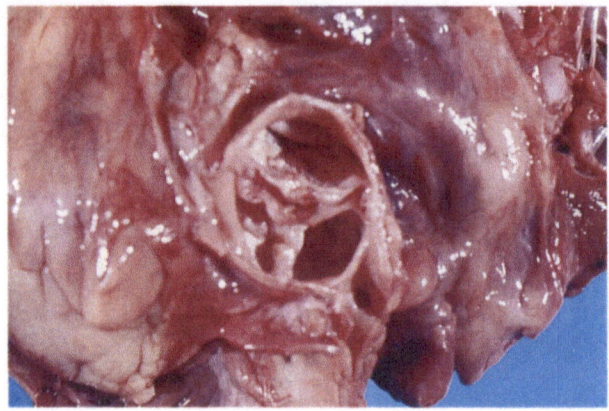

Figure 6.13 The aortic valve in chronic rheumatic heart disease viewed from above (the aorta). Valvar thickening and commissural fusion and foci of calcification are seen

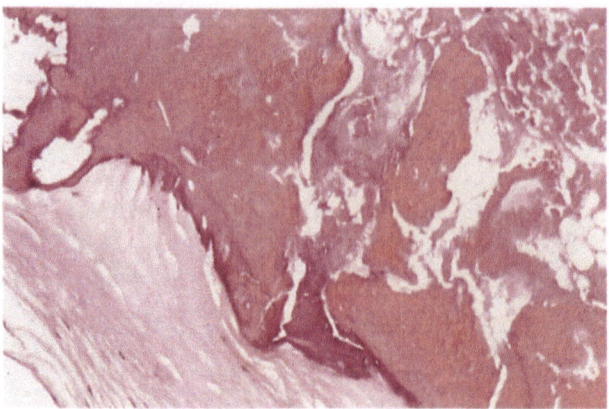

Figure 6.14 The architecture of the valve leaflet (bottom left of the photomicrograph) is severely distoreted. A large focus of calcification is illustrated. Inflammatory cells which are frequently seen are not conspicuous in this illustration.   H & E × 50

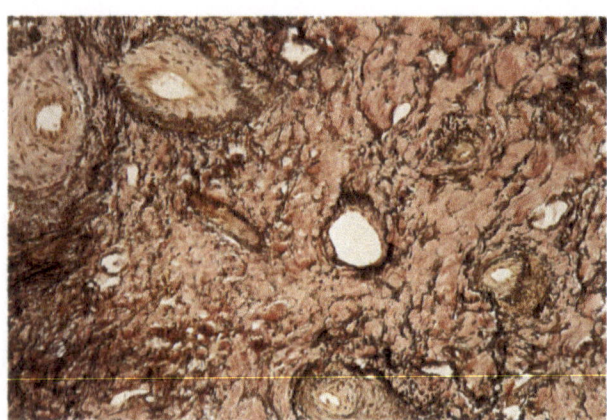

Figure 6.15 Several thick-walled capillary sized vessels are identified in this photomicrograph of the mitral valve affected by chronic rheumatic heart disease. This increased vascularity is typical in this condition. It also distinguishes acquired lesions of the valves due to inflammation from degenerative changes or congenital valvar anomalies.   Elastic van Gieson × 200

Infective Endocarditis

7

The term infective endocarditis is preferable to older terminology which indicated specific types of causal agents such as bacterial endocarditis. Infective endocarditis encompasses all possible infective agents that may involve the heart, especially the valves. Terms such as acute, subacute and chronic endocarditis should also be avoided as each discipline (clinicians, bacteriologists and histopathologists) attaches different meanings to these terms.

Despite modern techniques for establishing the clinical diagnosis and the introduction of new therapeutic agents, the number of patients dying as a result of infective endocarditis has remained steady over recent years (approximately 300 deaths are annually recorded in England and Wales)[1].

Infective endocarditis has remained a world-wide problem[2]. In the West the age of patients affected has increased from the third decade to the sixth decade, whereas in tropical countries such as Africa or India, the average age has remained low at around 28 years[3–5].

Males are more commonly affected than females, the ratio varying between 2 : 1 and 5 : 1. The predilection in men may be due to calcific aortic disease which becomes manifest as a result of longer life expectancy[6]. Rheumatic heart disease, which more frequently affects females, has decreased in recent years in the industrial countries but the pattern of infective endocarditis is also changing in the industrialized countries[7].

The incidence of post mortem series falls between 0.4 to 1.8% to 3.2% in Uganda. The incidence of morbidity is, of course, higher than the 300 cases dying in England and Wales as many patients survive following medical therapy and surgery.

Predisposing factors include congenital heart disease which before the introduction of antibiotics was in the region of 17.6%, but since the wider use of this type of therapy has been reduced to approximately 2%[1]. The type of congenital anomaly must, however, be considered. For example, an atrial septal defect in the region of the fossa ovalis is very rarely affected by infective endocarditis, whereas in the common atrio-ventricular canal type of defect, endocarditis is more frequently found.

As far as acquired heart disease is concerned, rheumatic heart disease has been the most prevalent. Although there is a decrease of rheumatic heart disease in industrialized countries, as late as the end of the 1970s chronic rheumatic heart disease accounted for some 70% of patients with infective endocarditis[3,8].

Classification

Infective endocarditis is best classified according to the infective organism into:

bacterial endocarditis
fungal endocarditis
Rickettsial endocarditis.

Valve cusps are usually first affected but when the process extends to involve adjacent cardiac walls, then the term 'mural endocarditis' is applied.

Localization of Vegetations on Valves

Vegetations usually start along the line of closure of heart valves, i.e. the atrial surface (deformed face) of the atrio-ventricular valves and on the ventricular sides of the semilunar valves. Localization has been explained by the work of Lepeschkin[9] who related the frequency of the valves involved to the average pressure on the valves. His findings are summarized below.

Table 7.1 Frequency of involvement of valves in relation to pressure on the valve

Valve	No. affected (%)	Average pressure on valve (mmHg)
Mitral	86	116
Aortic	55	72
Tricuspid	19.6	24
Pulmonary	1.1	5

Pathology

Bacterial Endocarditis

Any bacterium can affect the heart valves. *Streptococcus viridans* and *Staphylococcus aureus* head the list[10,11]. No macroscopic appearance is typical for a specific organism and caution must be exercised in ascribing an organism macroscopically to a vegetation. Vegetations vary in size and can attain large proportions which may interfere with the blood flow (Figure 7.1). The vegetations vary greatly in size and shape and often have a variegated appearance: yellow, red-brown or red in colour (Figure 7.2). Frequently they are extremely friable and examination must be undertaken with great care. Vegetations may extend over the whole surface of the valve leaflet and may also involve the under-surface (ventricular side) of the atrio-ventricular valves. Adjacent myocardial walls may also be involved. In cases of intercavitory communication, for example ventricular septal defect, the vegetations are located on the side of the lower pressure[12] (Figure 7.3).

Ulceration, perforation or aneurysm formation (Figure 7.4) of valve cusps also occur depending to some extent on the virulence of the organism. Accompanying

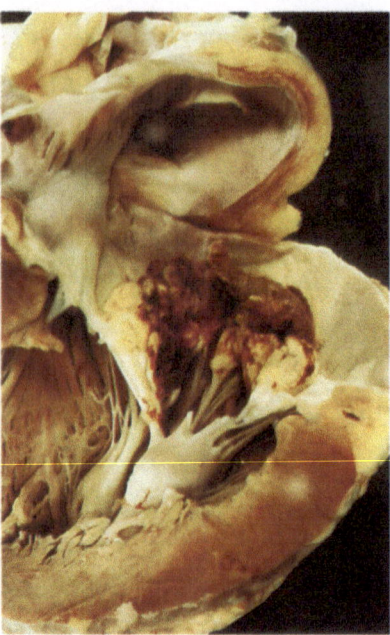

Figure 7.1 Infective endocarditis showing vegetations on the mitral valve, which have attained a large size, interfering with the flow of blood

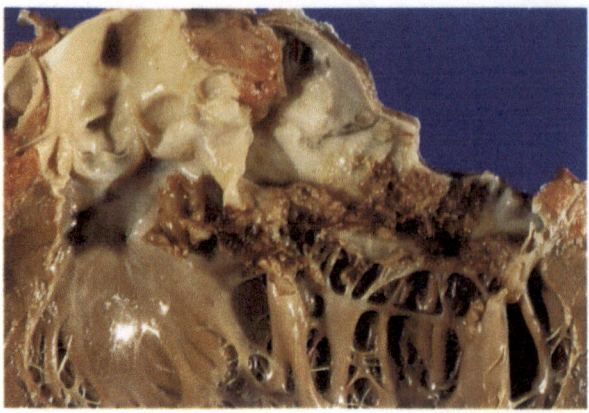

Figure 7.2 The vegetations, similar to Figure 7.1, also have a variegated appearance but in this case have extended to the adjacent endocardium

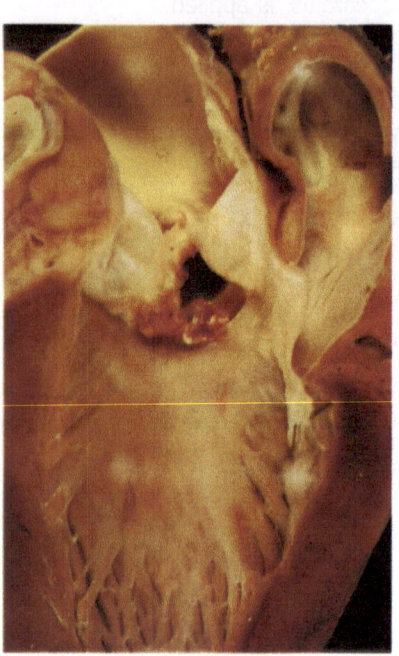

Figure 7.3 Ventricular septal defect complicated by infective endocarditis. The vegetations being located on the left ventricular side indicate significant pulmonary hypertension

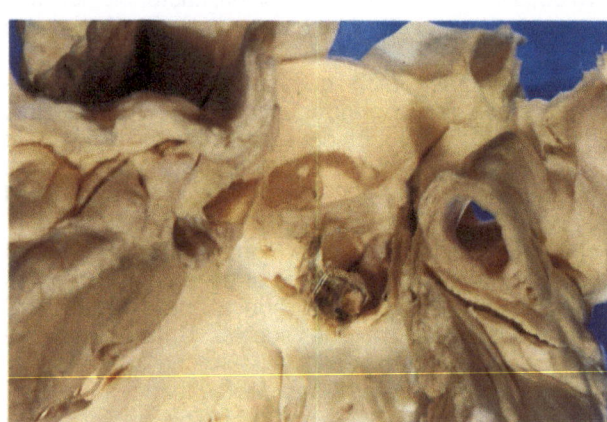

Figure 7.4 Ulceration and perforation from a patient with endocarditis due to *Staphylococcus aureus*

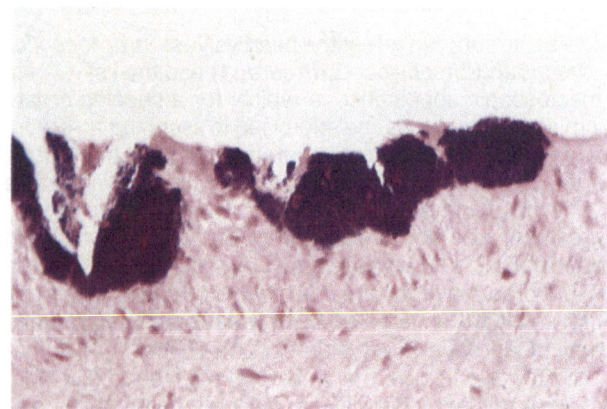

Figure 7.5 Clumps of bacteria can be seen superficially in the fibrin deposited on the valve leaflet. By the dark coloration on haematoxylin and eosin stain the bacteria would appear to be viable. H & E × 100

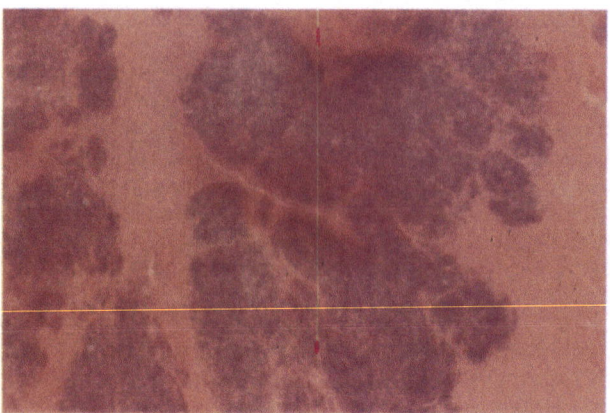

Figure 7.6 In this illustration the bacteria have a pale purple appearance suggesting non-viability (previous effective treatment). H & E × 400

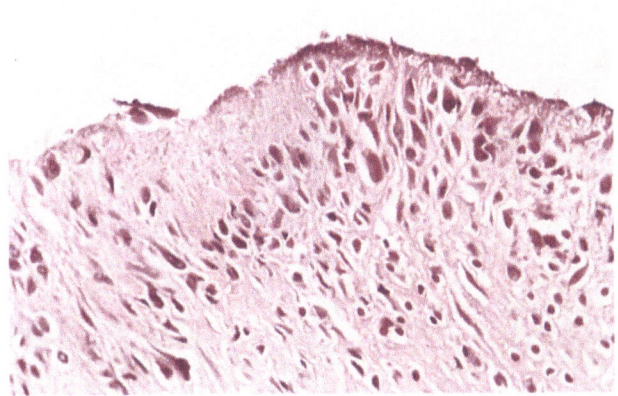

Figure 7.7 Reactive macrophages and chronic inflammatory cells are arranged in columns, the so-called 'palisading', at one time believed to be typical of *Streptococcus viridans*, from a patient with *Staphylococcus* infection. H & E × 100

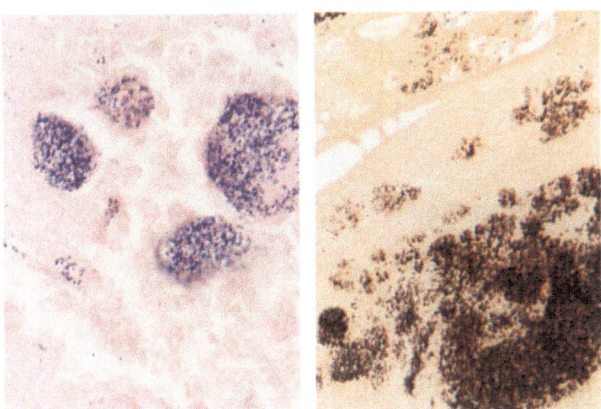

Figure 7.8a (left) Apparently viable bacteria but see Figure 7.8b. H & E × 200
Figure 7.8b (right) The granular appearance of the calcium deposit represents dead bacteria coated with calcium. Von Kossa × 200

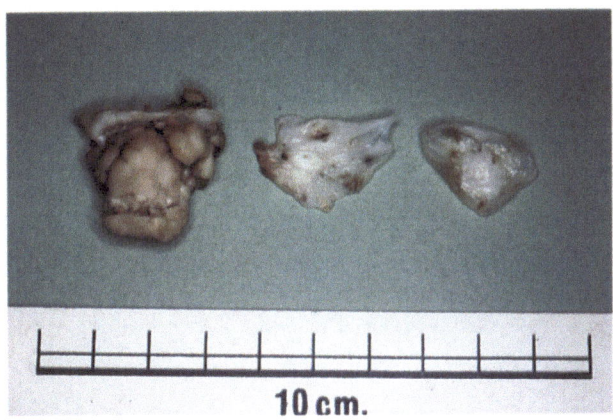

Figure 7.9 Fungal endocarditis showing the typically rounded, large vegetations on the left coronary leaflet (by kind permission of The Macmillan Press Ltd, London and Basingstoke)

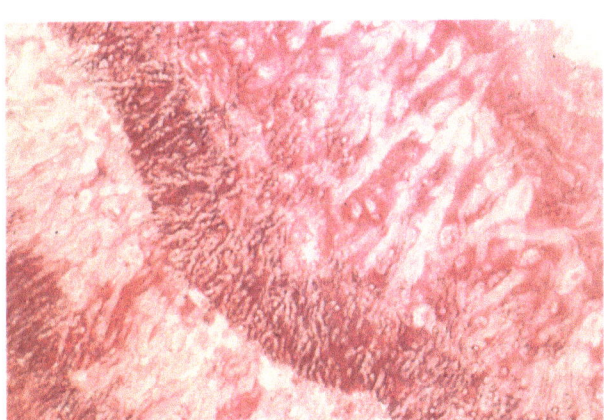

Figure 7.10 Part of the vegetation of fungal endocarditis stained with PAS. On haematoxylin and eosin staining fungus may be missed and the vegetation can be interpreted as consisting of fibrin only. PAS × 200

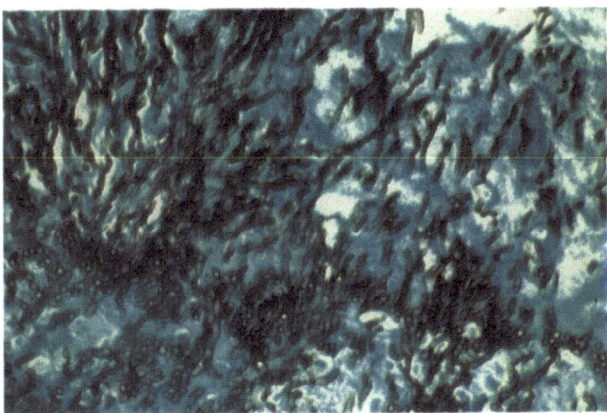

Figure 7.11 Fungal hyphae (*Aspergillus*) from the vegetation of fungal endocarditis. Grocott stain × 200

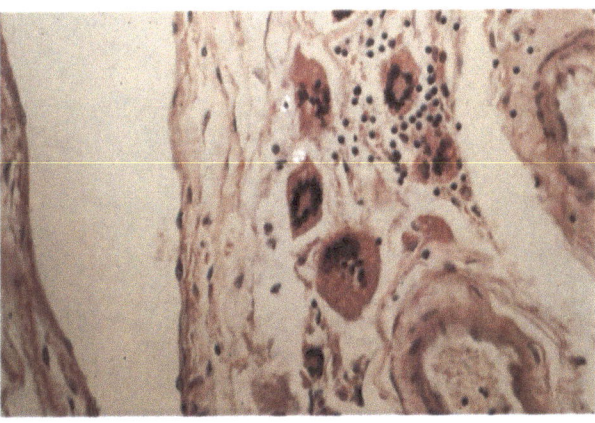

Figure 7.12 *Cryptococcus* having evoked a giant cell reaction and a sparse chronic inflammatory infiltrate. The Maltese cross is not starch but is the organism. H & E × 200

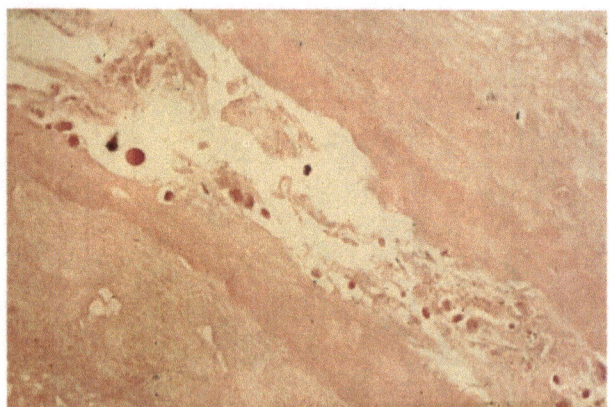

Figure 7.13 *Cryptococcus* taking up a positive reaction with muci-carmine × 200

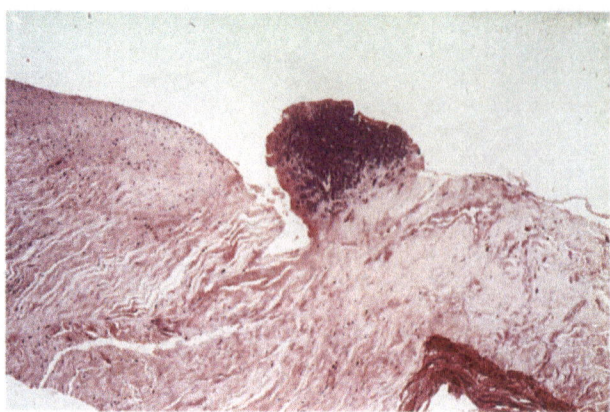

Figure 7.14 Q-fever endocarditis showing a small vegetation containing macrophages. H & E × 25

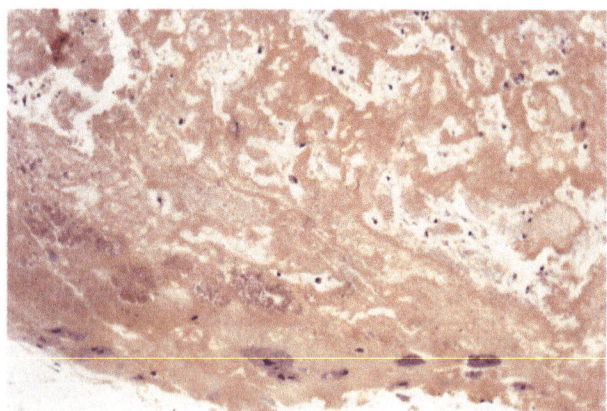

Figure 7.15 Vegetation from a patient with Q-fever endocarditis showing only a few macrophages (some of which contain rickettsiae). H & E × 200

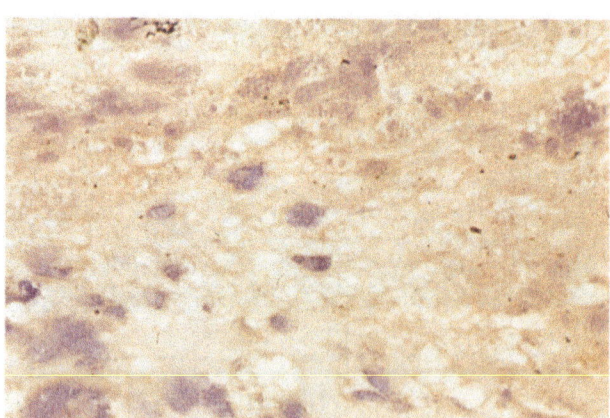

Figure 7.16 Rickettsial endocarditis, on haematoxylin and eosin staining the organism has a pale purple, granular appearance. H & E × 200

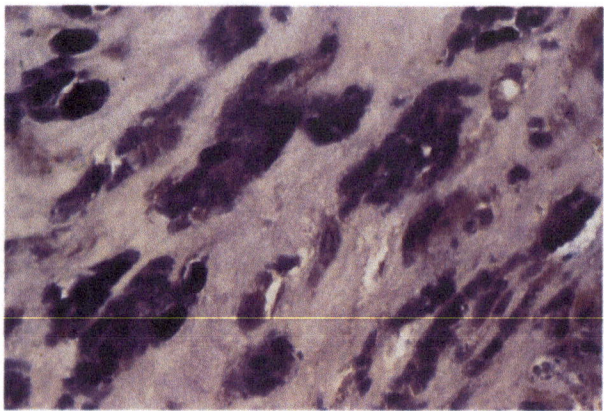

Figure 7.17 With Giemsa the blue–black bodies can be seen, many of which are contained in macrophages. Giemsa × 400

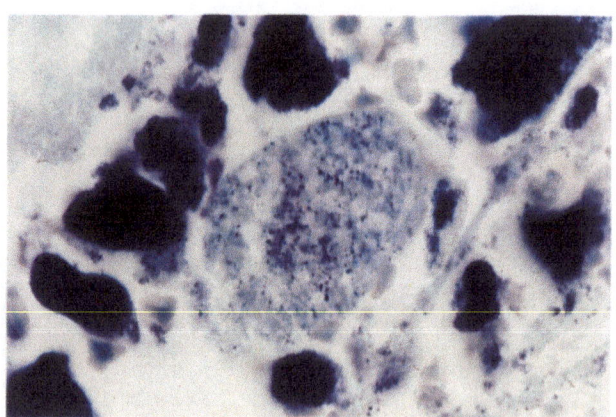

Figure 7.18 Pseudocysts are typical. Giemsa × 600

changes in the myocardium include pallor and flabbiness. Focal areas of necrosis which may represent small abscesses or myocarditis can often be discerned.

Histology Vegetations consist predominantly of fibrin and frequently of clumps of organisms. Cellular elements of the blood stream may also be found, particularly in crevices of the vegetation; thrombus superimposition is rare. Clumps of organisms are usually identified and on haematoxylin and eosin staining, may have a dark purple appearance which indicates viability of the organisms in previously untreated or ineffectually treated patients (Figure 7.5). To some extent effective treatment can be assessed since the bacteria will then show a pale blue discoloration only (Figure 7.6).

The underlying valve tissue is frequently oedematous, resulting in separation of collagen fibres and extensive destruction of the covering endothelial cells. Not infrequently, fibrin may extend into the valve leaflets making demarcation between the vegetation and the valve difficult to assess. An inflammatory reaction, neutrophilic in the early stages but later lymphocytic and mono-nuclear in type, which includes Anitschkow cells, can be found. At one time, the arrangement of reactive cells in columns, so-called 'palisading' was taken to be synonymous with *Streptococcus viridans* infection; but this is by no means always the case (Figure 7.7).

Increase of collagen tissue and later calcification or an increase in vascularity can also be found. Care must be taken not to confuse calcification with dead bacteria which are surrounded by a thin coat of calcium (Figure 7.8a). These, on haematoxylin and eosin staining, might suggest viable bacteria (Figures 7.8a and b).

Fungal Endocarditis

Any fungus can involve the heart valves but *Candida* and *Aspergillus* are those most commonly encountered[1].

Macroscopy Large, lobulated, frequently rounded vegetations are found (Figure 7.9), which are frequently extremely friable. In this form of endocarditis embolization of vegetations may be the presenting symptom.

Histology The vegetations consist of fibrin; there may be a sparse inflammatory reaction in the underlying valvar tissue. Special staining will show fungus (Figures 7.10 and 7.11) and the morphology of these help to distinguish the major groups.

Special mention must be made of *Cryptococcus* insofar that the organism invokes a giant cell reaction, gives rise to a Maltese cross on examination under crossed polaroids (Figure 7.12) and is mucicarmine positive (Figure 7.13). Valves are rarely affected by this organism.

Rickettsial Endocarditis (Q Fever)

This is of world-wide distribution and most frequently involves the aortic valve[13]. It affects man particularly in rural districts where exposure to cows, sheep, goats and wild rodents exists. The causative organism, *Coxiella burnetti*, is present in milk, birth fluids and placenta. Transmission occurs by ticks, drinking unpasteurized milk or by clothing worn by workers in close contact with animals. Diagnosis is achieved by tests in specialized centres. Depending on the number of passages in chick embryo yolk sac, two phases are recognized: patients with high titre of phases one and two indicate endocar-

ditis and presence of high titre of phase one suggests long-standing disease.

The vegetations tend to be small, granular, reddish-brown to white in colour and usually firmly adherent to the valve cusp. When ulceration of the valve occurs, the vegetations may assume large proportions and friability.

Histology The vegetations consist of fibrin and occasional macrophages (Figure 7.14). The underlying valve tissue may show little inflammatory reaction (Figure 7.15). Routine staining with haematoxylin and eosin may just show a peppering of pale blue tiny granules (Figure 7.16). Special stains such as Giemsa or Macchiavello are mandatory to define the infective organism (Figures 7.17 and 7.18).

Complications

Complications of infective endocarditis include congestive heart failure; rupture of cusps and chordae tendineae; aneurysm formation of the cusps, sinus of Valsalva, large vessels, ventricular and atrial walls; myocardial abscesses; pericarditis and emboli. Renal complications are focal glomerulonephritis, proliferative glomerulonephritis and pyelonephritis. Osler's nodes, neurological manifestation and blood changes complete the list[1].

References

1. Olsen, E. G. J. (1980). Infective endocarditis. In *The Pathology of the Heart*. Second Edition, p. 155. (London and Basingstoke: The Macmillan Press Ltd)

2. Olsen, E. G. J. (1985). Die Endokarditis – ein weltweites Problem. *Dtsch. Artzebl.*, **51/52**, 3855

3. Bayliss, R., Clarke, C., Oakley, C. M., Somerville, W., Whitfield, A. G. W. and Young, S. E. J. (1983). The microbiology and pathogenesis of infective endocarditis. *Br. Heart J.*, **50**, 513

4. Robinson, M. J. and Ruedy, J. .(1962). Sequelae of bacterial endocarditis. *Am. J. Med.*, **32,** 922

5. Datta, B. N. (1983). Cardiovascular disease in the Tropics. In Silver, M. D. (ed.). *Cardiovascular Pathology*, Vol. 2, (New York, Edinburgh, London, Melbourne: Churchill Livingstone)

6. Weinstein, L. and Rubin, R. H. (1973). Infective endocarditis. *Prog. Cardiovasc. Dis.*, **16**, 239

7. Steiner, I., Patel, A. K., Hutt, M. S. R. and Somers, K. (1973). Pathology of infective endocarditis, postmortem evaluation. *Br. Heart J.*, **35**, 159

8. Pelletier, L. L. and Petersdorf, R. G. (1977). Infective endocarditis: a review of 125 cases from the University of Washington Hospitals, 1963–1972. *Medicine, Baltimore*, **56**, 287

9. Lepeschkin, E. (1952). On the relation between the site of valvular involvement in endocarditis and the blood pressure resting on the valve. *Am. J. Med. Sci.*, **224**, 318

10. Roberts, W. C. (1978). Characteristic and consequence of infective endocarditis (active or healed or both) learned from morphologic studies. In Rahimtoda, S. H. (ed.). *Infective Endocarditis*. Vol. 55, p. 123. (New York: Grune and Stratton)

11. Hughes, P. and Gauld, W. R. (1966). *Bacterial endocarditis; a changing disease*. *Q. J. Med.*, **35**, 511

12. Rodbard, S. (1963). Blood velocity and endocarditis. *Circulation*, **27**, 18

13. Olsen, E. G. J. (1975). Q-fever endocarditis. In Harrison, C. V. and Weinbren, K. (eds). *Recent Advances in Pathology*, Vol. 9, p. 17. (Edinburgh, London, New York: Churchill Livingstone)

Myocarditis and Pericarditis

8

Myocarditis has been defined as:

An inflammatory process of the heart muscle due to known or unknown causes excluding damage secondary to vascular lesions, such as atherosclerosis or arteritides.

Of the many classifications that have been proposed that by Gore and Saphir, 1947[1], is still relevant and will be used with minor modifications. Myocarditis can be divided into four main groups.

(1) After infection; with or without endocarditis.

(2) With specific or characteristic anatomical structure or identifiable organism including:
rheumatic fever
tuberculosis
sarcoidosis
blastomycosis
Chagas' disease.

(3) Due to chemical poisons.
Drugs.
Physical agents.
Hypersensitivity states.

(4) Isolated; unassociated with any known illness.

Myocarditis is one of the most difficult diagnoses to make, clinically as well as morphologically. The onset may be sudden or insidious. Patients may die at any stage during the disease and the usual causes of death are referable to abnormalities of conduction or heart failure but death may also be sudden.

The incidence is also difficult to ascertain as reports usually come from referral centres. Nonetheless, on the reported series the incidence varies between 3.5%[2] and 9%[3].

Myocarditis after Infection (and with or without Endocarditis)

The following types of infection will be described: bacterial, viral, Rickettsial, fungal, protozoal and metazoal. For convenience of description and illustration, some types of myocarditis with specific morphology will also be included here.

Bacterial Myocarditis

Any bacterium may involve the myocardium. Bacterial myocarditis often occurs as an accompaniment to septicaemia. Macroscopically, the hearts of those patients who had died in congestive heart failure are hypertrophied and dilated and if the causative organism had been *Staphylococcus aureus*, abscesses may be found (Figure 8.1). Histology may often show a heavy inflammatory infiltrate and many Gram-positive organisms (Figure 8.2). Frequently, however, the infective agent cannot be identified.

Clumps of bacteria may occasionally be found at postmortem but these bacteria are confined to vessels in the myocardium without inciting any inflammatory infiltrate. These changes do not represent cardiac involvement during life but indicate postmortem proliferation of bacteria.

Diphtheritic myocarditis This condition which is now, fortunately, rare throughout the world deserves special mention. The organisms may damage the heart directly or through toxins, particularly when the conduction system is involved.

Myocarditis in tuberculosis, syphilis and Whipple's disease are examples of the type with specific or characteristic anatomical features.

Tuberculosis Involvement of the heart by tuberculosis shows three patterns.

(1) *Miliary type.*

(2) *Nodular type:* tuberculomas may be single or multiple and preferentially affects the right atrium. The typical changes of caseation, Langhans giant cells, epithelioid cells and a few chronic inflammatory cells can be observed (Figure 8.3).

(3) *Diffuse type:* chronic inflammatory cells and epithelioid cells are diffusely distributed throughout areas of the myocardium. The diagnosis is confirmed by identifying acid-fast bacilli.

Syphilis Gummata may be single or multiple and may vary in size from 2 mm to several centimetres. Changes of gumma include a central zone of necrosis surrounded by plasma cells and lymphocytes with occasional giant cells (Figure 8.4).

Whipple's disease Cardiac involvement in this condition is well recognized[4]. Histology shows PAS-positive granules in macrophages, associated with chronic inflammatory cells and foci of fibrosis in the myocardium. Pericarditis is a frequent accompaniment. Myocardial fibres show evidence of degeneration and valve deformities may mimic rheumatic fever. Electron microscopy shows rod-shaped bodies, similar in structure to those which have been found in the mucosa or in the small intestine (Figure 8.5).

Viral Myocarditis

Any virus may cause myocarditis. Myocardial involvement has been described with entero viruses, particularly Coxsackie B and A, polio virus and echovirus. Arbo viruses group A and B have also been noted. Other viruses such as rubella, cytomegalovirus, measles, varicella zoster, mumps, influenza and those causing hepatitis have also been described. Infectious mononucleosis may also cause myocarditis.

Coxsackie B virus is probably the most common. It was believed that replication of virus took place within the first 2 days following inoculation experimentally, and even though replication may differ in man, by the time patients have been investigated, which included sampling of endomyocardial tissue by bioptome, virus has seldom been identified in the myocardium[5]. The diagnosis is inferred by raised or rising titres.

In fulminant cases, frequently associated with pericardial involvement, the myocardium shows serpiginous reddish-purple depressions on cutting the ventricular walls (Figure 8.6) and histologically a non-specific chronic inflammatory infiltrate with necrosis of myocardial fibres adjacent to the widened interstitium is seen (Figure 8.7). In those cases with an insidious onset the first presenting features may be those of heart failure, indistinguishable from patients with dilated cardiomyopathy (see also Chapter 9).

The inflammatory infiltrate is usually sparse, though occasionally heavy. In view of the modern therapeutic approaches with corticosteroids and immunosuppressive agent such as azothiaprin, recognition of the stage of myocarditis is essential.

Definition

The following definition of myocarditis and classification of its stages have been proposed[6]. Myocarditis is now defined as:

> The presence of inflammatory cells in the myocardium with evidence of fraying of adjacent myocardial fibres but without concomitant sequential fibre necrosis (as can be seen in ischaemic heart disease).

This definition is for *active myocarditis* (Figure 8.8). Judging from the morphology, these patients would be suitable for therapy. Sequential biopsies have permitted definition of the resolving stages.

Healing myocarditis This is the term employed when widening of the interstitium is found, in which a variable number of inflammatory cells are identified and in which occasional foci of fraying (necrosis) may still be present. Fraying may be absent but the inflammatory cells are in intimate contact with the myocardial fibres. There is usually a minimal to mild increase in interstitial fibrous tissue (Figure 8.9). In these patients, therapy may be of use and should be instigated if the clinical state demands it.

Healed myocarditis In these instances the increase in interstitial fibrous tissue is moderate to severe. Foci of fibrous replacement may be present but in these areas the inflammatory cells are at a distance from the cardiocyte cell margin. Features of hypertrophy and dilatation are also present (Figure 8.10).

Re-definition

More recently the above definition and classification have been amended and expanded at a conference of a group of pathologists who met in Dallas in 1984 (to be published).

Counting of chronic inflammatory cells has been of no value. The diagnosis is made not only by the presence of inflammatory cells, but also by the changes in adjacent myocardial fibres. Numerical evaluation of foci of fraying (necrosis) has also not proved to be helpful in view of the variable and focal nature of myocarditis.

Neutralizing antibody titres to Coxsackie B virus are found in some patients with myocarditis but in other patients no inflammatory cells are present and all that is found is a hypertrophied, dilated myocardium. These patients also have shown titres in significant dilutions[7]. A third group of cases with myocarditis has been found in which no neutralizing antibody titres to Coxsackie B virus have been established. The development of molecular biological techniques to produce a Coxsackie B-specific DNA probe has shown evidence of virus in all these groups[8].

This complex subject has also been extensively investigated by other approaches and in view of a significant number of patients showing, in addition, preferential binding of IgG and IgA and evidence of a cell-mediated immune abnormality and evidence of cytotoxicity, together with defective T suppressor cell function, the conclusion has been reached that in a significant number of patients with dilated cardiomyopathy an infectious–immune mechanism is likely[7] (see also Chapter 9).

Care and uniformity of interpretation of biopsy tissue is essential. As the inflammatory infiltrate is usually sparse, and in view of the fact that chronic inflammatory cells can occur in normal myocardium, a clear definition and concept for diagnosis of myocarditis is essential. Differentiation from ischaemic heart disease and early myocardial infarction can also be difficult. Figure 8.11a illustrates early myocardial infarction, lymphocytes constituting the major cellular infiltrate but the nuclei have disappeared in myocardial fibres, whereas, in myocarditis nuclei in fibres adjacent to the inflammatory infiltrate are preserved. The structure of the myocardial fibres is also normal (Figure 8.11b).

Mumps, vaccinia, influenza, virus causing hepatitis, rabies and psittacosis may all show myocarditis but the morphological changes are non-specific. The myocardium is rarely involved in infectious mononucleosis and death is very rarely attributable to myocarditis. The interstitial cell infiltrate contains typical large lymphocytes.

Rickettsial Myocarditis

Epidemic (louse-borne) and non-epidemic (tick-borne) typhus fever may involve the heart. The interstitial inflammatory infiltrate consists of chronic inflammatory cells and eosinophils (Figure 8.12). Q-fever endocarditis may involve the myocardium although this association is very rare (Figure 8.13).

Fungal Myocarditis

This form of myocarditis is rarely seen in the industrial countries and usually occurs in patients on immunosuppressive therapy or in patients with immunological deficiencies. Any fungus may be involved but *Candida* and *Aspergillus* are the most frequently encountered. Apart from a non-specific chronic inflammatory infiltrate the microcolonies of yeast cells forming radially arranged pseudorosettes are often seen in micro-abscesses (Figure 8.14a and b). Occasionally no inflammatory reaction may be present. The lesions may be discernible to the naked eye, nodules being haphazardly distributed throughout the myocardium. Figure 8.15 is an illustration of an aspergilloma.

Blastomycosis, actinomycosis, histoplasmosis, coccidioidomycosis and phycomycetosis may all involve the heart. Cryptococcosis can also cause myocarditis.

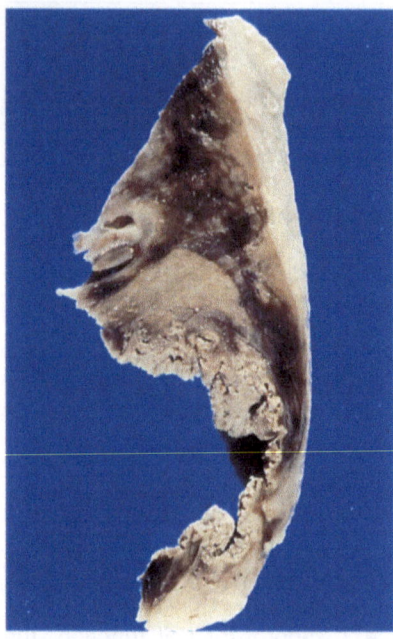

Figure 8.1 *Staphylococcus aureus* infection involving the heart, resulting in abscess formation. Part of the left ventricular wall also shows evidence of extensive myocarditis (haemorrhagic areas)

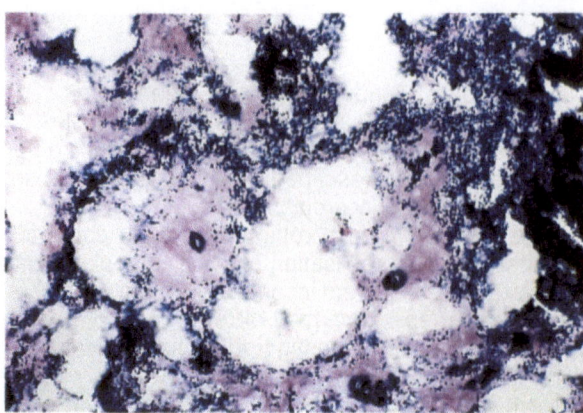

Figure 8.2 Photomicrograph from the region of the abscess shown in Figure 8.1. Staphylococci abound. H & E × 400

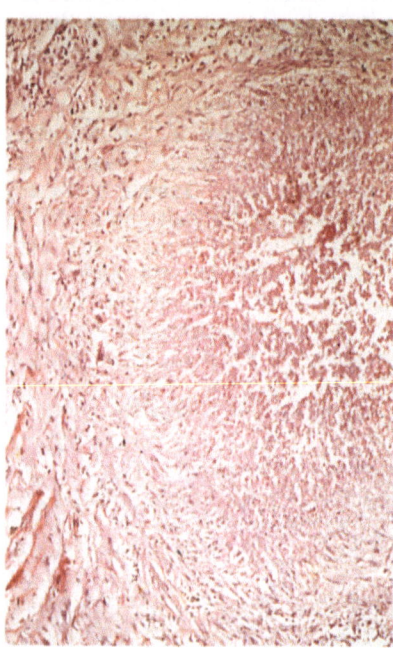

Figure 8.3 Nodular tuberculosis in the right atrial myocardium. Typical caseation in the centre surrounded by epithelioid cells and an occasional giant cell is seen. H & E × 50 (By courtesy of Professor Kinare, Bombay)

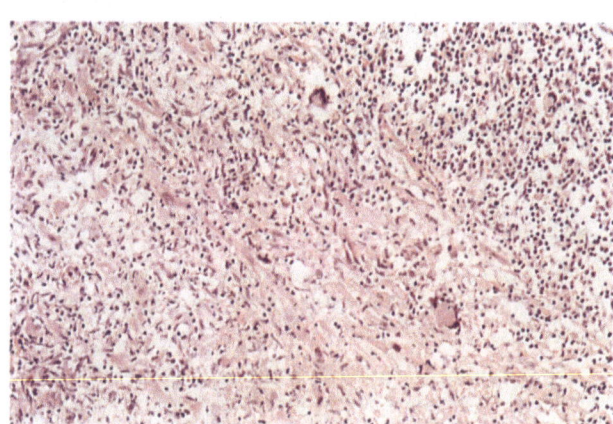

Figure 8.4 Photomicrograph of gumma in the left ventricular myocardium. The zone of necrosis extends from the centre of the illustration to the left lower border and is surrounded by a mantle of chronic inflammatory cells. A few giant cells are seen close to the necrotic area. H & E × 50

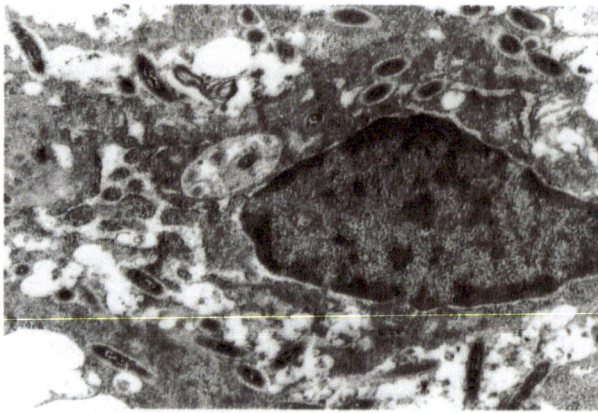

Figure 8.5 Electron micrograph of Whipple's disease showing rod-shaped bodies in a histiocyte with vacuolated cytoplasm, from a patient described in *Gastroenterology*, 1986, who had clinical cardiac involvement. Lead citrate and uranyl acetate × 20 000 (By kind permission and courtesy of Professor D. J. Evans)

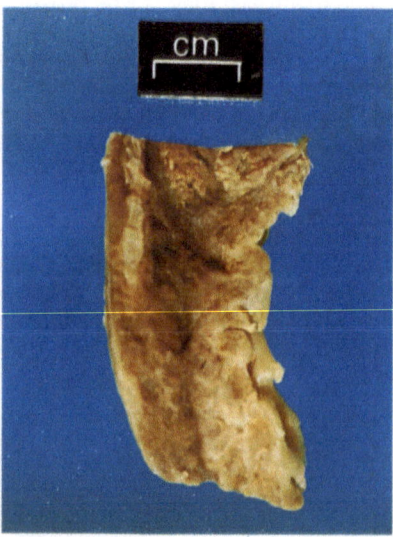

Figure 8.6 Part of the left ventricular wall showing serpiginous haemorrhagic depressions indicative of necrosis due to myocarditis

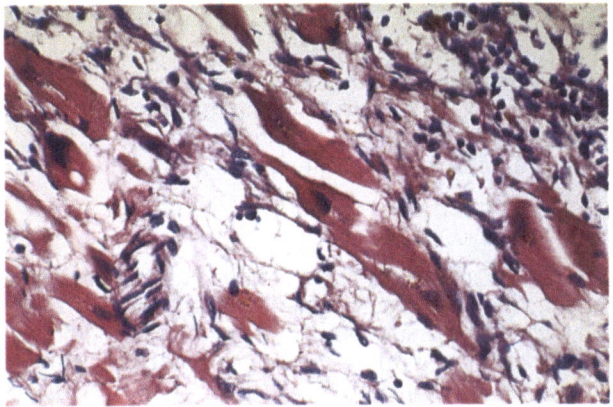

Figure 8.7 Viral myocarditis. Myocytolysis and some necrosis of myocardial fibres adjacent to the chronic inflammatory infiltrate, almost entirely lymphocytic, can be identified. Despite these changes myocardial fibres have retained their nuclei. H & E × 200

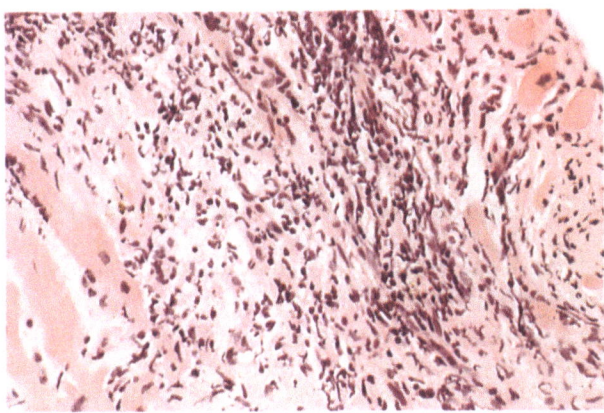

Figure 8.8 Active myocarditis (see definition in text). H & E × 100

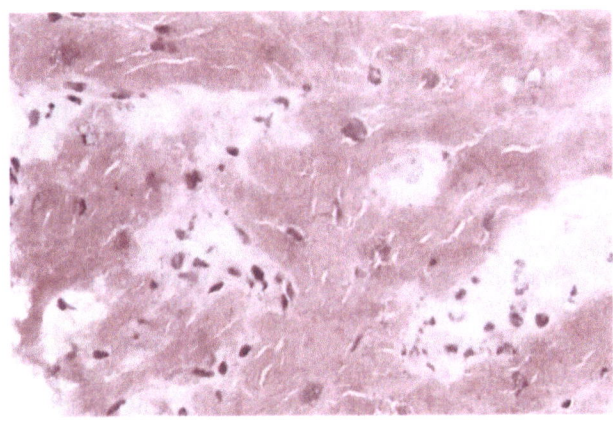

Figure 8.9 Healing myocarditis. In the widened interstitium a sparse chronic inflammatory cell infiltrate is shown. The inflammatory cells are in intimate contact with myocardial fibres, occasionally giving rise to a 'moth-eaten' appearance of the contour of the fibres. Some increase in interstitial collagen tissue is found (frozen section). H & E × 400

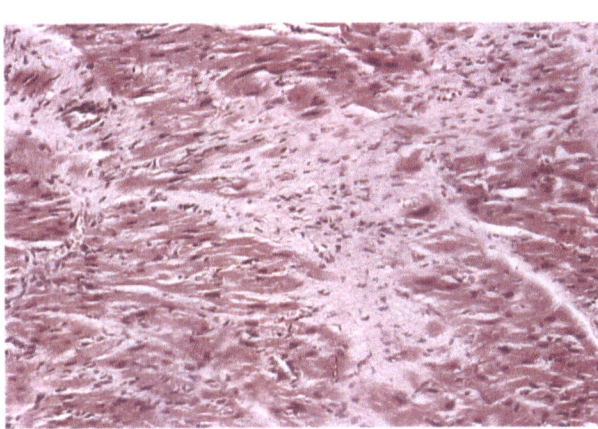

Figure 8.10 Healed myocarditis. The centre of the illustration is occupied by an area of fibrous replacement in which chronic inflammatory cells can still be identified. If this had been the patient's first endomyocardial biopsy, myocarditis, at this late stage, could only be surmised. H & E × 50

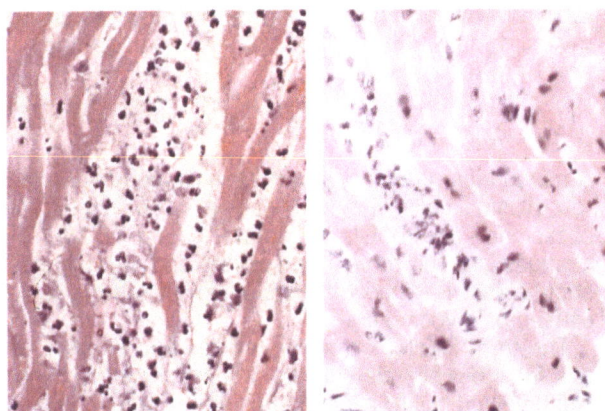

Figure 8.11a (left) Recent myocardial infarction showing a mixed cellular infiltrate rich in lymphocytes. The myocardial fibres show hyaline change and no nuclei. In contrast, **Figure 8.11b (right)** shows preservation of the structural integrity of myocardial fibres adjacent to the inflammatory cells with preservation of their nuclei. These appearances distinguish myocarditis from infarction. Distinction may be difficult in small samples obtained by bioptome. H & E × 200 (a and b)

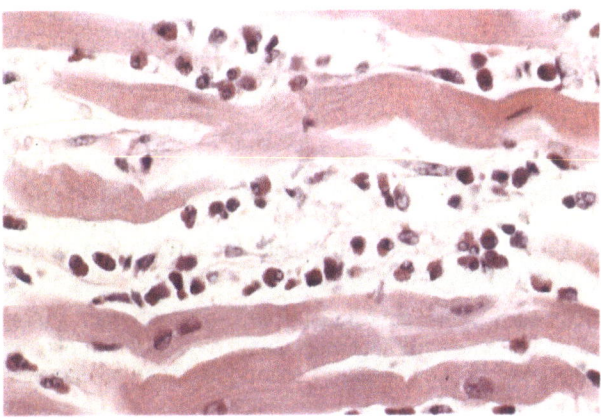

Figure 8.12 Typhus fever involving the heart showing an inflammatory cell infiltrate including some eosinophils. These changes are not morphologically specific. H & E × 400

Protozoal Myocarditis

Toxoplasmosis can occur in neonates or at any age. Macroscopically no specific features are identifiable and those illustrated for viral myocarditis apply. Histologically, myocarditis with a mixed inflammatory infiltrate is found. Rarely, cysts crowded with Toxoplasma can be identified, not infrequently in areas without an inflammatory infiltrate (Figure 8.16).

Chagas' disease This disease, which may affect the heart or the alimentary tract, is almost confined to the South American continent with 35 000 000 people at risk of infection. Transmission to man is mediated through bugs belonging to the triatomid family. Clinically, three phases are recognized[9,10].

Acute phase: In the acute phase signs and symptoms suggestive of myocarditis are found, together with oedema of one or both eyes, skin rashes and enlargement of the liver and spleen. Myocarditis is present in this stage. Foci of fibrosis may also be identified. The diagnostic features are pseudo-Leishmanic cysts (Figure 8.17a and b; Figure 8.18).

Latent phase: The latent phase follows and may last for 10 to 20 years. Little is known of the pathology at this stage.

Chronic phase: The chronic phase may be further subdivided into three stages. Firstly, no symptoms may be experienced but rhythm disturbances can occur. Dizziness and syncope may occur in some patients. The second stage is characterized by cardiomegaly, and the third stage by congestive heart failure and thrombo-embolic complications.

In the chronic phases the heart is hypertrophied and dilatation of all cardiac chambers is found. Lymphatic hyperplasia, outlining the epicardial vessels, can be striking (Figure 8.19). Characteristically an apical aneurysm is found (Figure 8.20). The myocardium may show interstitial fibrosis but occasional foci of chronic inflammatory cells may also be found. Pseudocysts can be found by painstaking search.

The exact mechanism of the pathogenesis of Chagas' disease is still under debate but vascular, toxic, inflammatory, neurogenic and immunological pathways have been suggested. Extreme neuronal depletion in right atrial strips between the venae cavae have been found (Figure 8.21).

African trypanosomiasis, malaria (*Plasmodium falciparum*) and rarely an amoebiasis myocarditis may be found.

Metazoal Myocarditis

Hydatid cysts due to *Echinococcus granulosus* results in multiple cysts involving the myocardium with a strong fibrous reaction which includes a chronic inflammatory infiltrate. The worm and part of a wall of a cyst is illustrated in Figure 8.22a and b.

Filariasis A myocarditis rich in eosinophils is characteristic (Figure 8.23). *Onchocerca* have been implicated as being causally related to endomyocardial fibrosis[11] (see Chapter 9).

Trichinosis (trichiniasis) The products of degenerating larvae may induce a myocarditis.

Chemical Poisons – Physical Agents

In 0.7% of cases of carbon monoxide poisoning the heart may be severely involved, the papillary muscles, the interventricular septum and the conduction system being particularly affected[12]. Apart from epicardial ecchymoses and myocardial haemorrhages, muscle necrosis and a neutrophil infiltrate are also found.

Irradiation Injury

Therapeutic irradiation in cases of malignant neoplasm, for example of lung and breast, may lead to necrosis of the myocardium and an inflammatory reaction, although the pericardium is more vulnerable. Vascular damage may be striking[13] (Figure 8.24).

Drugs

Drug sensitivity to a number of agents is recognized. Mechanisms involved include the direct effects of toxins on the myocardium or on small blood vessels, causing necrotizing arteritis, and effects mediated by immune pathways (allergy or hypersensitivity). Pathogenetic mechanisms can overlap.

Toxic effects The many drugs that are known to have adverse effects on the myocardium include immunosuppressive agents, antihypertensive agents, amphetamine, barbiturates, emetine and many others. Myocardial necrosis with myocarditis consisting of chronic inflammatory cells can be found. The changes appear to be dose-dependent (Figure 8.25).

Antineoplastic agents have a direct toxic effect. These agents include adriamycin, daunorubicin, rubidazone and carminomycins. Although these agents do not evoke myocarditis their cardiotoxicity acting in synergy with irradiation or drugs can evoke myocarditis.

Immune-mediated pathways Drugs, including sulphonamides, penicillin, streptomycin, tetracycline, phenylbutazone and methyldopa may incite an inflammatory infiltrate, often rich in eosinophils. A granulomatous reaction may also occur.

Isolated Myocarditis

Not infrequently myocarditis occurs unassociated with any other disease process elsewhere in the body. In these cases and, because the aetiology is unknown, the term 'isolated myocarditis' is employed. An incidence of 0.35% has been reported[14]. Another group of investigators from Jamaica have reported 102 cases of isolated myocarditis in 3000 autopsies[15]. Three morphological types are recognised.

Diffuse Myocarditis

A mixed inflammatory infiltrate consisting of lymphocytes, plasma cells, mononuclear cells, eosinophils and occasional neutrophils is found (Figure 8.26). The changes are therefore non-specific and the diagnosis should only be made by excluding all other possible causes of myocarditis.

The term Fiedler's myocarditis has been attached to this form but has also included some cases with giant cell myocarditis. To avoid confusion the term should be abandoned.

Granulomatous Myocarditis

See Figure 8.27. This form is rare and may be difficult to diagnose. Giant cell follicles together with discrete chronic inflammatory cells are typical and the lesions are focally distributed throughout the myocardium. The distinction from giant cell myocarditis (see below) may be difficult. Although tuberculosis and gummata have specific features, these entities should be excluded before making such a diagnosis.

Other causes of myocarditis which could result in a granulomatous reaction include leprosy, brucellosis, fungal infections, histoplasmosis and coccidioidomycosis, protozoal infection and Leishmaniasis. Berylliosis may also be associated with a granulomatous reaction. This form of myocarditis should only be diagnosed if no possible link exists with such conditions.

Sarcoidosis This is also characterized by granulomatous change in the myocardium and it is therefore convenient to describe it here. Myocarditis in sarcoidosis is another example of the type with characteristic morphology. An excellent clinical account and description of postmortem findings has been given[16]. Disturbances of conduction and heart failure are important signs and symptoms occurring in affected patients. Death may be sudden. The diagnosis is confirmed by a Kveim test (which is frequently positive) and by tuberculin tests, which are often negative.

Macroscopically, fibrous areas may be discernible with the naked eye; the involvement may be massive, particularly in the septal region. Ventricular aneurysms may occur. Sarcoid nodules resemble tuberculosis but caseation is absent. Lymphocytes are fewer and giant cells tend to be larger (Figures 8.28a and b). A histological classification has been suggested[17]. Exudative, granulomatous, combined and fibrotic forms are recognised. The fibrotic form is illustrated in Figure 8.29.

The aetiology is uncertain. An immunological pathogenetic pathway (a delayed type of hypersensitivity) has been suggested. Raised abnormal immunoglobulins have been found and circulating B and T lymphocytes are diminished[18].

Giant Cell Myocarditis

This is the third and last type of isolated myocarditis. In addition to a diffuse type of myocarditis, isolated giant cells, particularly at the margin of myocytic necrosis, are scattered throughout affected areas of the myocardium. Large multinucleate giant cells of myogenic origin (Figure 8.30a and b), giant cells resembling the Langhans type and foreign body giant cells, as well as Touton giant cells have all been recognized in giant cell myocarditis.

The association of isolated giant cell myocarditis and thyroiditis has been repeatedly reported.

Patients with isolated myocarditis and a prominent increase in heart weight had a normal thymus/body weight ratio, whilst in patients with a normal or slight increase in heart weight, increased ratios were noted. Thymic weights between 60 and 90 g were recorded[19]. An immunological process seems likely.

Pericarditis

The occurrence of inflammation of the pericardium (an incidence of 6% has been cited[20]) may be secondary to diseases elsewhere in the body and, not infrequently, may accompany or be accompanied by myocarditis. Pericarditis may also occur in an isolated form.

Pericarditis is divided into two main groups. (This classification is modified from that of El-Maraghi[21].)

(1) Primary pericarditis which is unassociated with any other disease process in the body.

(2) Secondary pericarditis:

(i) Following bacterial, fungal or viral infection.
(ii) In association with recognized disease processes. These include:
rheumatic fever
uraemia
infarction
surgical intervention
trauma
neoplasm.

Morphological Changes

The pericardium reacts to various agents or disease processes in a limited way. Basic changes consist of fibrin deposition and fluid accumulation. Pericardial effusion is present when more than 50 ml of fluid is present. It may be straw-coloured (hydropericardium), bloody (haemopericardium), or milky (chylopericardium, due to obstruction of the thoracic duct). Cellular elements may also be involved. Healing takes place by fibrosis resulting either in discrete adhesions or sheets of fibrous tissue which may culminate clinically in constriction. Calcification may occur[22].

Diagnostic features may be identifiable, for example, granulomata in rheumatic fever or tuberculosis, or in certain fungal infections such as *Coccidioides immitis*.

Primary or secondary neoplasms may be a cause of pericarditis. Cholesterol crystals may abound in cholesterol pericardial effusion (gold paint pericardial effusion). Haemorrhagic pericarditis usually accompanies neoplastic involvement of the pericardium, as, for example, in lymphoma, leukaemia, mesothelioma, and carcinoma of the lung or breast (Figure 8.31).

In isolated forms of pericarditis the basic components are also seen and these will be briefly described. Macroscopically the pericardium is shaggy and may be haemorrhagic (Figure 8.32). It resembles other forms of serous or fibrinous pericarditis. Histologically, oedema, and chronic inflammatory cells, rich in lymphocytes but also in plasma cells and other mononuclear cells, are found (Figure 8.33). Fibrin deposition may be extensive. Vascularity is increased (Figure 8.34). Virus has been implicated as being causally related to the isolated form of pericarditis.

For bacterial or fungal infections any organism may give rise to pericarditis[23] and, depending on the type of organism, the pericarditis may be seropurulent and large numbers of neutrophils may be present.

In tuberculosis, fibrinous pericarditis is the first stage and resembles fibrinous pericarditis from other disease processes such as rheumatic fever. The second stage is characterized by an effusion and thickening, lymphocytes abound and typical tubercles may be found[24]. The third stage, the stage of healing, shows increasing fibrosis and fibrocaseous lesions and tubercles (Figures 8.35a and b) but these gradually disappear as healing progresses, resulting in sheets of fibrous tissue which may clinically result in constriction (Figure 8.36)[23].

In rheumatic fever, fibrinous or serofibrinous pericarditis is found with a mixed cellular infiltrate and Aschoff nodules. Healing by fibrosis results either in 'milky spots' or adhesions (Figure 8.37).

In uraemia, fibrin deposition may be severe but a sparse inflammatory cell response is typical. Hydropericardial or haemopericardial effusions may be found[25].

Virus infection resembles primary pericarditis. Myocarditis is a frequent accompaniment[26]. Any virus affecting the myocardium may also affect the pericardium.

Pericarditis associated with infarction also results in fibrinous pericarditis (Figure 8.38), particularly when the

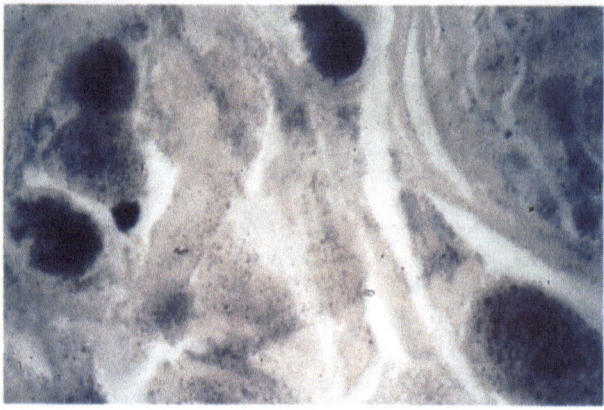

Figure 8.13 Q-fever myocarditis showing a pseudocyst (bottom right of the illustration), Rickettsiae in macrophages and necrotic myocardial fibres. This scattering of organisms may be found in tissue sections after rupture of a pseudocyst.   Giemsa × 800

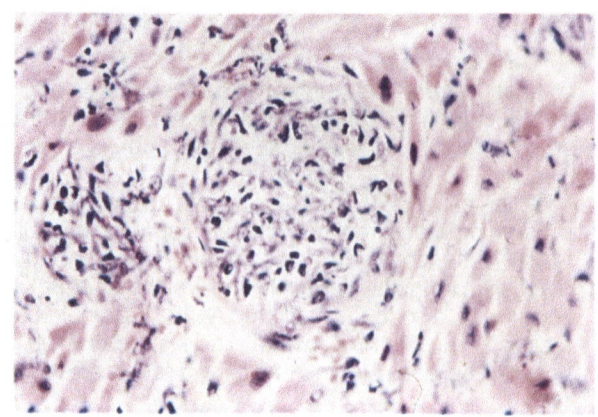

Figure 8.14a Fungal myocarditis. Micro-colonies of fungi may form pseudo-rosettes.   H & E × 200

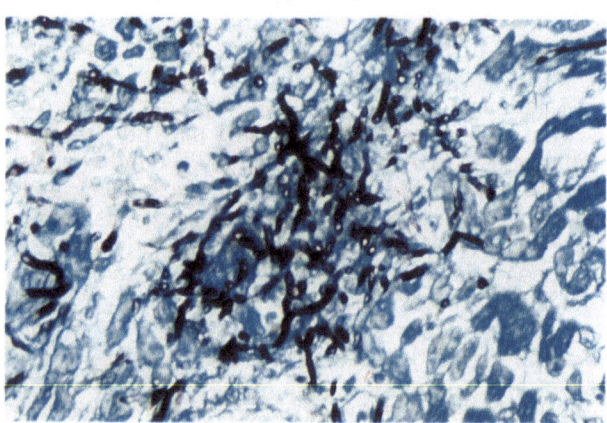

Figure 8.14b From the same case as Figure 8.14a, stained by Grocott's technique × 200

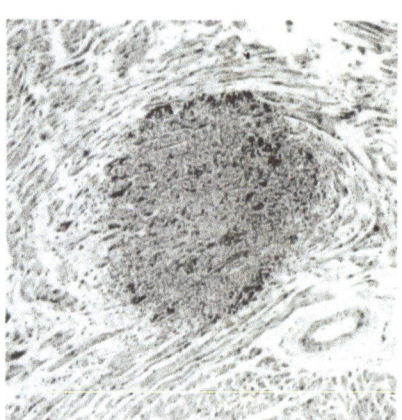

Figure 8.15 Illustration of an aspergilloma   × 100 (By permission of The Macmillan Press Ltd)

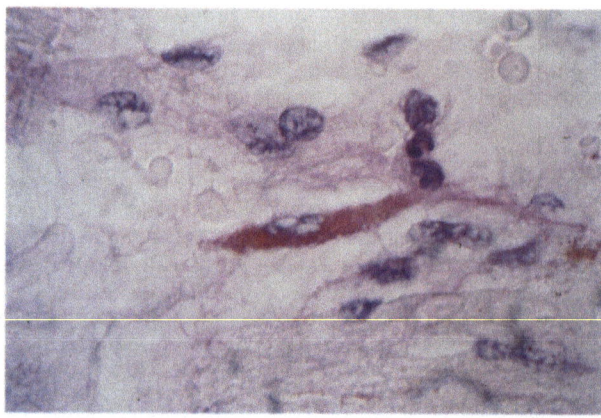

Figure 8.16 Toxoplasmosis. The organisms can be seen in a necrotic myocardial fibre in an area devoid of inflammatory cells. PAS × 600

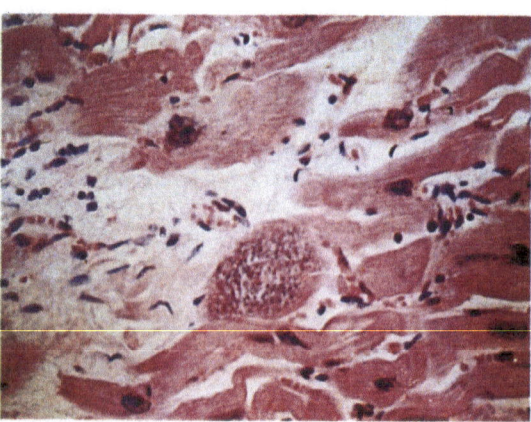

Figure 8.17a Illustration of a pseudo-leishmanic cyst in a myocardial fibre close to the centre of the illustration together with a sparse chronic inflammatory cell infiltrate near the pseudocyst. H & E × 400

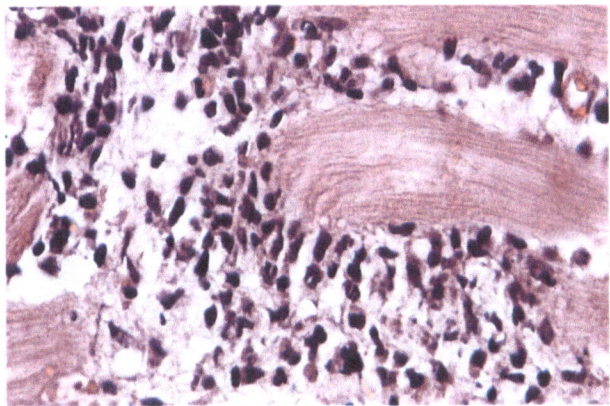

Figure 8.17b A severe, non-specific chronic inflammatory cell infiltrate is seen close to the area illustrated in Figure 8.17a, devoid of pseudocysts. H & E × 600

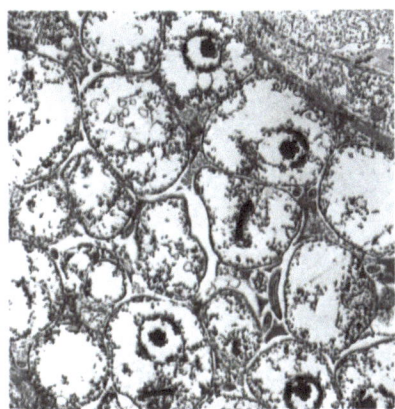

Figure 8.18 Electron micrograph of *Trypanosoma cruzi*. Lead citrate and uranyl acetate × 25 000

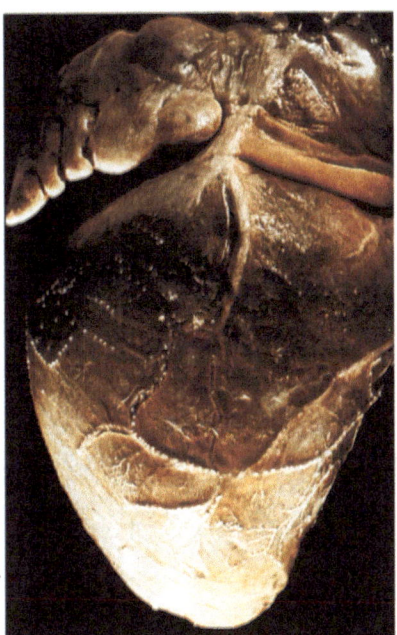

Figure 8.19 Surface view of the heart showing lymphatic hyperplasia in a heart affected by Chagas' disease in the chronic phase

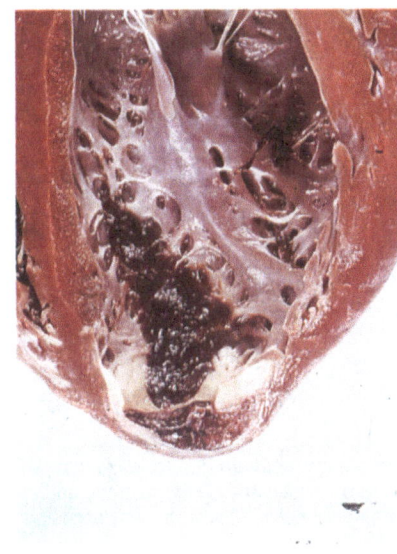

Figure 8.20 Part of the left ventricle has been sectioned to show the characteristic apical aneurysm in chronic Chagas' heart disease. Thrombus is superimposed

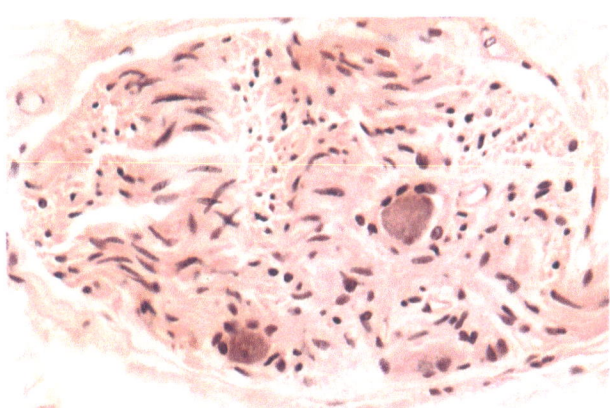

Figure 8.21 Severe neuronal depletion in the right atrium (between venae cavae) is found in chronic Chagas' heart disease. The surviving neurones are widely separated by connective tissue in which some chronic inflammatory cells can also be seen. H & E × 400

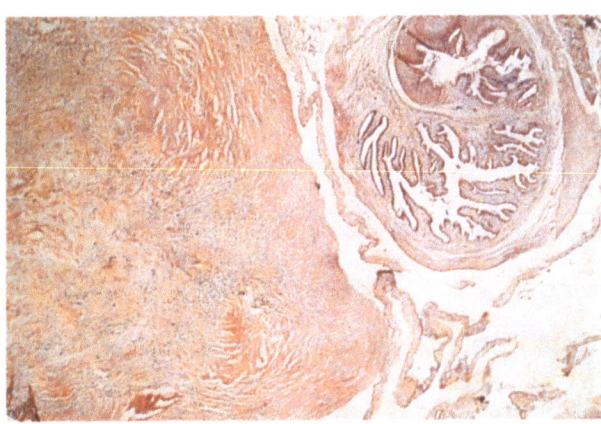

Figure 8.22a Cross-section of *Ecchinococcus granulosus* in the heart. H & E × 25

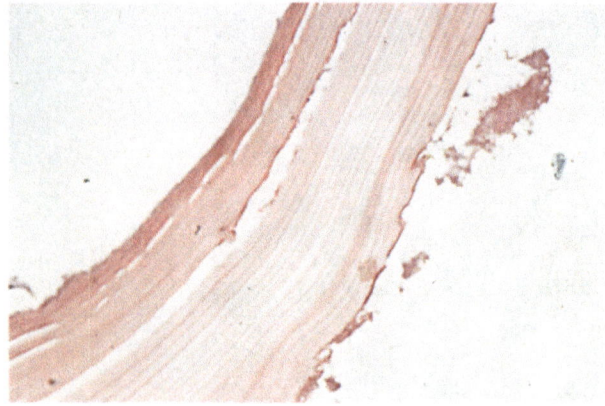

Figure 8.22b   Part of the wall of a hydatid cyst.   H & E × 50

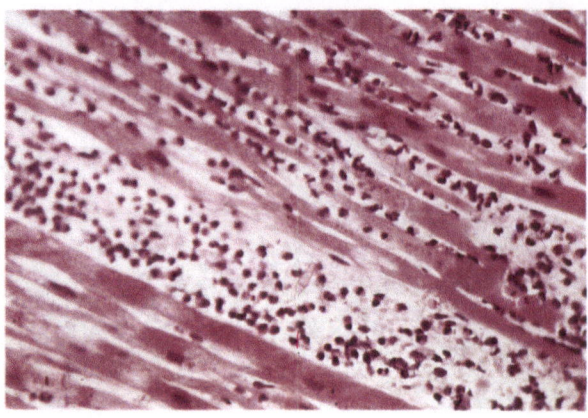

Figure 8.23   An eosinophilic myocarditis due to *Onchocerca*. H & E × 200

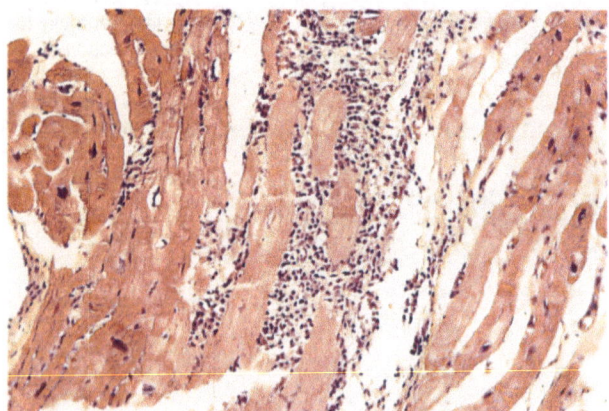

Figure 8.24   Damage to the myocardium due to irradiation. The muscle fibres in the centre of the illustration are necrotic and are surrounded by inflammatory cells including an occasional eosinophil.   H & E × 100

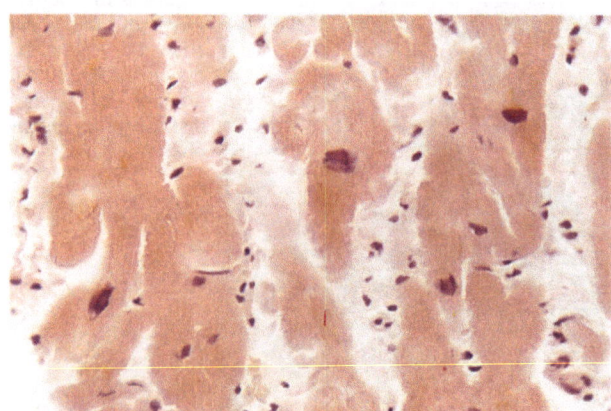

Figure 8.25   A low grade inflammatory cell infiltrate attributable to amphetamine dependence.   H & E × 400

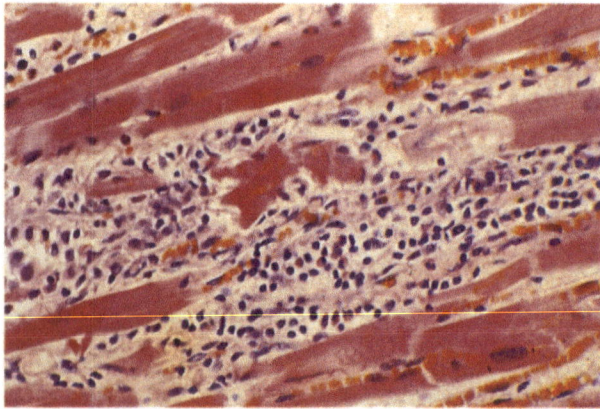

Figure 8.26   Isolated myocarditis of the diffuse type is illustrated. The cellular infiltrate is mixed. Necrosis of myocardial fibres is seen in the centre of the photomicrograph. Distinction from an infarcted area may be extremely difficult, particularly on small tissue samples obtained by bioptome.   H & E × 250

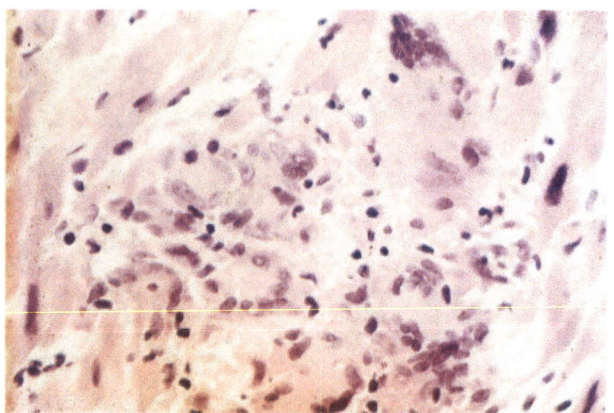

Figure 8.27   Granulomatous myocarditis. A giant cell granuloma occupies the centre of the photomicrograph. Hypertrophied, attenuated myocardial fibres can be seen surrounding the granuloma. No cause could be established and therefore the term isolated granulomatous myocarditis can be applied.   H & E × 300

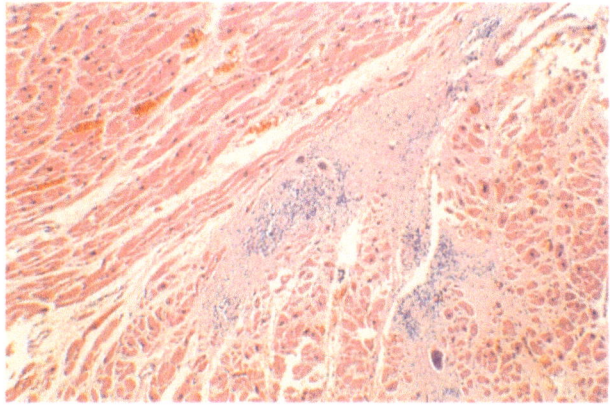

Figure 8.28a Sarcoidosis involving the myocardium. In the centre of the illustration fibrous areas can be seen containing inflammatory cells.   H & E × 50

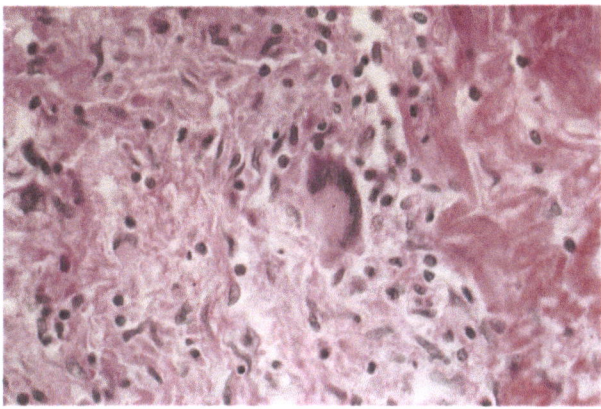

Figure 8.28b Close-up view of a granuloma of sarcoid.   H & E × 300

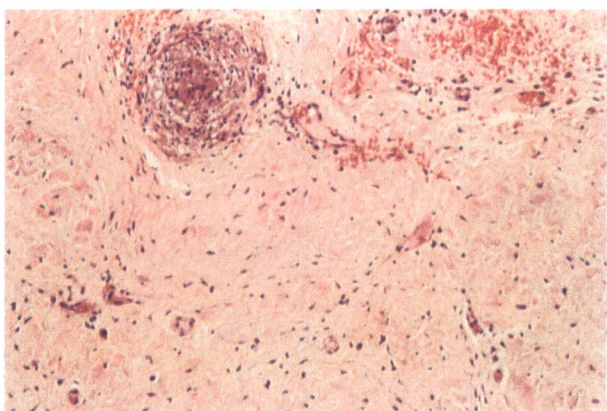

Figure 8.29 Illustrates the fibrotic form of sarcoid of the heart. The entire area is occupied by fibrous tissue containing a few chronic inflammatory cells. An occasional granuloma can be recognized in the upper region of the photomicrograph   H & E × 50

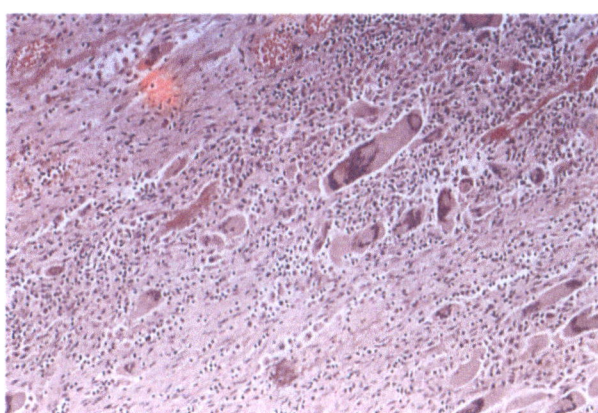

Figure 8.30a Isolated giant cell myocarditis. Apart from a diffuse distribution of inflammatory cells, giant cells are scattered throughout the area, clearly recognizable, even at a low power of magnification   H & E × 50

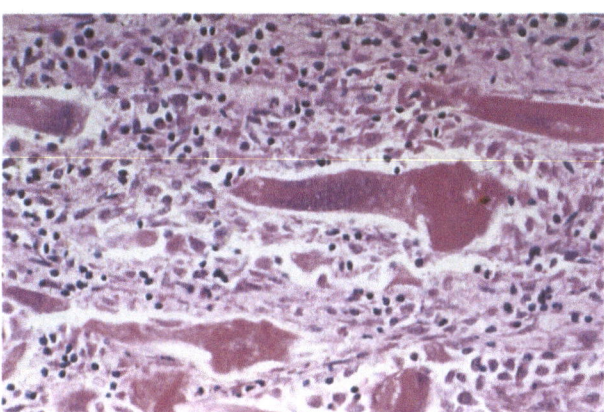

Figure 8.30b High power view of giant cells which, by their eosinophilic cytoplasm, suggests a myogenic origin. The nuclei at the left pole of the largest giant cell in the centre of the photomicrograph are believed to represent an attempt of regeneration of the affected myocardial cell   H & E × 250

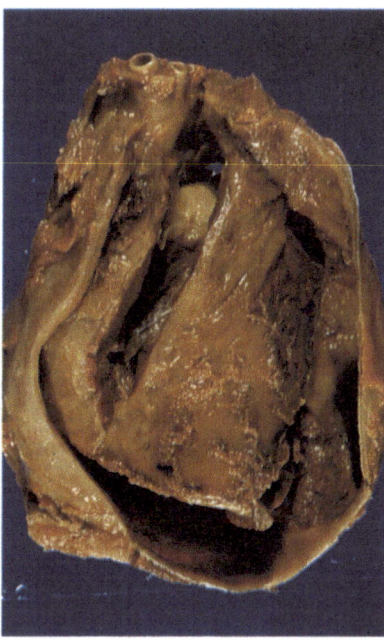

Figure 8.31 Haemorrhage and blood clot are seen in the pericardium, in this case due to secondary deposits in the pericardium of carcinoma of the breast

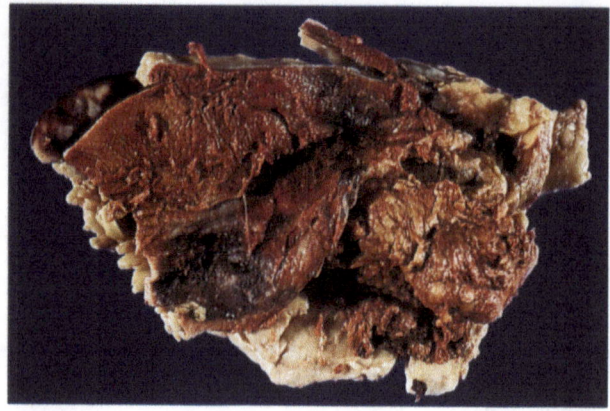

Figure 8.32 Fibrinous pericarditis. Fibrin gives the pericardium a shaggy lining. Haemorrhagic areas are clearly seen. From a patient with the isolated form of pericarditis

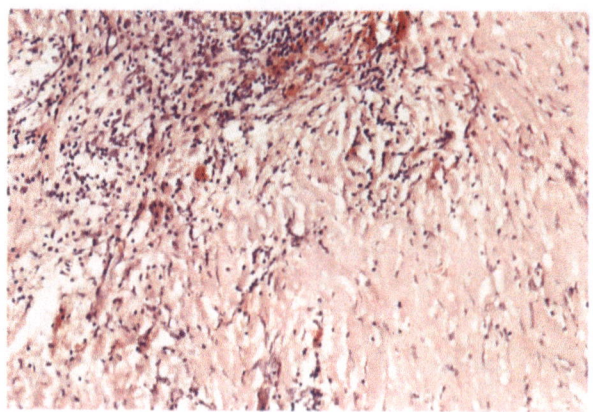

Figure 8.33 Fibrinous pericarditis. This view shows loosely arranged collagen fibres (separated by oedema) and chronic inflammatory cells. H & E × 50

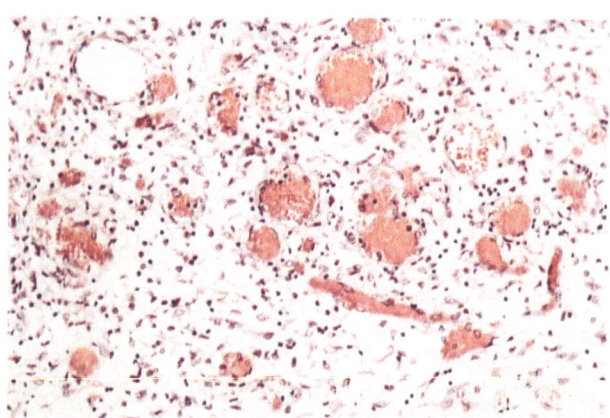

Figure 8.34 Fibrinous pericarditis. This view shows loosely arranged collagen fibres (separated by oedema), chronic inflammatory cells and an increase in vascularity. H & E × 50

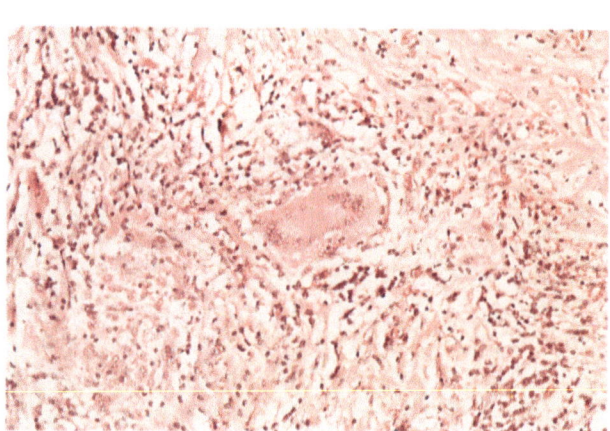

Figure 8.35a Tuberculous pericarditis. Typical granulomata occupy the illustration. H & E × 50

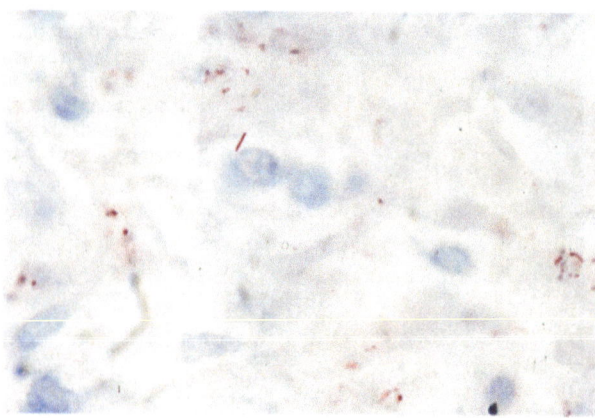

Figure 8.35b Acid-fast bacilli are demonstrated. Ziehl–Neelsen × 600

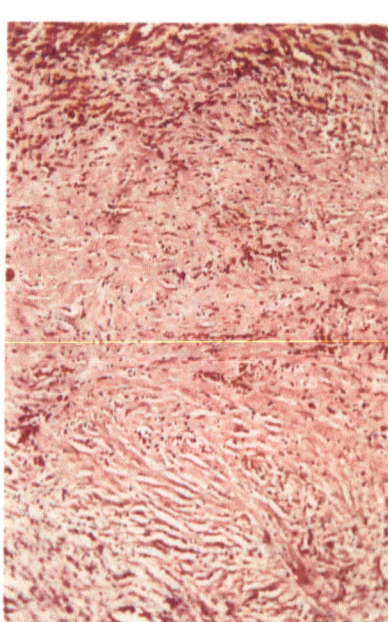

Figure 8.36 Healed tuberculous pericarditis. The pericardium consists of fibrous tissue in which occasional chronic inflammatory cells may be found. Some fibrin superimposition is also seen. At this stage the changes are entirely non-specific and in this patient, constrictive pericarditis resulted. H & E × 25

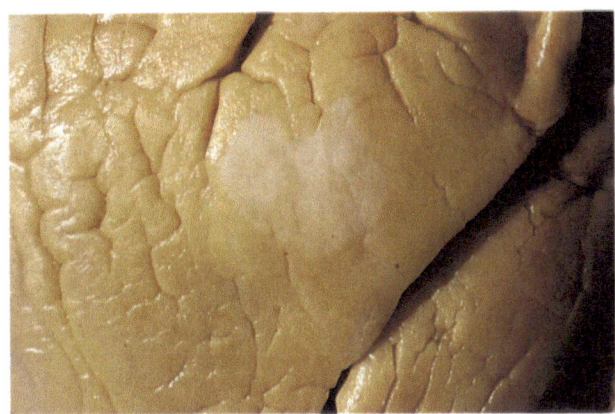

Figure 8.37 Healed rheumatic pericarditis. All that has remained is a fibrous area to which the term 'milky spot' has been applied

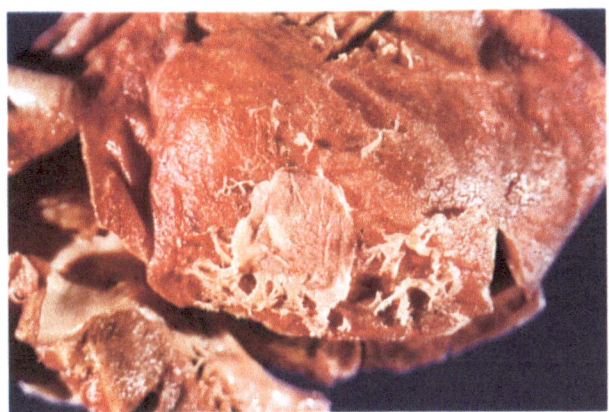

Figure 8.38 Fibrinous pericarditis in infarction. The epicardium is haemorrhagic. Fibrin deposition giving a shaggy appearance to the pericardium is clearly seen

sub-epicardium is involved. Post-pericardiotomy syndrome shows similar changes and resembles Dressler's syndrome.

References

1. Gore, I. and Saphir, O. (1947). Myocarditis. A classification of 1,402 cases. *Am. Heart J.*, **34**, 827

2. Moritz, A. R. and Zamcheck, N. (1946). Sudden and unexpected death of young soldiers. *Arch. Pathol.*, **42**, 459

3. Saphir, O. (1960). In Gould, S. E. (ed.) *Pathology of the Heart*, Second Edition, p. 779. (Springfield, Ill.: Charles C. Thomas)

4. McAllister, H. A. and Fenoglio, J. J. (1975). Cardiac involvement in Whipple's disease. *Circulation*, **52**, 152

5. Abelmann, W. (1978). In discussion, 'congestive cardiomyopathy'. *Postgrad. Med. J.*, **54**, 509

6. Olsen, E. G. J. (1981). Panel discussion. In Goodwin, J. F., Hjalmarson, A. and Olsen, E. G. J. (eds) *Congestive Cardiomyopathy*, Kiruna, Sweden, 1980. p. 122. (Molndal, Sweden: AB Hassle)

7. Olsen, E. G. J. (1983). Myocarditis – a case of mistaken identity? *Br. Heart J.*, **50**, 303

8. Bowles, N. E., Archard, L. C., Richardson, P. J. and Olsen, E. G. J. (1986). Detection of Coxsackie-B-virus-specific RNA sequences in myocardial biopsy samples from patients with myocarditis and dilated cardiomyopathy. *Lancet*, **i**, 1120

9. Puigbo, J. J., Valecillos, R., Hirschhaut, E., Giordano, H., Boccalandro, I., Suarez, C. and Aparicio, J. M. (1977). Diagnosis of Chagas' cardiomyopathy. Non-invasive techniques. *Postgrad. Med. J.*, **53**, 527

10. Amorim, D. S. (1978). Special problems in 'COCM', South America. *Postgrad. Med. J.*, **54**, 462

11. Ive, F. A. and Brockington, I. F. (1966). Endomyocardial fibrosis and filariasis. *Lancet*, **i**, 212

12. Hadley, M. (1952). Coal-gas poisoning and cardiac sequelae. *Br. Heart J.*, **14**, 534

13. Ali, M. K., Khahil, K. G., Fuller, L. M., Leachman, R. D., Sullivan, M. P., Loh, K. K., Gamble, J. F. and Shullenberger, C. C. (1976). Radiation-related myocardial injury. Management of two cases. *Cancer*, **38**, 1941

14. Corby, C. (1960). Isolated myocarditis as a cause of sudden obscure death. *Med. Sci. Law*, **1**, 23

15. Hayes, J. A. and Summerell, J. M. (1966). Myocarditis in Jamaica. *Br. Heart J.*, **28**, 172

16. Fleming, H. A. (1974). Sarcoid heart disease. *Br. Heart J.*, **36**, 54

17. Matsui, Y., Iwai, K., Tachibana, T., Fruie, T., Shigematsu, N., Isumi, T., Homma, A. H., Mikami, R., Hongo, O., Hiraga, Y. and Yamamoto, M. (1976). Clinicopathological study on fatal myocardial sarcoidosis. *Ann. N.Y. Acad. Sci.*, **278**, 455

18. Tannenbaum, H., Rocklin, R. E., Schur, P. H. and Sheffer, A. L. (1976). Immunological identification of subpopulations of mononuclear cells in sarcoid granulomas. *Ann. N.Y. Acad. Sci.*, **278**, 136

19. Okuni, M., Yamada, T., Mochizuki, S. and Sakurai, I. (1975). Studies on myocarditis in childhood, with special reference to the possible role of immunological process and the thymus in the chronicity of the disease. *Jpn. Circulation J.*, **39**, 463

20. Griffith, G. C. and Wallace, L. (1953). The etiology of pericarditis. *Dis. Chest*, **23**, 282

21. El-Maraghi, N. R. H. (1983). In Silver, M. D. (ed.) *Cardiovascular Pathology*. Vol. 1, p. 134. (New York, Edinburgh, London, Melbourne: Churchill Livingstone)

22. Roberts, W. C. and Spray, T. L. (1976). Pericardial heart disease: a study of its causes, consequences and morphologic features. *Cardiovasc. Clin.*, **7**, 11

23. Olsen, E. G. J. (1980). Pericarditis and pericardial effusions. In *The Pathology of the Heart*. Second Edition, p. 200. (London and Basingstoke: The Macmillan Press Ltd)

24. Gabriel, L. and Sheburne, J. C. (1977). 'Acute' granulomatous pericarditis. A clinical and hemodynamic correlate. *Chest*, **71**, 473

25. Lowy, A. C. and Boyd, L. J. (1960). Some clinical aspects of uremic pericarditis. *Exp. Med. Surg.*, **18**, 90

26. Burch, G. E. (1976). Acute viral pericarditis. *Cardiovasc. Clin.*, **7**, 149

Cardiomyopathies

9

Much controversy has centered around the topic of cardiomyopathies since the term was coined by Brigden in 1957[1]. The difficulty has been a tendency to use the term indiscriminately. To overcome the confusion the World Health Organization together with the International Society and Federation of Cardiology set up a Task Force. Their recommended definition and classification will be used[2].

Cardiomyopathies are defined as heart muscle diseases of unknown cause and are classified into three groups:

dilated cardiomyopathy
hypertrophic cardiomyopathy
restrictive cardiomyopathy.

Dilated Cardiomyopathy

This disease may occur at any age but usually affects patients over the age of 35 years[3]. The illness may be preceded by an upper respiratory infection. Signs and symptoms of congested heart failure, including dyspnoea, oedema and cough may first bring the patient to the physician. Chest pain may also be experienced[4]. The symptoms may progress rapidly. Prognosis is usually poor once heart failure has occurred. Unexpected death may occur at any time during the illness.

Familial cases have been described. Though the natural history is not known, chest radiographs undertaken for a variety of reasons including insurance purposes have shown that enlargement of the heart shadow is all that may be present. It is for this reason that the term 'dilated cardiomyopathy' is to be preferred to 'congestive cardiomyopathy'.

In advanced cases all chambers are severely dilated (Figure 9.1), though dilatation confined to the right side of the heart has been described[5]. Heart weights are often more than twice normal, yet despite the hypertrophy measurements of wall thicknesses may be within normal limits, due to the severe dilatation that is usually present. Endocardial thickening is usual, and is non-specific in type and distribution (Figure 9.2). Thrombus is superimposed in more than half the patients (Figure 9.3). The coronary arteries are usually normal. In as much as death can occur at any stage, hypertrophy alone or accompanied by some dilatation may be all that can be found (Figure 9.4)[6]. The diagnosis is made when all causes that could result in a hypertrophied, dilated heart are excluded.

Histology

The myocardial fibres are in normal alignment and in patients with severe dilatation and/or congestive symptoms the myocardial fibres show nuclear evidence of hypertrophy, consisting of pyknosis or vesicular changes but the diameter of the fibres is often normal (up to 15 μm diameter; see also Chapter 1) or may even be less than normal. This dissociation of nuclear changes and diameter of myocardial fibres is due to stretching (Figure 9.5). Interstitial fibrous tissue may be focally increased or may be widespread, particularly in the subendocardial region (Figure 9.6). Foci of fibrous replacement of myocardial fibres may also be found (Figure 9.7). The intramural vessels are usually normal (Figure 9.8), but occasionally a mild degree of intimal fibrosis may be present. This is interpreted as being secondary rather than a primary change causally related to dilated cardiomyopathy. The endocardium may be focally thickened to a severe degree with varying prominence of the smooth muscle component (Figure 9.9). When severe dilatation and heart failure have not been present, radiologically and clinically, hypertrophy alone with or without some evidence of dilatation may be found. All these changes are non-specific and at this level of investigation infiltrative diseases and other causes which could give rise to dilatation and hypertrophy must be excluded[6].

With the increasing use of the bioptome to obtain fresh endomyocardial tissue by biopsy, histochemical examination has been undertaken. In these cases substances such as glycogen and succinic dehydrogenase may be increased, normal or decreased, depending on the duration and the severity of heart failure (Figure 9.10 a and b, Figure 9.11 a and b)[7].

Electron Microscopy

The myocardial fibrils are in regular alignment and changes of hypertrophy are observed consisting of an increase in mitochondria to more than one per two sarcomeres (Figure 9.12). Crenellation of nuclear membranes, prominence of the Golgi apparatus and focal accumulation of glycogen can all be seen and are similar to the changes of hypertrophy (see also Chapter 2). In addition, intercellular spaces contain varying degrees of collagen fibrils (Figure 9.13). The capillaries are usually normal (Figure 9.14), though oedema of their walls may be found (Figure 9.15), probably as an artefact of the process of recovery of endomyocardial biopsies[6].

Varying degrees of degeneration can be observed including cristolysis, dissolution of actin and myosin, and the presence of myelin figures (Figure 9.16). Membrane bound vesicles as well as accumulation of lipofuscin granules can also be observed (Figure 9.17 a and b). Comparative studies, using a scoring system relating degenerative changes to length of history or haemodynamic features, as well as to prognosis has resulted in conflicting reports. In our experience no significant correlation could be established but a trend that patients

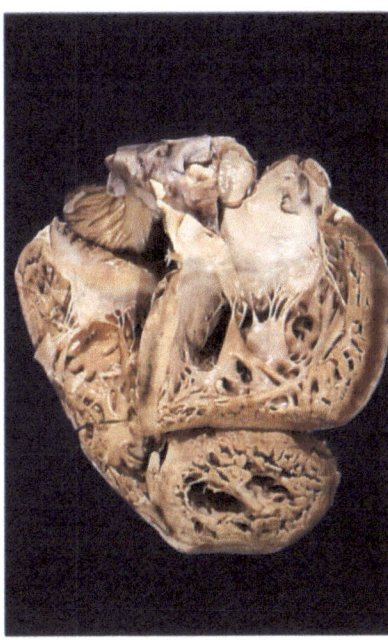

Figure 9.1 Dilated cardiomyopathy. All cardiac chambers are exposed, showing dilatation. Despite the hypertrophy the myocardial walls may be normal in thickness. This is due to dilatation

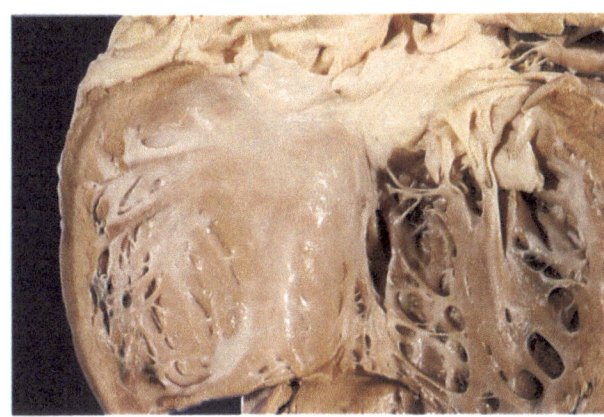

Figure 9.2 Close-up view of the left ventricle showing endocardial thickening in the outflow tract

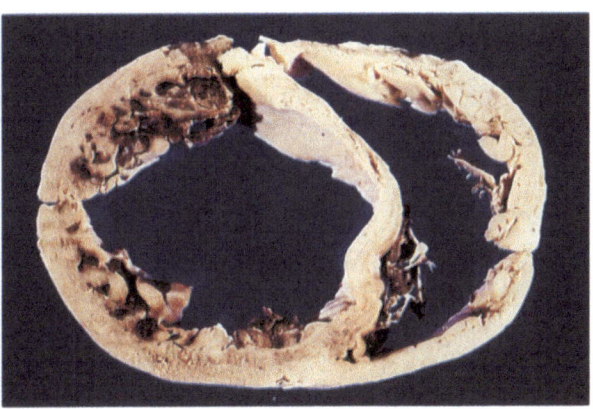

Figure 9.3 Transverse section of the severely dilated ventricles, showing thrombus superimposition

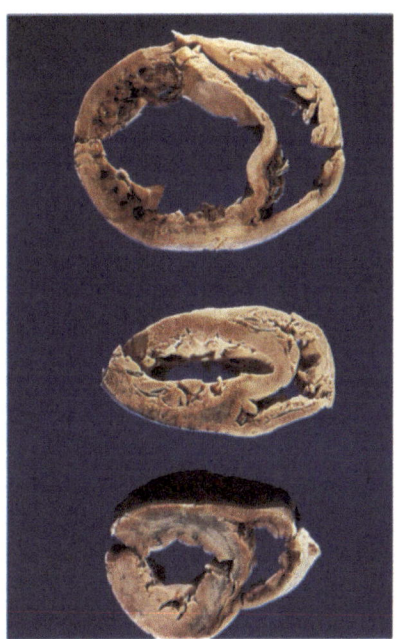

Figure 9.4 Three transverse sections from ventricles of patients clinically diagnosed as having dilated cardiomyopathy, showing severe dilatation (upper transverse section) with normal ventricular walls, some dilatation with a mild increase in ventricular wall thickness (middle section), and hypertrophy alone with minimal dilatation of the ventricle (lower section)

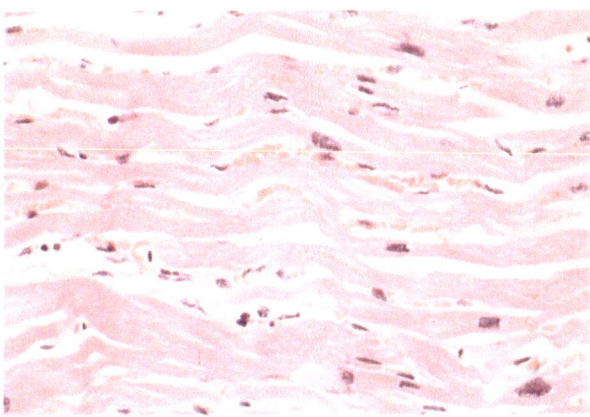

Figure 9.5 Histological section of hypertrophied myocardial fibres in almost parallel alignment, showing nuclear changes of hypertrophy (vesicular changes), pyknosis and blunting of the nuclear poles. The diameter of the myocardial fibres is normal. This dissociation is due to stretching. H & E × 100

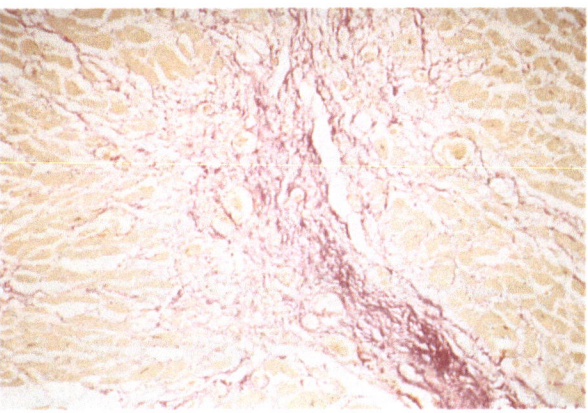

Figure 9.6 Interstitial fibrosis. There is an increase in collagen tissue (in red) between the myocardial fibres. Miller's elastic van Gieson × 50

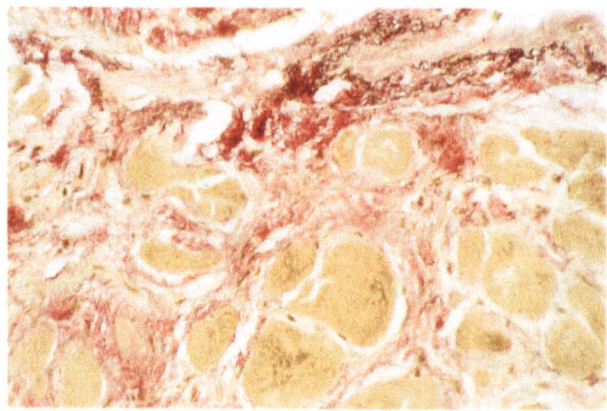

Figure 9.7 Sub-endocardial region showing, apart from interstitial fibrosis, foci of collagen tissue which has replaced myocardial fibres. Miller's elastic van Gieson × 400

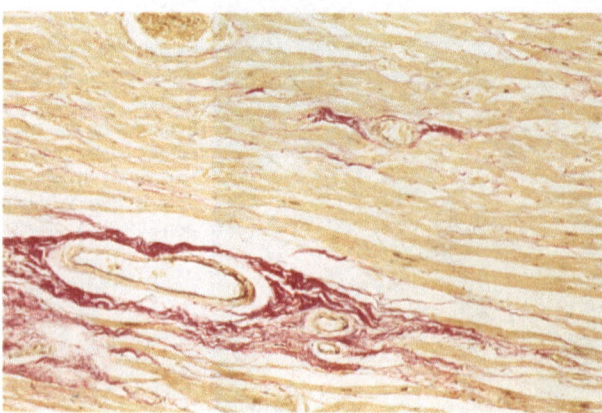

Figure 9.8 Normal arterioles in patients with dilated cardiomyopathy. Miller's elastic van Gieson × 75

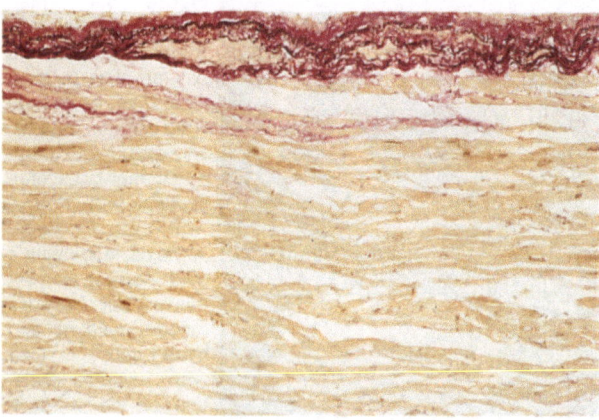

Figure 9.9 Endocardial thickening to a mild degree. Note the focal smooth muscle prominence in the endocardium. Miller's elastic van Giesen × 75

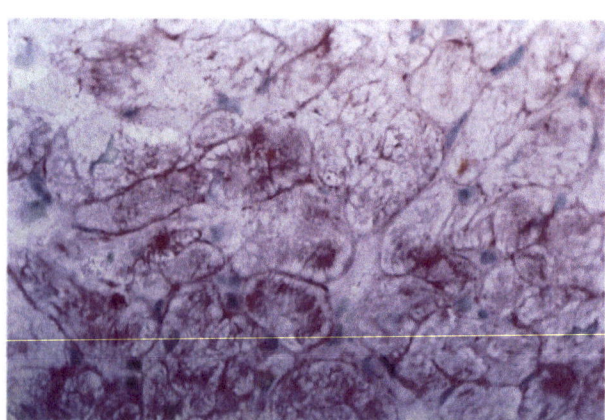

Figure 9.10a A focal increase in glycogen. PAS × 400

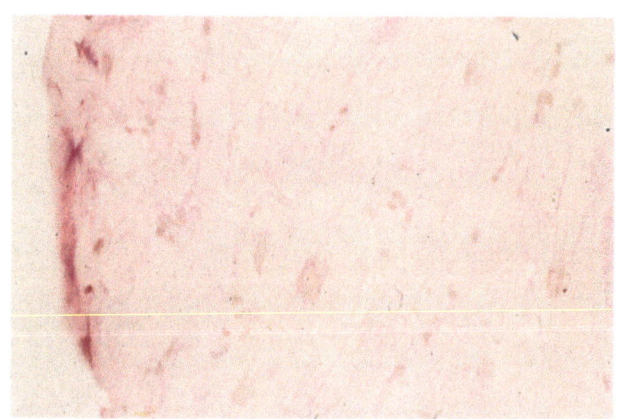

Figure 9.10b Diffuse decrease of glycogen. PAS ×.400
Both Figures 9.10a and b come from patients with dilated cardiomyopathy

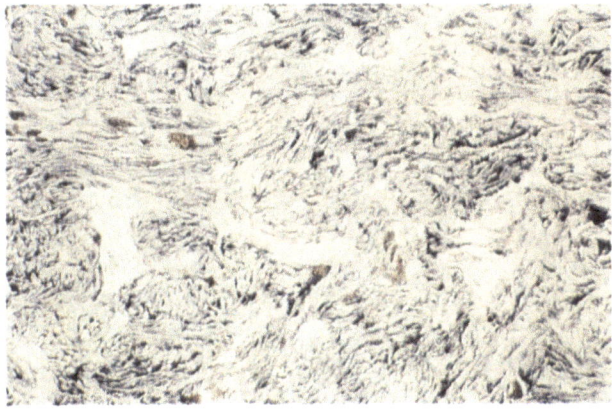

Figure 9.11a A focal increase of succinic dehydrogenase. MTT × 250

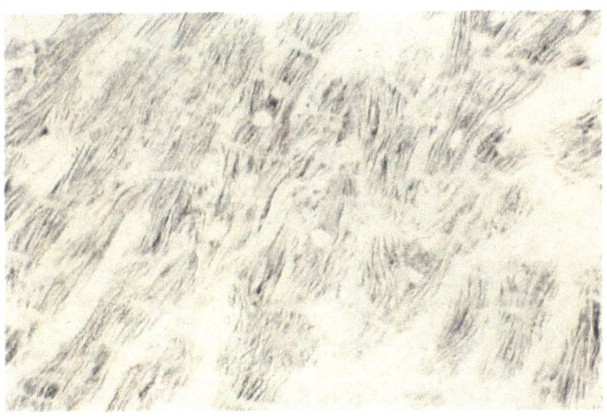

Figure 9.11b A focal decrease of succinic dehydrogenase. MTT × 250
Both Figures 9.11a and b are from patients with dilated cardiomyopathy

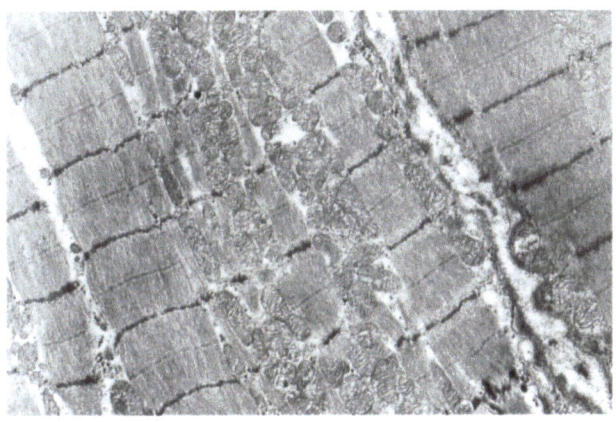

Figure 9.12 Electron micrograph of myocardial fibrils in parallel alignment showing more than one mitochondrion per two sarcomeres. Uranyl acetate and lead citrate × 5900

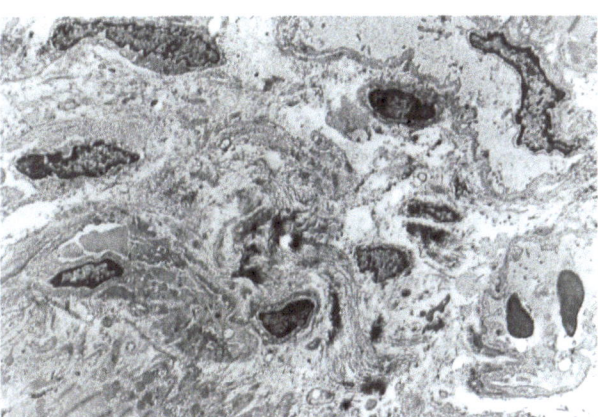

Figure 9.13 The widened interstitium contains numerous collagen fibrils showing the typical periodicity. Several capillaries are included in this electron micrograph. Uranyl acetate and lead citrate × 2800

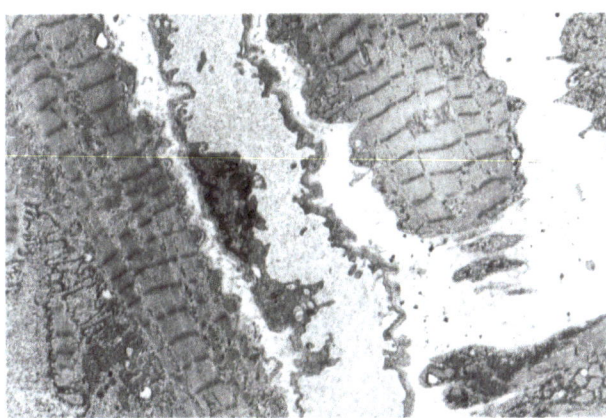

Figure 9.14 Electron micrograph of a normal capillary. Uranyl acetate and lead citrate × 2200

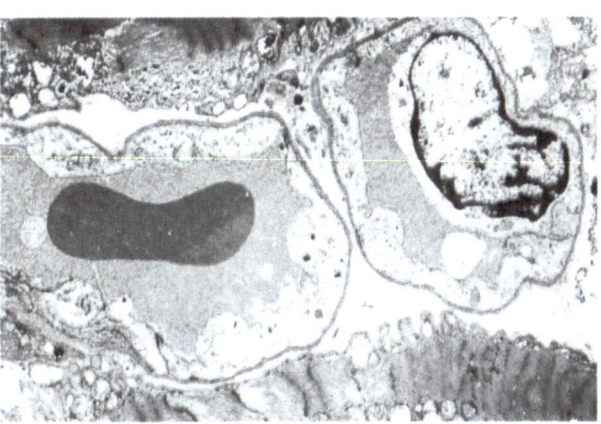

Figure 9.15 Two capillaries, both showing oedema of their walls. Uranyl acetate and lead citrate × 4500

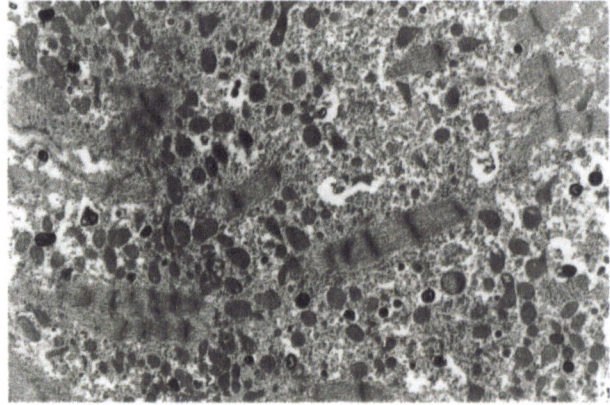

Figure 9.16 Degenerative changes of the myocardium, showing cristolysis of the mitochondria and focal dissolution of actin and myosin, as well as myelin figures.   Uranyl acetate and lead citrate × 4500

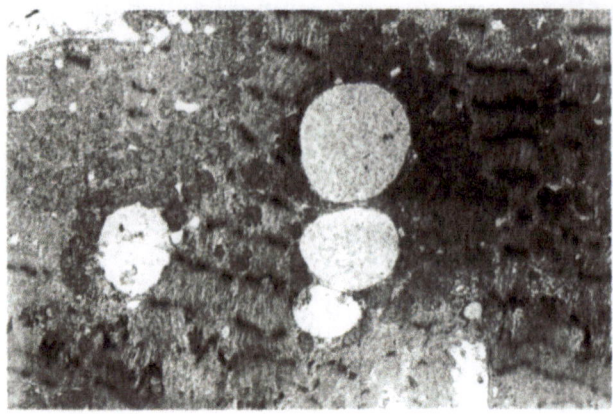

Figure 9.17a Electron micrograph of membrane bound vesicles. Uranylacetate and lead citrate × 5900

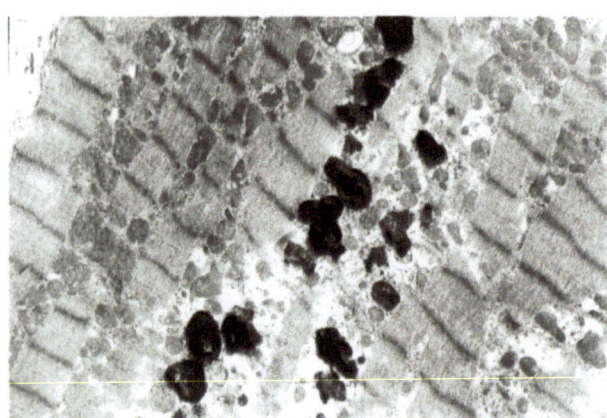

Figure 9.17b Lipofuscin granules.   Uranyl acetate and lead citrate × 5900

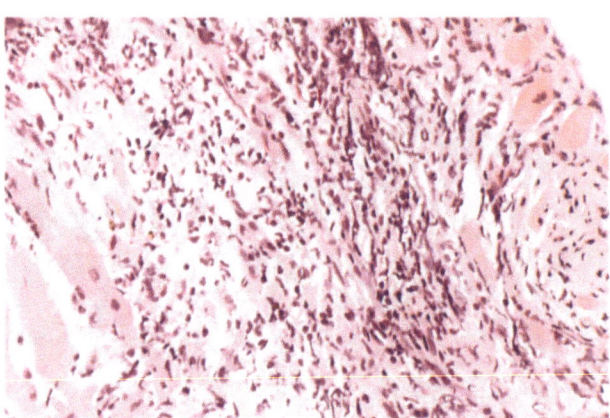

Figure 9.18 Photomicrograph showing evidence of active myocarditis in a patient clinically suspected of dilated cardiomyopathy.   H & E × 250

Figure 9.19 Diagrammatic representation of the area between the venae cavae (hatched) which is serially sectioned for neuronal counts

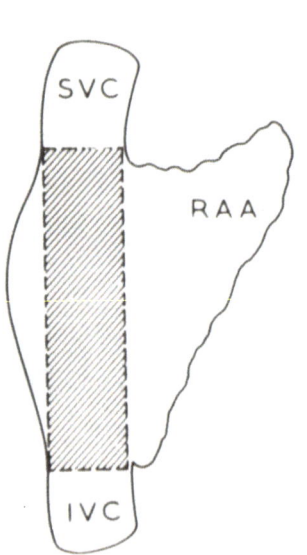

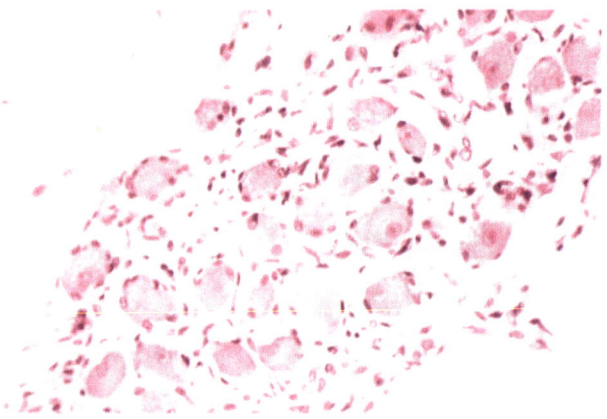

Figure 9.20 A normal neuronal arrangement. The cells are separated by a few strands of connective tissue.   H & E × 100

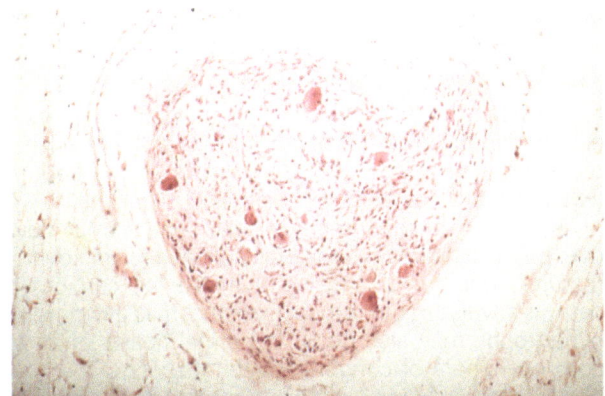

Figure 9.21 Neuronal cells in a patient with dilated cardiomyopathy, severely reduced in number and widely separated by connective tissue. H & E × 25

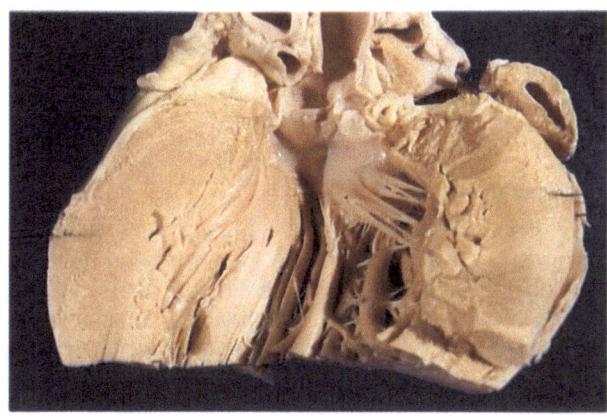

Figure 9.22 Hypertrophic cardiomyopathy where the maximal bulge is beneath the aortic valve

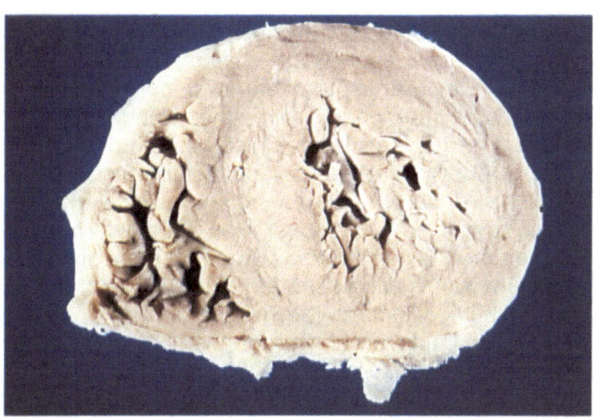

Figure 9.23 Transverse section of the ventricle showing concentric hypertrophy. Histology shows changes of hypertrophic cardiomyopathy

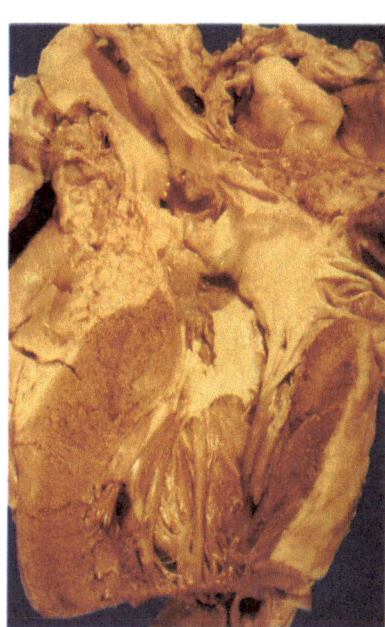

Figure 9.24 The left ventricle has been displayed to show endocardial thickening beneath the aortic valve forming a 'mirror image' of the anterior mitral valve leaflet, which has been deflected to the right

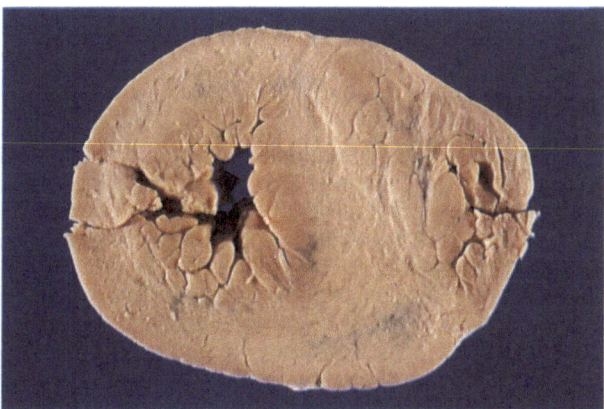

Figure 9.25 Transverse section of the ventricles showing the maximum bulge of the interventricular septum midway between the apex and the aortic valve. In the asymmetrically thickened interventricular septum the appearance of watered silk can be discerned

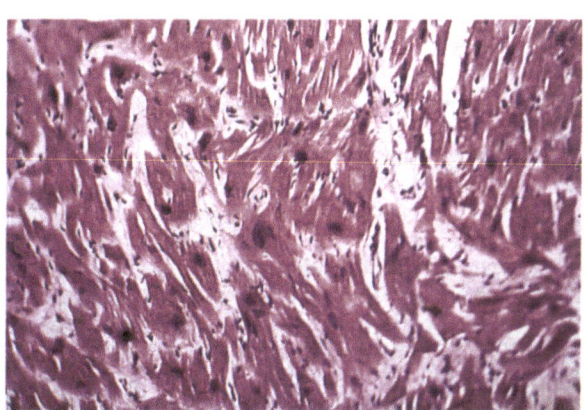

Figure 9.26 The myocardial fibres are in disarray, exemplified by short runs and severe hypertrophy of myocardial fibres separated by cellular connective tissue. H & E × 100

with more severe degenerative changes have a worse prognosis has been established[8].

Aetiology

The aetiology of dilated cardiomyopathy is by definition unknown but various suggestions have been made including deficiency of succinic dehydrogenase, small vessel disease, autoimmune disturbances, viral infection and T lymphocyte anomalies. These have previously been summarized[9].

Reference to an upper respiratory tract infection before symptoms of dilated cardiomyopathy become manifest has already been made. Examination of endomyocardial biopsy, on patients suspected of this type of cardiomyopathy, has shown that in a proportion of patients changes of myocarditis in the active, healing or healed phases are evident (see Chapter 8) (Figure 9.18). Simultaneous viral microneutralization studies have shown high titres of antibody to Coxsackie B virus in those patients with evidence of myocarditis; but even if myocarditis is present they are not invariably raised. Alternatively, high titres may be found in some patients in whom no evidence of myocarditis is seen. Recent studies have suggested that as there are a significant number of patients with dilated cardiomyopathy showing evidence of myocarditis, an infectious immune mechanism may be operative[10]. It furthermore demonstrates that dilated cardiomyopathy is likely to have a multifactorial aetiology. It has also been suggested, on examining strips of right atrial muscle between the venae cavae (Figure 9.19), that a reduction in neuronal cells is present in a significant number of patients with dilated cardiomyopathy (Figures 9.20 and 9.21). The recent findings of virus RNA in endomyocardial tissue obtained by bioptome has added a new dimension to our concept of dilated cardiomyopathy and its associated myocarditis (see Chapter 8).

Hypertrophic Cardiomyopathy

The older British nomenclature 'hypertrophic obstructive cardiomyopathy' has now been revised as the previous term implied that obstruction is an essential part of the clinical manifestations. Experience has shown that obstruction is incidental and that the underlying haemodynamic change is failure of diastolic compliance[12]. The controversy as to whether true obstruction is present or not is as yet unsolved. Obstruction may dominate the clinical picture, which includes dyspnoea, angina and syncope. Signs and symptoms of mitral valve insufficiency are not infrequently present. Sudden death is, unfortunately, fairly common. A familial incidence has been well established[13].

Whether or not obstruction has played a clinical role, macroscopic changes are characterized by asymmetric hypertrophy of the interventricular septum, which can be striking and may be as much as three times thicker than the already hypertrophied free left ventricular wall (Figure 9.22)[14]. The maximal bulge of the septum may be at the apex, in the mid-region of the septum or beneath the aortic valve. Concentric forms are also recognized (Figure 9.23). The asymmetric thickening of the septum displaces the anterior papillary muscle, which interferes with the normal function of the mitral valve apparatus resulting in mitral insufficiency. The bulge of the septum and abnormal mitral valve movement may become manifest as a mirror image of endocardial thickening of the anterior mitral valve leaflet on the septal wall (Figure 9.24)[15]. Systolic pockets may be

identified if obstruction has been significant during the natural history of the disease. Cross-section of the ventricles frequently shows whorling, giving the appearance of watered silk in the thickened areas of the septum (Figure 9.25)[15].

Asymmetry of the interventricular septum may however be mild and for this reason caution in relying on this feature alone for diagnosing hypertrophic cardiomyopathy is advised. It has been shown that mild asymmetric hypertrophy may also occur in normal hearts or as an accompaniment of congenital heart disease.

Histology

Histological examination shows disarray of myocardial fibres, consisting of short runs (Figure 9.26) and an interlacing pattern occurring in the same areas (Figure 9.27), as well as extremely severe hypertrophy, bizarre-shaped nuclei, often surrounded by a clear zone (the so-called perinuclear halo) and interstitial fibrosis which may be rich in chronic inflammatory cells (Figure 9.28). Disarray alone (Figure 9.29) is not a reliable indicator but it has been suggested that if this is widespread it constitutes a characteristic appearance[16]. It must be remembered that even if the changes are confined to the interventricular septum areas of normally aligned fibres may be interspersed. A diagnostic index has been proposed for each of the five histological criteria (short runs of fibres interrupted by connective tissue, large bizarre nuclei, fibrosis, degenerating muscle with disappearing myofibrils and disorganized 'whorling' muscle). A maximum of 3 points are awarded for each of the five features which is expressed as 100%. When the index exceeds 50% diagnosis can reliably be made[17].

Large accumulation of glycogen is characteristic and aids diagnosis (Figure 9.30) but other substances such as succinic dehydrogenase, non-specific esterases (Figure 9.31) or phosphatases, though increased, may merely reflect the degree of hypertrophy and are not of diagnostic value.

Electron Microscopy

The myocardial fibrils run in all directions (Figure 9.32). Frequent abnormal intra- and inter-fibrillar connections (Figure 9.33) are found forming a network of fibrils. In addition to the severely increased numbers of mitochondria between adjacent sarcomeres, reflecting severe hypertrophy, focal accumulation or 'mitochondriosis' is found (Figure 9.34)[14].

Aetiology

The aetiological suggestions for this type of cardiomyopathy have been summarized[7]. As far as diagnosis is concerned, if asymmetric hypertrophy is severe it is likely that hypertrophic cardiomyopathy is present. This is confirmed by histological investigation, which includes histochemical assessment of glycogen. In surgically excised tissue or on endomyocardial biopsy examination, histological changes together with glycogen, as well as electron microscopy will establish the diagnosis with certainty. Diagnosis by electron microscopy alone is not reliable because of the size of the sample and also disarray is known to accompany hypertrophy due to known causes.

Hypertrophic Cardiomyopathy 'Without Obstruction'

As has already been stated 'obstruction' is believed to be incidental, even though it may dominate the clinical picture. In some patients 'obstruction' has never been of clinical importance and for descriptive purposes hypertrophic cardiomyopathy 'without obstruction' has been retained by some workers.

Despite the absence of obstruction, asymmetry of the interventricular septum may be present. At one time it was believed that in cases with obstruction the abnormal fibres were predominantly located in the thick interventricular septum, extending to varying degrees into the anterior and posterior left ventricular wall (Figure 9.35). By contrast, in cases 'without obstruction' the same abnormal fibres were focally distributed in a haphazard fashion throughout the ventricular walls including the free left ventricular wall (Figure 9.36). This distribution unfortunately does not always correlate with clinical symptoms and cases 'with obstruction' have been found to have a 'non-obstructive' pattern[18] and *vice versa*.

Restrictive Cardiomypathy

Under this term endomyocardial fibrosis, described by Davies in 1948[19] and for a long time believed to be confined to the tropical and subtropical zones, and Löffler's endocarditis parietalis fibroplastica have been included. The latter condition was described by Löffler in 1936[20] and was found to be associated with an eosinophilia and believed to be confined to the temperate zone. Retrospective morphological studies have shown that both conditions belong to the same disease spectrum[21].

Macroscopically, the striking feature is the extremely thick endocardium, which may be several millimetres thick. Left (38%), right (11%) or both ventricles (51%) may be involved[22]. When the left ventricle is involved, usually the inflow tract, apex and part of the outflow tract are affected but when the region of the anterior mitral valve leaflet is reached the thick endocardium ends abruptly in a thick rolled edge (Figure 9.37). Thrombus is frequently superimposed. The papillary muscles and the posterior mitral valve leaflet are also not uncommonly affected. This pattern is usual but five different patterns of distribution have been described[22]. In cases of right ventricular involvement the apex becomes progressively obliterated by fibrous tissue and an area of fibrosis beneath the tricuspid valve constitute characteristic sites (Figure 9.38). Thrombus is frequently superimposed. Fibrous septae extending into the underlying myocardium may be striking. They usually extend to the innner third of the myocardial wall but may reach the epicardial zone of the myocardium (Figure 9.39).

Histology

Histologically, beneath the thrombus or fibrin superimposition a layer of collagen tissue, often dense, is seen, beneath which loose connective tissue in which dilated blood channels and some inflammatory cells, including eosinophils, may be found. This latter region is also referred to as the granulation tissue layer (Figure 9.40). It is from this region that septae extend into the underlying myocardium. Calcification may be found in the thick endocardium (Figure 9.41)[21].

Pathogenetic Mechanism

In the retrospective study, already cited[21], 90 patients who had died with endomyocardial disease were studied. Eosinophilia was usually associated with and attributable to conditions such as polyarteritis nodosa, hypersensitivity states, asthma, or malignant tumours in approximately 25%. In another 25% the cases were ascribed to eosinophilic leukaemia but in half of the patients the cause for eosinophilia could not be ascertained.

Morphologically three major stages, dependent on the length of history between onset of symptoms and death, could be established. The necrotic stage (average length of history 5 weeks) showed, macroscopically, some depression of the ventricular walls indicative of myocarditis (Figure 9.42) and, histologically, myocarditis rich in eosinophils (Figure 9.43). Periarteritis was also frequently present (Figure 9.44). The thrombotic stage was reached after average duration of the history of 10 months where thrombus superimposition could be slight (Figure 9.45) or extreme (Figure 9.46) obliterating the entire affected ventricular cavity. Histologically some endocardial thickening was already present and the severe thrombus superimposition was easily identified (Figure 9.47). Intramural vessels frequently contained thrombotic material (Figure 9.48).

After an interval of $2\frac{1}{2}$ years between onset of symptoms and death the fibrotic stage was evident, showing identical changes to those already described. Figure 9.49 illustrates the fibrous thickness at electron microscopic level. On histological examination the intramyocardial vessels showed non-specific intimal thickening only (Figure 9.50). The cases belonging to the fibrotic stage were then compared with cases of endomyocardial fibrosis from Uganda, Nigeria and Brazil and no differences could be identified. It was, therefore, concluded that endomyocardial fibrosis and Löffler's endocarditis parietalis fibroplastica belonged to the same disease spectrum, the origin of which could be traced back to the presence of eosinophils in the myocardium[21].

Further study on the morphology of eosinophils has shown that, in cases with cardiac involvement, abnormalities consisting predominantly of vacuolation and degranulation of the eosinophils were present (Figure 9.51). These abnormal eosinophils can easily be identified in blood films (Figure 9.52). It was furthermore established that if 15% of the circulating eosinophils were degranulated endomyocardial disease was associated[23]. Figure 9.53 illustrates degranulated eosinophils at electron-microscopic level.

Similar features have been found in various parts of the world. The diagnosis can now be established early. If on blood film examination significant numbers of eosinophils are degranulated and on assessment of serum cationic proteins (normal average 46 µg/l) these are raised, endomyocardial biopsies have been found to be positive. Treatment with corticosteroids and immunosuppressive agents can then be instituted. If the patient is first seen in the fibrotic stage surgery consisting of decortication of the thick endocardium has yielded good results (Figure 9.54).

There is now good evidence for the unitarian theory of this disease, though claims that arteritis affecting organs other than the heart is present in cases in the temperate zones in association with eosinophilia have been made. The reason for the apparent discrepancy is that if cases in the tropics are found in the early stages an arteritis is also present, together with abnormal eosinophils, but once the fibrotic stage is reached, whether cases are examined in the tropics or the temperate zones, non-specific intimal change is all that can be diagnosed. Unfortunately when patients reach the physician in the tropics the fibrotic stage has usually become manifest.

Differences in clinical aspects have also been formulated[24]. These differences may well have a common

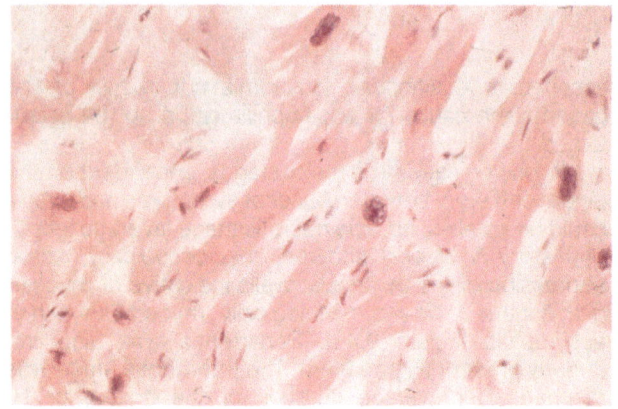

Figure 9.27 Interlacing myocardial fibres from a patient with hypertrophic cardiomyopathy. This interlacing pattern was widespread.   H & E × 250

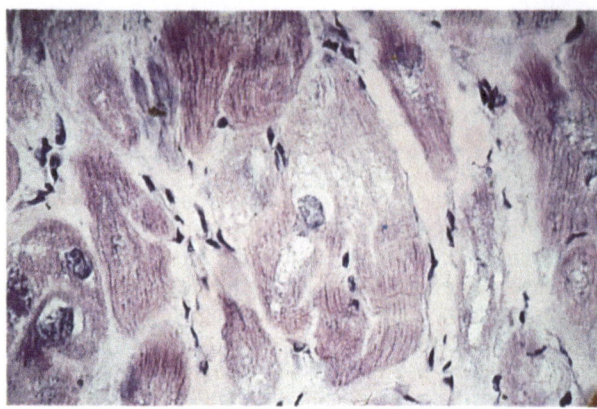

Figure 9.28 Extremely hypertrophied myocardial fibres with nuclei bizarre in outline (bottom left). The perinuclear halo is well illustrated in the centre, where disintegrating myofibrils can be identified towards the top of the halo, giving a 'moth-eaten' appearance.   H & E × 250

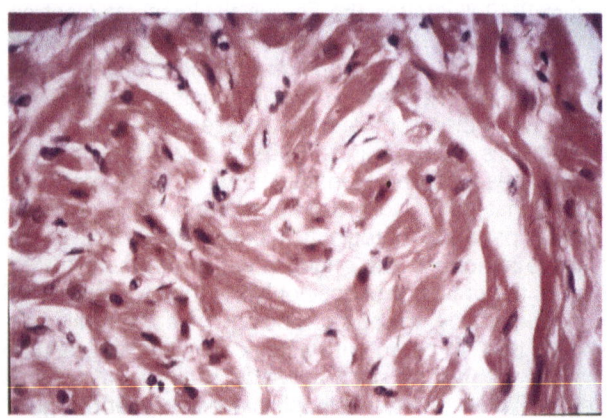

Figure 9.29 Disarray of myocardial fibres but without any additional features characteristic of hypertrophic cardiomyopathy. This photomicrograph comes from a patient with tetralogy of Fallot from the right ventricular outflow tract.   H & E × 150

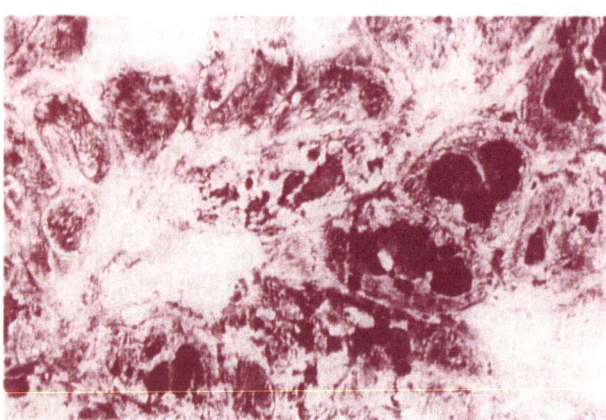

Figure 9.30 Immense accumulation of glycogen resulting in pooling in the perinuclear areas.   PAS × 250

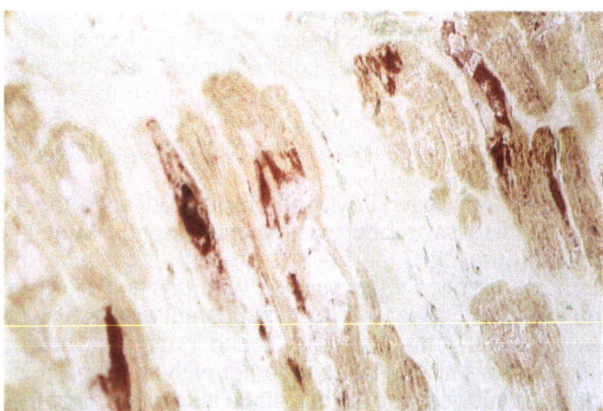

Figure 9.31 Focal accumulation of non-specific esterases in hypertrophic cardiomyopathy × 250

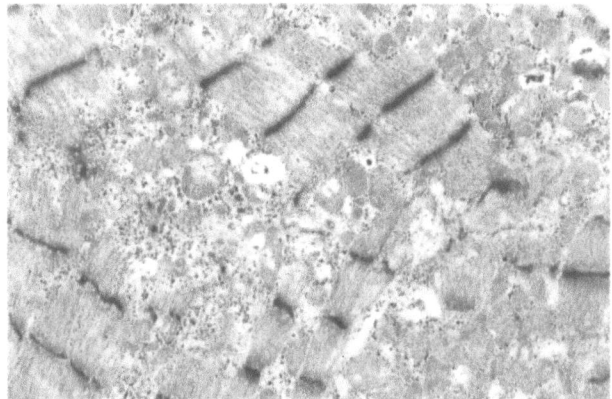

Figure 9.32 The myocardial fibrils run in all directions in hypertrophic cardiomyopathy but can also be observed in 'ordinary' hypertrophy. Uranyl acetate and lead citrate × 5900

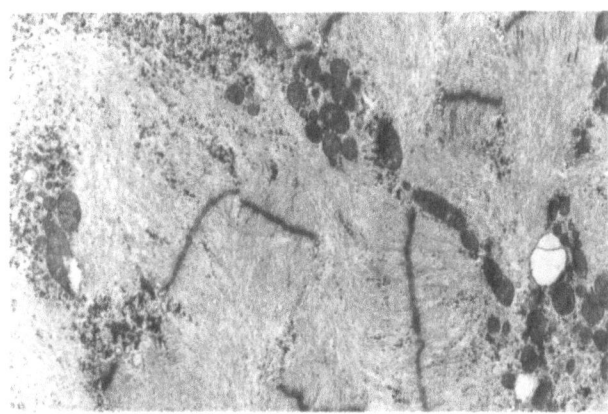

Figure 9.33 Interlacing myofibrils. When these areas are widespread, the possibility of hypertrophic cardiomyopathy being present can be entertained at this level of examination. Uranyl acetate and lead citrate × 5900

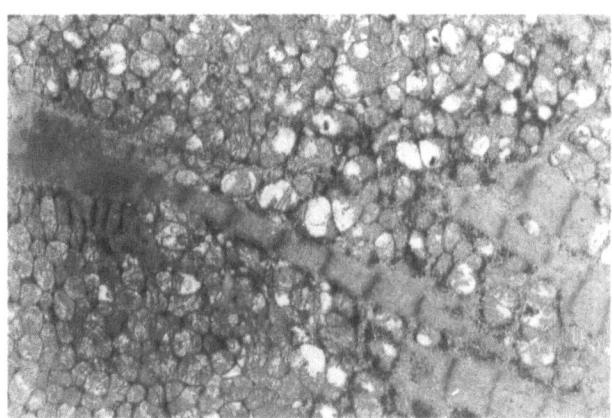

Figure 9.34 Severe accumulation of mitochondria between myocardial fibrils, several of which show varying degrees of cristolysis. This can be referred to as mitochondriosis. Uranyl acetate and lead citrate × 5900

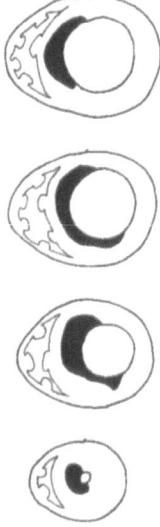

Figure 9.35 Diagrammatic representation of hypertrophic cardiomyopathy 'with obstruction'. The abnormal fibres are principally confined to the asymmetrically thickened interventricular septum but extending for varying distances into the anterior and posterior left ventricular walls

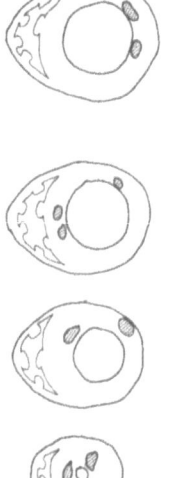

Figure 9.36 Diagrammatic representation of hypertrophic cardiomyopathy 'without obstruction'. Identical abnormal myocardial fibres are haphazardly, focally distributed throughout the myocardial walls

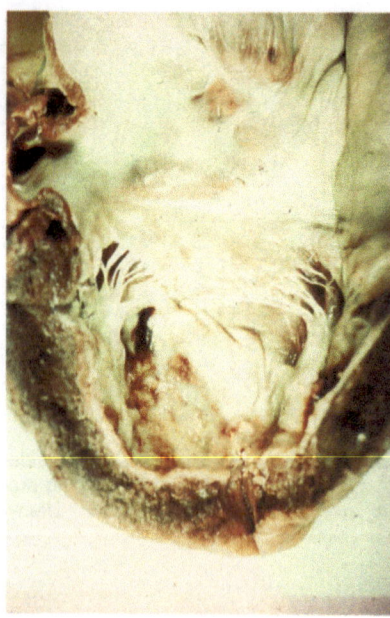

Figure 9.37 The left ventricular cavity is cut to show the severely thickened endocardium. Both papillary muscles are involved in the endomyocardial fibrotic process. The thick rolled edge beneath the margin of the anterior mitral valve leaflet can clearly be seen. Fibrous septae can be seen, extending into the myocardium

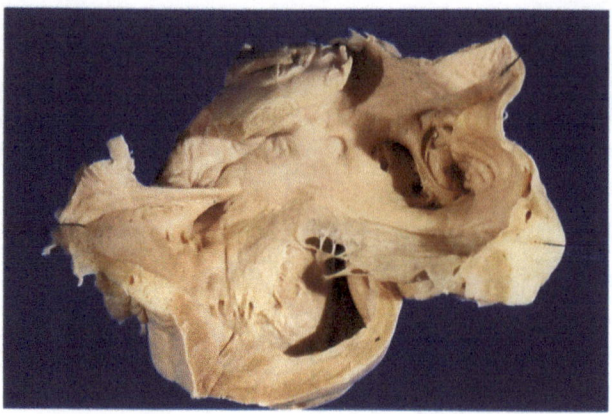

Figure 9.38 The right ventricle has been opened to show the apex obliterated by thick fibrous tissue. This thick endocardium can also be seen beneath the tricuspid valve

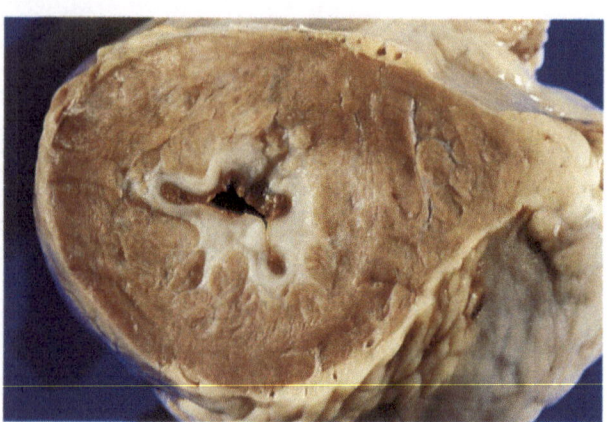

Figure 9.39 Cross-section of the ventricles showing severe endocardial thickening of the left ventricular cavity. The septae extending into the underlying myocardium can clearly be seen. The right ventricular cavity is not shown at this level of sectioning because it is also involved by the endomyocardial fibrotic process. (By courtesy of Dr Guy Neil)

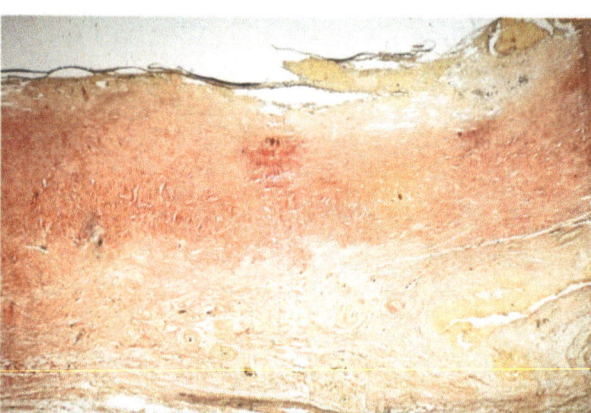

Figure 9.40 The thickened endocardium is arranged in layers. Beneath the layer of fibrin a dense collagen tissue layer follows. The deepest layer, the granulation tissue layer, consists of loosely arranged connective tissue containing several vascular channels. From this layer the septae extend into the underlying myocardium. Elastic van Gieson × 50

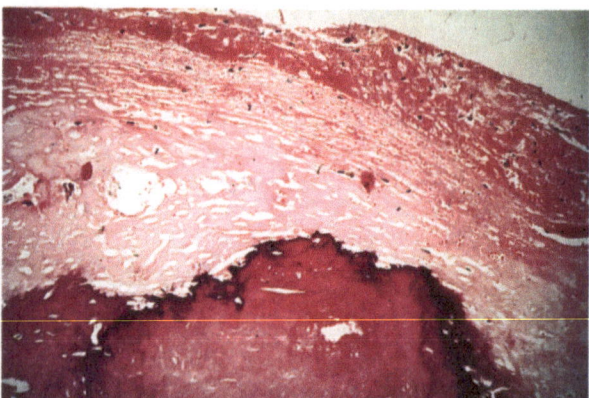

Figure 9.41 In the collagen tissue layer of the thick endocardium an area of calcification is present. H & E × 100

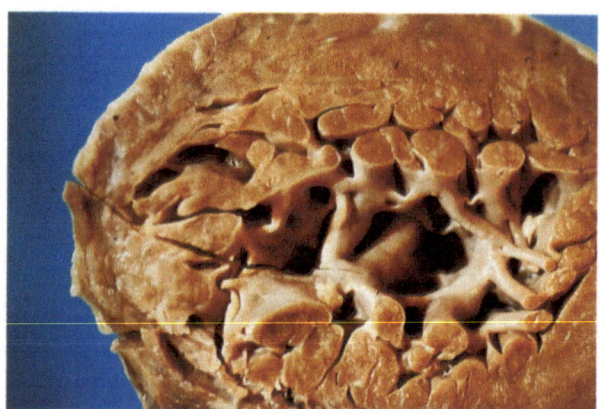

Figure 9.42 Transverse section of the left ventricle showing various sized areas of depression, particularly prominent in the sub-endocardial areas

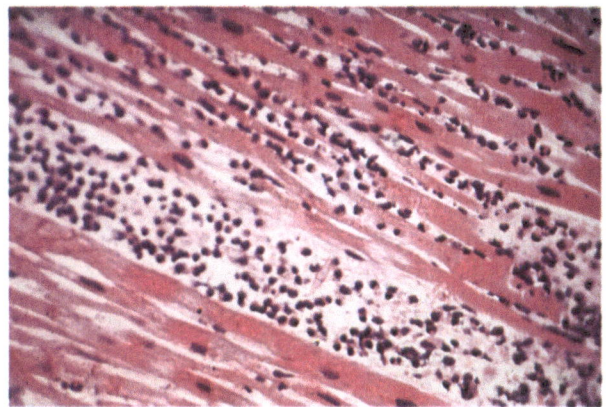

Figure 9.43 A section from one of the depressed areas showing myocarditis. The inflammatory infiltrate is rich in eosionphils. A Charcot Leyden crystal can be identified. H & E × 200

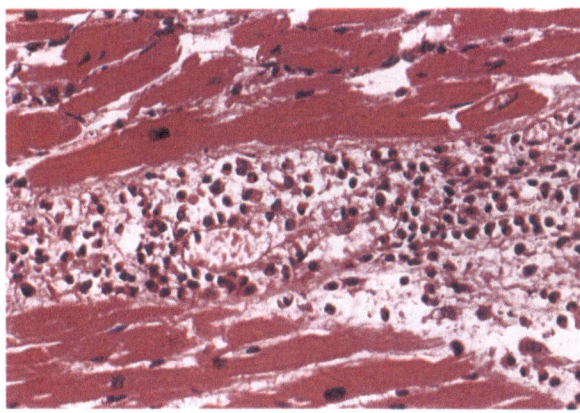

Figure 9.44 A small vessel in the myocardial interstitium shows periarteritis. The inflammatory infiltrate is rich in eosinophils. H & E × 250

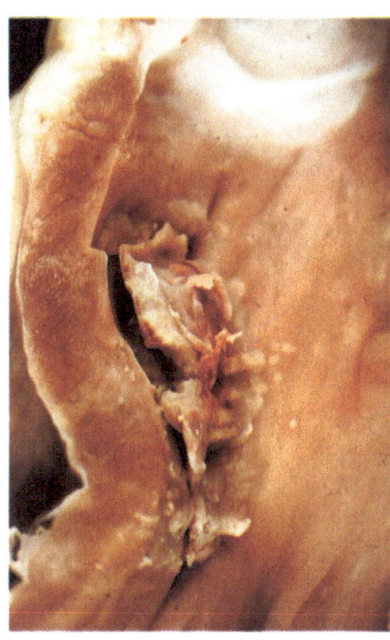

Figure 9.45 The left ventricular outflow tract has been cut to show some thrombus superimposition. The endocardium is not yet severely thickened. (By courtesy of Dr U. Baandrup)

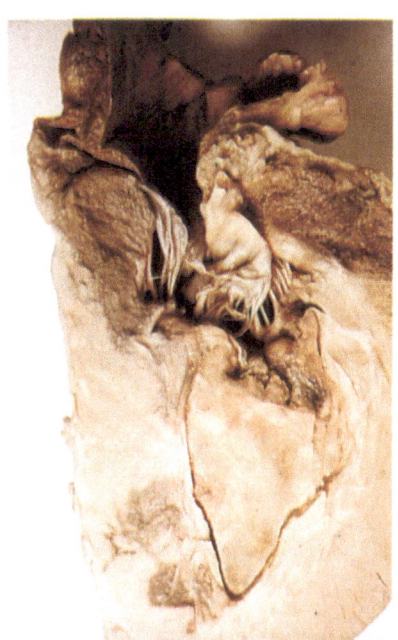

Figure 9.46 The left ventricular cavity is totally obliterated by thrombus. Endocardial thickening can already be noted. (By courtesy of Dr M. Batata)

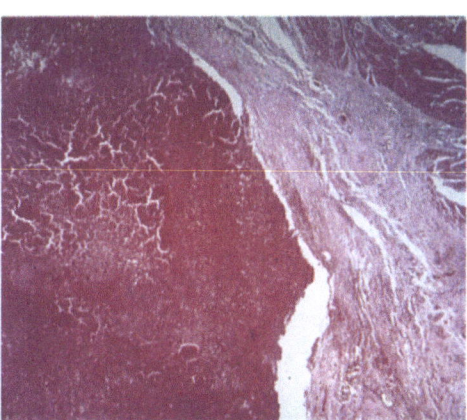

Figure 9.47 The endocardium is already considerably thickened but the zonal layering is still not fully established. The left half of the photograph is occupied by thrombus. H & E × 25 (See also Figure 9.46)

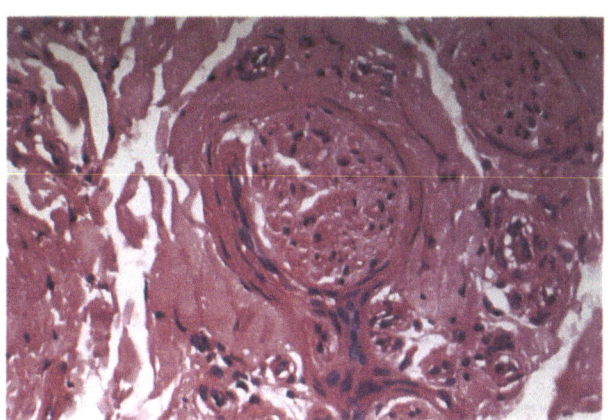

Figure 9.48 The vascular lumen is obliterated by thrombus. The perivascular infiltrate has largely disappeared. H & E × 200

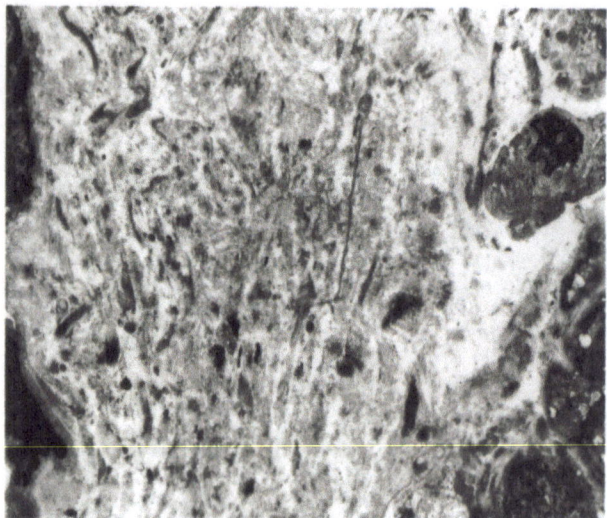

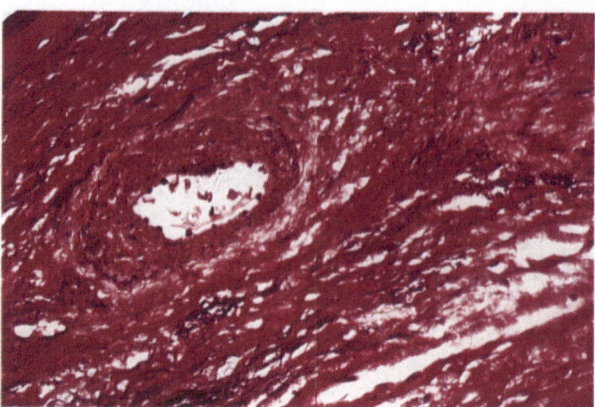

Figure 9.50 The non-specific initital thickening is all that can be identified in the intramural vessels of the heart in the fibrotic stage of the disease process. H & E × 50

Figure 9.49 Electron micrograph of the thick endocardium showing the features noted histologically. The collagen bundles run in all directions. A fibroblast is seen. Uranyl acetate and lead citrate × 3600

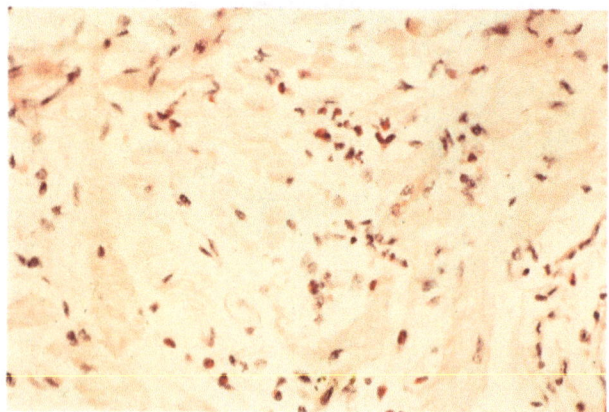

Figure 9.51 Tissue sample from a patient in the necrotic phase of endomyocardial disease, showing evidence of myocarditis with several abnormal eosinophils. Carbol chromotrope × 150

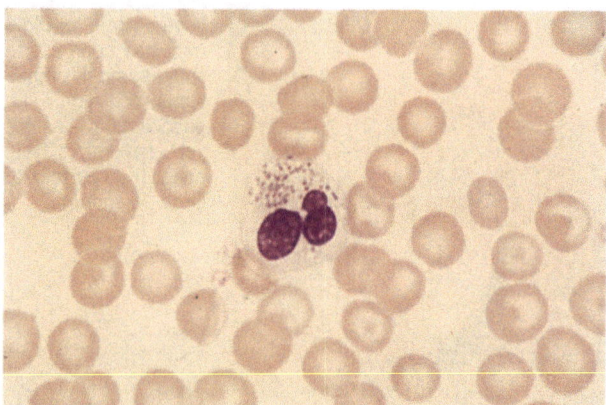

Figure 9.52 Blood film from the same patient clearly showing vacuolation and degranulation. May–Grünwald–Giemsa × 1000

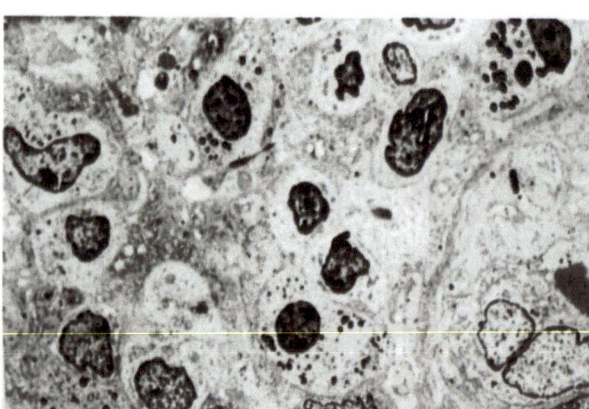

Figure 9.53 Severe degranulation of a clump of eosinophils. Several eosinophils are devoid of granules, which are difficult to identify on semi-thin sections or histology. Uranyl acetate and lead citrate × 3600

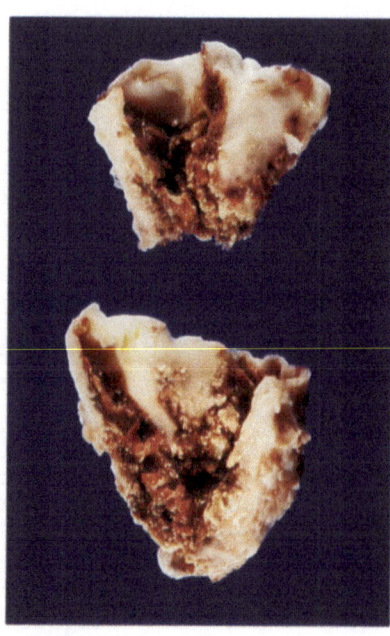

Figure 9.54 Surgical specimen of decorticated thick endocardium. (By courtesy of Dr John Davies)

denominator which could possibly be ascribed to malnutrition affecting the cases in the tropics.

The pathogenetic mechanism is likely to be that a stimulus (either due to infection, parasites, malignancy or for unknown reasons) leads to an unmasking of Fc receptors. Phagocytic activity and binding to IgG or C3b coated particles becomes enhanced. These stimulated cells by virtue of the microcirculation reach the heart and through peroxidases and other noxious substances produce myocarditis. The granules consisting, among other things, of cationic proteins are thrombogenic. Thus the necrotic and thrombotic phases are explained. The fibrotic stage is the phase of healing[23].

References

1. Brigden, W. (1957). Uncommon myocardial diseases. The noncoronary cardiomyopathies. *Lancet*, **2**, 1179

2. Report of the WHO/ISFC Task Force (1982). Report on the definition and classification of cardiomyopathies. *Br. Heart J.*, **44**, 672

3. Cockshott, W. P., Thorpe, G. J. and Ikeme, A. C. (1967). Radiological aspects of heart muscle disease in Nigerian adults. *Circulation*, **36**, 460

4. Goodwin, J. F. (1975). Myocardial diseases. *Medicine*, (2nd series), **25**, 1286

5. Fitchett, D. H., Sugrue, D. D., MacArthur, C. G. and Oakley, C. M. (1984). Right ventricular dilated cardiomyopathy. *Br. Heart J.*, **51**, 25

6. Olsen, E. G. J. (1981). Pathology of congestive cardiomyopathy. In Goodwin, J. F., Hjalmarson, A. and Olsen, E. G. J. (eds). *Congestive Cardiomyopathy*. Kiruna, Sweden 1980, p. 66. (Mölndal, Sweden: A. B. Hässle)

7. Olsen, E. G. J. (1978). Special investigations of COCM: Endomyocardial biopsies (morphological analysis). *Postgrad. Med. J.*, **54**, 486

8. Baandrup, U., Florio, R. A., Roters, F. and Olsen, E. G. J. (1981). Electron microscopic investigation of endomyocardial biopsy samples in hypertrophy and cardiomyopathy. A semiquantitative study in 48 patients. *Circulation*, **63**, 1289

9. Olsen, E. G. J. (1980). In *The Pathology of the Heart*. 2nd Ed., p. 317. (London and Basingstoke: The Macmillan Press Ltd)

10. Olsen, E. G. J. (1983). Myocarditis – a case of mistaken identity? *Br. Heart J.*, **50**, 303

11. Amorin, D. S. and Olsen, E. G. J. (1982). Assessment of heart neurons in dilated (congestive) cardiomyopathy. *Br. Heart J.*, **47**, 11

12. Goodwin, J. F. (1970). Congestive and hypertrophic cardiomyopathies. A decade of study. *Lancet*, **1**, 731

13. Henry, W. L., Clark, C. E. and Epstein, S. E. (1973). Asymmetric septal hypertrophy (ASH): the unifying link in the IHSS disease spectrum. Observation regarding its pathogenesis, pathophysiology and course. *Circulation*, **47**, 827

14. Olsen, E. G. J. (1980). The pathology of idiopathic hypertrophic subaortic stenosis (hypertrophic cardiomyopathy). A critical review. *Am. Heart J.*, **100**, 553

15. Davies, M. J., Pomerance, A and Teare, R. D. (1975). Pathological features of hypertrophic obstructive cardiomyopathy (HOCM). *J. Clin. Pathol.*, **27**, 529

16. Maron, B. J. and Roberts, W. C. (1979). Quantitative analysis of cardiac muscle cell disorganization in the ventricular septum of patients with hypertrophic cardiomyopathy. *Circulation*, **59**, 689

17. Van Noorden, S., Olsen, E. G. J. and Pearse, A. G. E. (1971). Hypertrophic obstructive cardiomyopathy. A histological, histochemical and ultrastructural study of biopsy material. *Cardiovasc. Res.*, **5**, 118

18. Edwards, W. D., Zakheim, R. and Mattioli, L. (1977). Asymmetric septal hypertrophy in childhood. Unreliability of histologic criteria for differentiation of obstructive and nonobstructive forms. *Hum. Pathol.*, **8**, 277

19. Davies, J. N. P. (1948). Endomyocardial necrosis. A heart disease of obscure aetiology in Africans. M.D. Thesis, University of Bristol

20. Löffler, W. (1936). Endocarditis parietalis fibroplastica mit Bluteosinophilie ein eigenartiges Krankheitsbild. *Schweiz. Med. Wschr.*, **17**, 817

21. Brockington, I. F. and Olsen, E. G. J. (1973). Löffler's endocarditis and Davies' endomyocardial fibrosis. *Am. Heart J.*, **85**, 308

22. Shaper, A. G., Hutt, M. S. R. and Coles, R. M. (1968). Necropsy studies of endomyocardial fibrosis and rheumatic heart disease in Uganda. *Br. Heart J.*, **30**, 391

23. Olsen, E. G. J. and Spry, C. J. F. (1979). The pathogenesis of Löffler's endomyocardial disease and its relationship to endomyocardial fibrosis. In Yu, P. N. and Goodwin, J. F. (eds.). *Progress in Cardiology*. Vol. 8, p. 281. (Philadelphia: Lea & Febiger)

24. Davies, J., Spry, C. J. F., Vijayaraghavan, G. and de Souza, J. A. (1983). A comparison of the clinical and cardiological features of endomyocardial disease in temperate and tropical regions. *Postgrad. Med. J.*, **59**, 179

Neoplasms of the Heart and Pericardium **10**

Neoplasms of the cardiovascular system are identical to tumours elsewhere in the body and the reader is referred to specialized texts. Tumours of the heart and pericardium are exceedingly rare. An incidence of 0.028% has been reported[1]. The ratio of malignant to benign neoplasms in the heart is 1 : 3 and in the pericardium 1 : 1[2].

One of the largest referral centres is the Armed Forces Institute of Pathology in Washington DC and in their published Fascicle[3] the following tumours are discussed and illustrated. Many of these neoplasms are extremely rare; only some of them are discussed in this chapter.

The extensive list set out in Table 10.1 serves as a classification of primary tumours of the heart and pericardium; that in Table 10.2 serves the same purpose for primary tumours of the major blood vessels.

Benign Tumours of the Heart and Pericardium

Myxoma

The most commonly encountered neoplasm is myxoma. The tumours may be single or multiple and are most frequently located in the intra-atrial septum of the left atrium in the region of the fossa ovalis but they may occur in other sites, for example the right atrium and ventricles[4].

Macroscopically, myxomas are usually globular, polypoid and frequently pedunculated (Figure 10.1). They are of greyish appearance but may have a dark brown surface when haemorrhage has occurred. Thrombus may be superimposed.

Histologically, the tumour consists of a homogenous eosinophilic matrix with slightly basophilic clear zones which surround vascular or cellular elements (Figure 10.2). These are usually sparse, polyhedral in shape and occasionally aggregated in small clusters. Stellate cells

Table 10.1 Primary tumours and cysts of the heart and pericardium

Benign	Malignant
Myxoma	Mesothelioma
Papillary fibroelastoma	Angiosarcoma
Papilloma of the epicardium	Rhabdomyosarcoma
Rhabdomyoma	Fibrosarcoma and Malignant fibrous histiocytoma
Fibroma	Malignant lymphoma
Lipomatous hypertrophy of the atrial septum	Extraskeletal osteosarcoma
Lipoma	Malignant nerve sheath tumours
Haemangioma	Malignant teratoma
Varix	Thymoma
Blood cyst	Other malignant cardiac tumours
Mesothelioma of the atrio-ventricular node	Leiomyosarcoma
Teratoma	
Bronchogenic cyst	
Pericardial cyst	
Tumours stimulating pericardial cyst	
Other benign cardiac tumours	
Granular cell tumour	
Hamartoma	
Heterotopic tissue	
Leiomyoma	
Lymphangioma	
Neurofibroma	

Table 10.2 Primary tumours of the major blood vessels

Large veins	Large arteries
Leiomyoma	Malignant tumours of:
Leiomyosarcoma	pulmonary artery
	aorta
	large arteries
	Intimal fibroplasia

and fibrocytes are found. Elastic fibres may also be seen, especially around vascular spaces. Fibrin, haemosiderin (Figure 10.3) and red blood cells may be identified which are secondary to trauma. Foci of calcification can occasionally be encountered[5] (Figure 10.4).

Histochemically, the stroma of the tumour stains positive with PAS and Alcian Blue (Figure 10.5). Metachromasia with thionin has also been reported.

Rhabdomyoma

Rhabdomyomas are the most frequently encountered primary tumours of the heart in the young (below the age of 15 years[3]. They are nearly always multiple and are most commonly sited in the left and right ventricles or atria but are never encountered on heart valves. In about half of the cases part of the tumour may be intracavitary (Figure 10.6).

Macroscopically, rhabdomyomas vary in size from a few millimetres to several centimetres in diameter and have a whitish to yellowish appearance.

Histologically, the tumours are circumscribed (Figure 10.7) but not encapsulated and compress surrounding myocardial fibres. Rhabdomyoma cells are large and may measure up to 80 μm in diameter and are characterized by centrally placed cytoplasmic masses with thin extensions which reach the cell border. These masses may contain nuclei. To these appearances the term 'spider cells' has been applied and is considered to be pathognomonic of rhabdomyomas[6] (Figure 10.8). Not infrequently the cytoplasmic masses are eccentrically placed and are compressed against the cell wall. From these, cytoplasmic projections also traverse the cell spaces. Myofilaments can always be found but may require careful search (Figure 10.9). The 'empty' spaces are seen, on staining with haematoxylin and eosin, to be filled with glycogen.

The nature of the tumours is controversial. Three major views have been expressed. (For a review of the subject see Hudson, 1965[7]).

(1) They are harmartomous.

(2) Their cell origin is the Purkinje fibre.

(3) The cells represent a localized form of cardiac glycogenesis.

Fibromas

These tumours are derived from fibroblasts and are usually single. They resemble fibromas encountered elsewhere in the body. All ages and both sexes are affected and they are often found in the young. Fibromas are most commonly located in the anterior wall of the left ventricle and the interventricular septum and may compress the bundle of His[8]. Symptoms depend on the site of the tumours and there may be 'incidental' findings post mortem.

Macroscopically, the tumours are firm, greyish in colour, and may attain a large size (10 cm or more). Dystrophic calcification in the centre of the tumour may occur.

Histologically, fibromas are non-encapsulated and strands of tumour may extend into the surrounding myocardium. The tumours are composed of interlacing cellular fibrous tissue (Figure 10.10 a and b). In larger tumours the cellular elements are confined to the periphery whereas the centre is then composed of hyalin collagen tissue. Cystic degeneration and calcification[9] are found in these areas.

Haemangiomas

These are exceedingly rare. The tumours are composed of vascular channels lined by endothelial cells and supporting stroma[3]. A capillary haemangioma is illustrated in Figure 10.11. Macroscopically, they are haemorrhagic.

Papillary Tumours

Although the nature of these tumours has also been controversial[10], it is believed that they are related to Lambl's excrescences and form as a result of fibrin deposition.

Macroscopically, the tumours are composed of many grey strands, some of which may be exceedingly long, resembling sea anemones. They are usually found on valves but may extend on to the chordae tendineae (Figure 10.12), the papillary muscles or on to the walls of the ventricles.

Histologically, the core usually consists of connective tissue and elastic-like material. More superficially the strands consist of loose basophilic tissue and fibrin (Figure 10.13).

Malignant Tumours of the Heart and Pericardium

Mesotheliomas

These are classified as malignant neoplasms of the pericardium. The so-called benign mesotheliomas are considered to be reactive mesothelial hyperplasia[3]. In recent years the mesotheliomas have become the most frequently encountered tumours in many reported series.

Criteria for diagnosis have been established by several authorities[3,11]. The criteria include:

tumour strictly localized to the pericardium without penetration of the wall;
only metastases to lymph nodes;
no other primary tumours;
complete autopsy examination of those cases that had died.

McAllister and Fenoglio[3] have defined morphological criteria such as cellular regularity and histological variability including tubules, solid cords of malignant cells and spindle cells imitating fibroblasts. Histochemically, an intra- and extracellular positive staining reaction, with colloidal iron or Alcian Blue, is also included in the list of criteria.

Macroscopically, the tumours are diffuse covering both surfaces of the pericardium and occluding the pericardial cavity. Very rarely may these tumours be solitary.

Histologically, three major types are recognized.

(1) *The fibrous type.* This is the most commonly encountered type. The bulk of the tumour is composed of fibrous tissue but occasionally some tubular elements can be found (Figure 10.14).

(2) *The epithelial type.* This may show either a tubular pattern (Figure 10.15) or a papillary pattern. Cleft formation may also be encountered or the tumour may consist of solid epithelial cords.

(3) *Mixed fibrous and epithelial type.* A mixture of fibrous and epithelial types are also encountered (Figure 10.16).

Sarcomas

All the malignant tumours listed at the beginning of this chapter have been reported. A rhabdomyosarcoma is illustrated in Figures 10.17–10.20. These neoplasms are also multiple and it is often difficult to ascertain the primary sites. The pericardium is involved in approximately half of the cases. A portion of the tumour is always intramyocardial (Figure 10.17).

Macroscopically, the tumours are nodular, brownish in colour and necrotic in the centre. Histologically, pleomorphism of the cellular elements is found (Figure 10.18) including strap cells, racket-shaped cells, rounded cells and 'spider cells' (Figure 10.19).

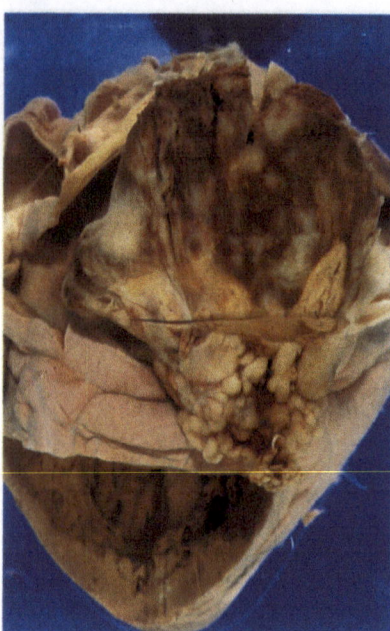

Figure 10.1 Left atrial myxoma arising from the interatrial septum and filling the atrial cavity

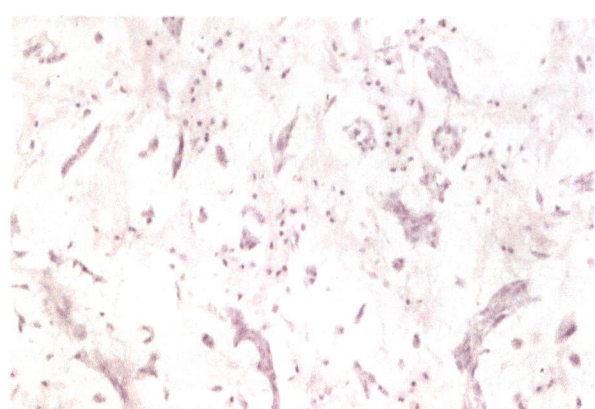

Figure 10.2 Photomicrograph of a myxoma showing clear zones around vascular and cellular elements. The matrix of the tumour is eosinophilic.   H & E × 100

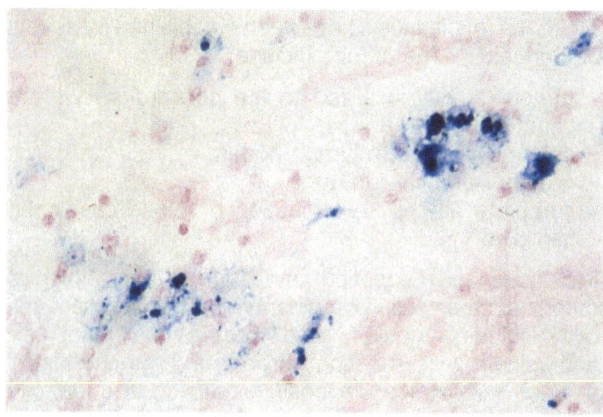

Figure 10.3 Haemosiderin granules in the myxoma are taken up by macrophages. Haemosiderin occurs as a result of haemorrhage into the tumour due to trauma, especially when the tumour is pedunculated.   Perl's reaction × 150

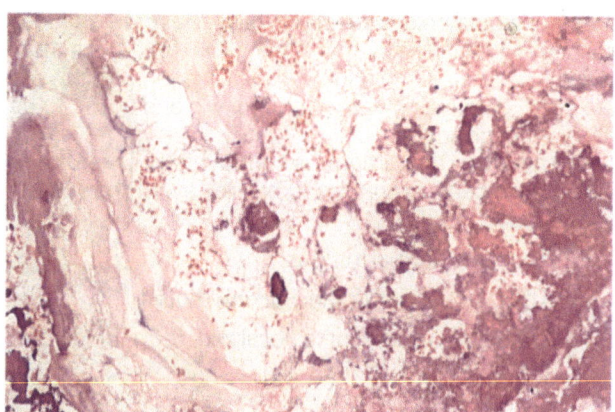

Figure 10.4 Calcification (dystrophic) has occurred in this myxoma.   H & E × 50

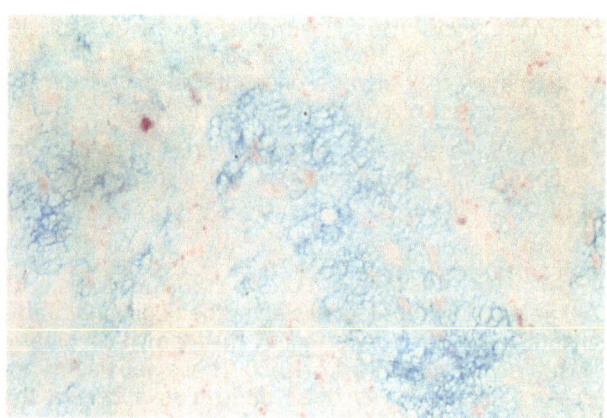

Figure 10.5 The stroma of a myxoma shows mucopoly-saccharides.   Alcian Blue × 100

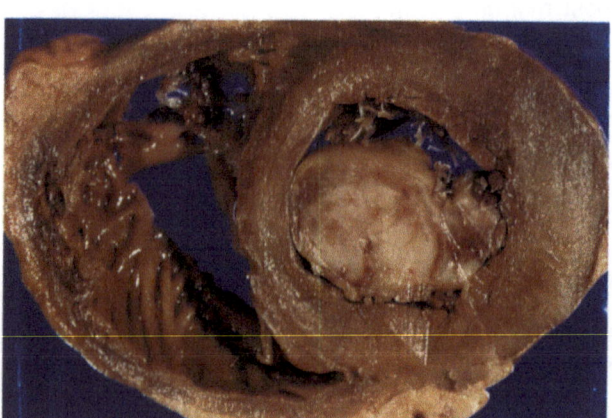

Figure 10.6 Cross-section of a rhabdomyoma. In this illustration the tumour is intracavitary but a large intramyocardial portion was seen in other sections. The tumour has a whitish appearance

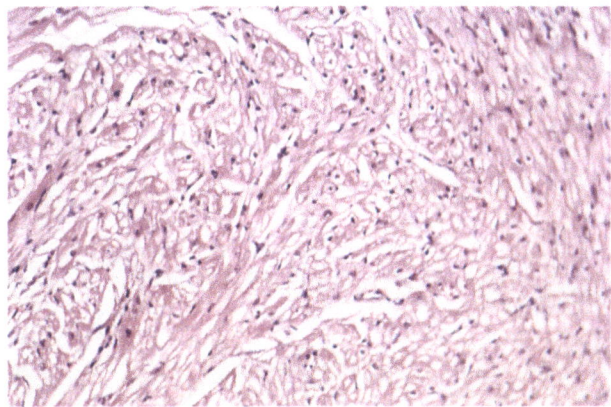

Figure 10.7 General view of a rhabdomyoma showing tumour cells arranged in interlacing bundles. The tumour cells have a 'lace-like' appearance. H & E × 50

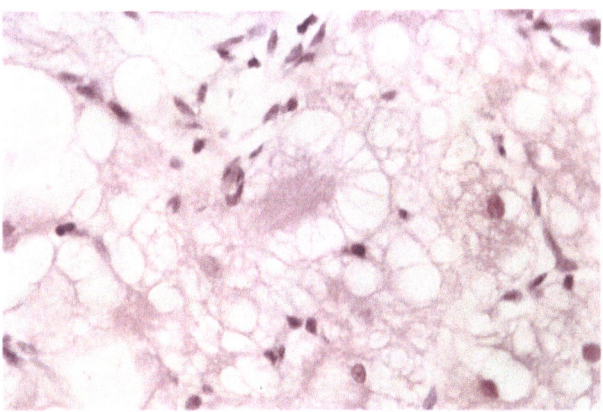

Figure 10.8 Rhabdomyoma cells often have a centrally placed cytoplasmic mass from which fine projections emanate. The cells have been referred to as 'spider cells'. H & E × 600

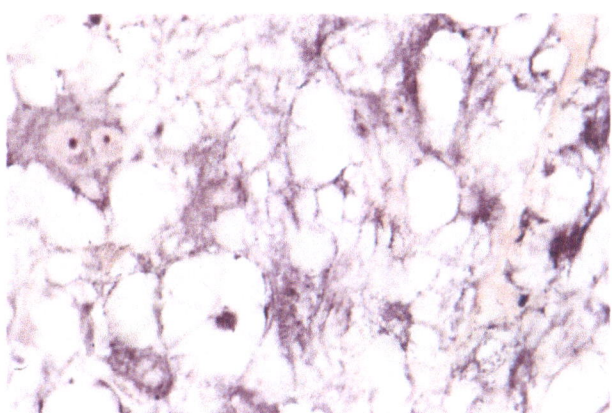

Figure 10.9 Myofilaments can always be found in rhabdomy-omas (towards the lower margin of the centre of the illustration). Phosphotungstic acid–haematoxylin × 400

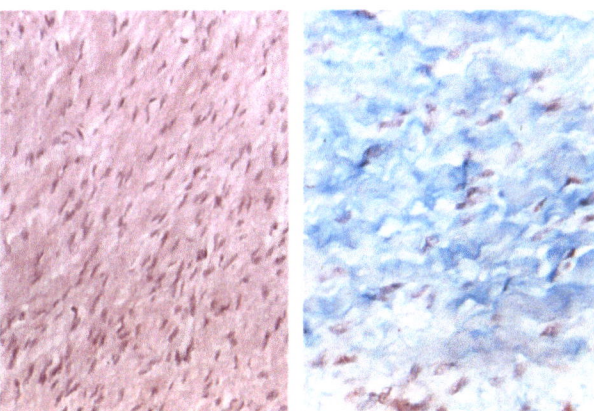

Figure 10.10a (left) Interlacing bundle of cellular fibrous tissue charactizes a fibroma. In cases of large tumours the centre is composed of hyaline collagen tissue and cystic degeneration is common. H & E × 50

Figure 10.10b (right) The same tumour as Figure 10.10a. Collagen tissue stains blue with Masson's trichrome × 50

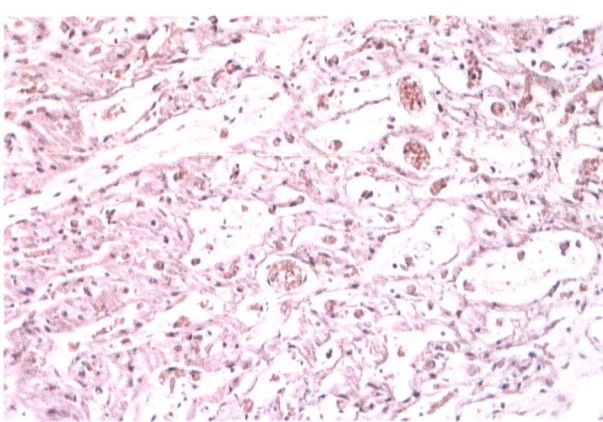

Figure 10.11 A capillary haemangioma consisting of capillary-sized vascular channels tightly packed with little stroma interven-ing. The tumour was found in the left ventricular myocardium close to the endocardium. H & E × 100

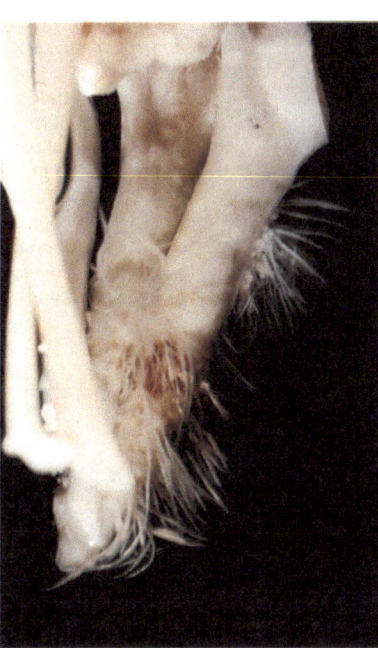

Figure 10.12 Papillary tumour on thickened chordae tendineae (due to chronic rheu-matic heart disease). The large grey strands have been likened to sea-anemones

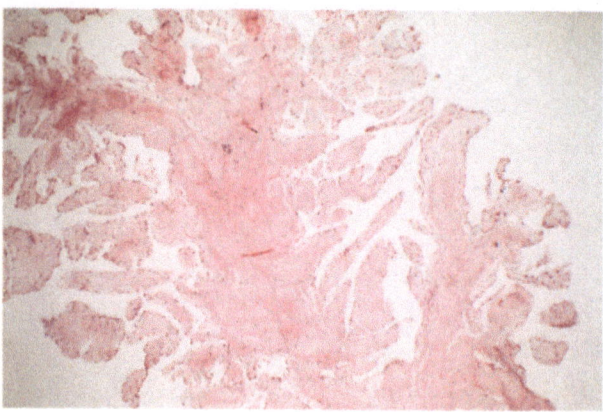

Figure 10.13 Photomicrograph of a papillary tumour consisting of connective tissue and fibrin. The strands are lined by endothelial cells. H & E × 25

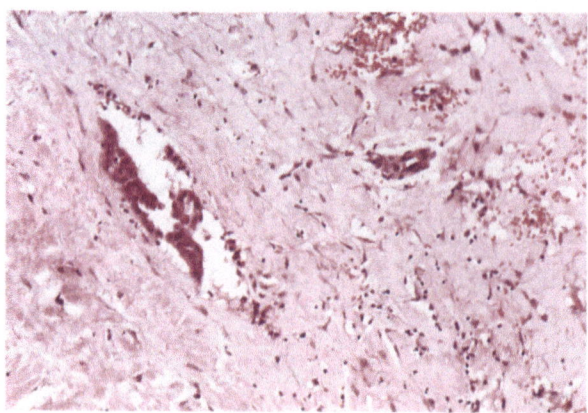

Figure 10.14 Mesothelioma in which fibrous tissue is the dominant tumour constituent. Occasional tubular elements may be found. H & E × 50

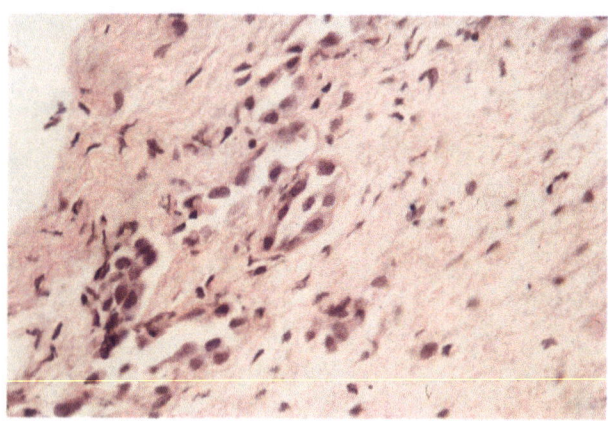

Figure 10.15 A tubular pattern predominates in this illustration of a mesothelioma. H & E × 200

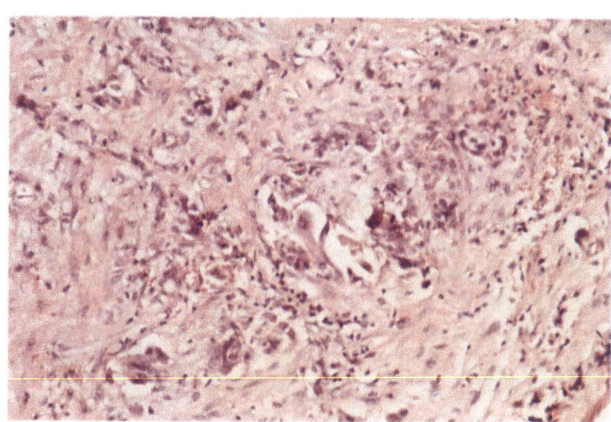

Figure 10.16 'Mixed' type of mesothelioma. Epithelial cellular elements, some of which show a tubular pattern are surrounded by fibrous stroma. H & E × 100

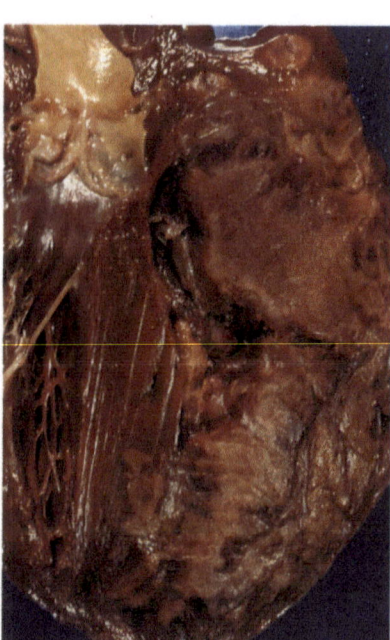

Figure 10.17 A rhabdomyosarcoma showing a predominantly intracavitary (left ventricular) position. The intramyocardial part is clearly seen in the cut free left ventricular wall. The tumour is of a brown appearance. Some foci of necrosis can also be seen

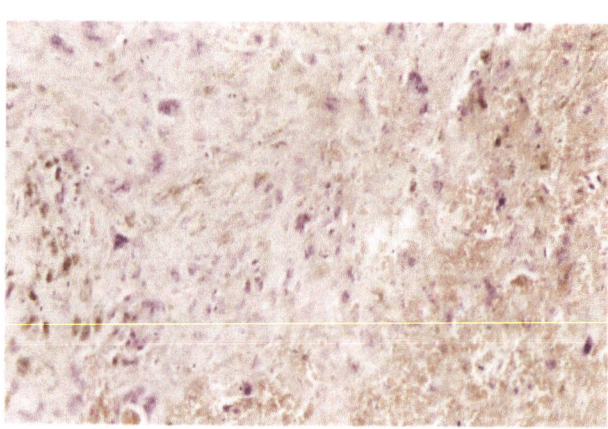

Figure 10.18 Photomicrograph of a rhabdomyosarcoma showing pleomorphic cellular constituents. H & E × 50

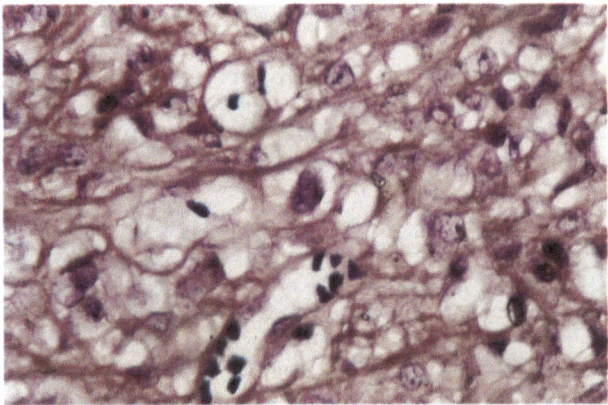

Figure 10.19 Rhabdomyosarcoma showing typical spider cells. The nucleus is placed in the centre of the cell, from the thin rim of cytoplasm fine projections can be seen. H & E × 400

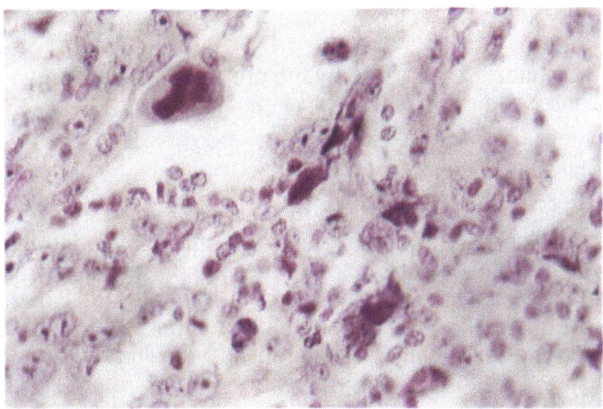

Figure 10.20 Rhabdomyoblasts are found in rhabdomyosarcoma. This cell determines the type of the sarcoma which in cases of poor differentiation may be difficult to categorize. Phospho-tungstic acid–haematoxylin × 400

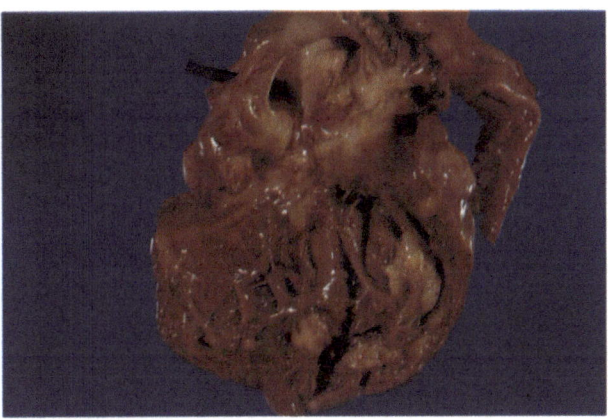

Figure 10.21a Illustration of a reticulum cell sarcoma of the heart

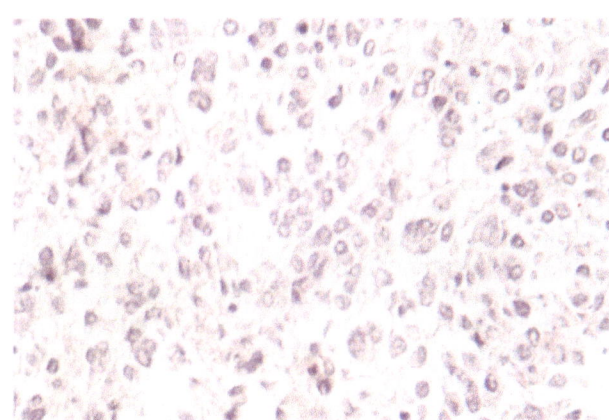

Figure 10.21b The reticulum cell sarcoma of Figure 10.21a. H & E × 100

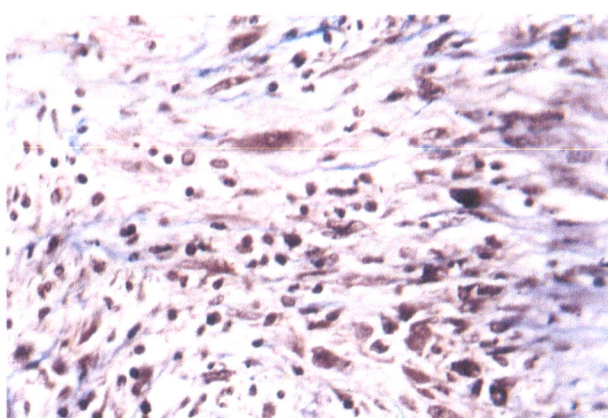

Figure 10.22 Photomicrograph of a leiomyosarcoma. The inter-lacing bundles of cells have a red-purple appearance when stained with Masson's trichrome stain × 100

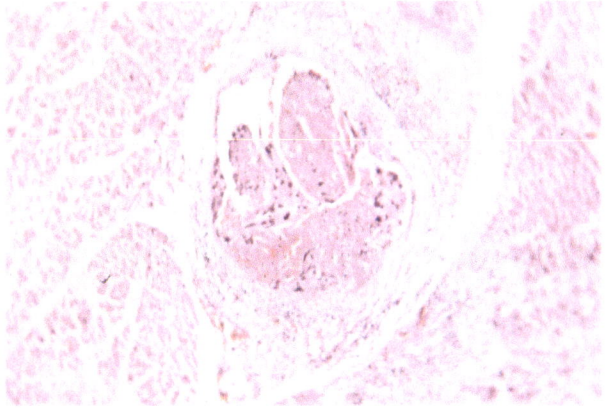

Figure 10.23 Tumour embolus (chorion carcinoma) in the left ventricular myocardium. H & E × 50

Diagnosis is achieved by the presence of rhabdomyoblasts[3] (Figure 10.20).

Malignant Lymphoma

The heart and pericardium may secondarily be involved by malignant lymphoma. These tumours confined to the heart and, therefore, primary are rare. A reticulum cell sarcoma confined to the heart is illustrated in Figure 10.21 a and b. Although some pleomorphism exists the cells are fairly uniform, resembling reticulum cells.

Leiomyosarcoma

These tumours are derived from smooth muscle and they are also extremely rare in the heart and pericardium. Histologically, the tumours are composed of interlacing cords of elongated cells with nuclei which are often blunted at their poles. The cytoplasm has a red-purple appearance with Masson's trichrome stain (Figure 10.22).

Secondary Tumours of the Heart and Pericardium

These are 13–39 times more common than the primary type of tumours. Bronchial and breast carcinoma, lymphoma and malignant melanomas head the list of the reported cases[12]. Pericardial and myocardial secondary deposits occur with approximately the same frequency but this depends on the primary tumour. For example, leukaemia favours the myocardium while bronchial carcinomas, on the other hand, involve the pericardium often by direct extension. Endocardial involvement including heart valves seems to be most frequently encountered in the tricuspid valve[13] but has also been documented in the mitral valve[14].

A secondary chorion carcinoma is illustrated in Figure 10.23.

In conclusion, on the topic of primary benign and malignant tumours of the heart and pericardium and of metastatic deposits, all features described in tumours encountered elsewhere in the body are also seen in the heart and pericardium. This includes pleomorphism, abnormal mitoses and invasion of the lymphatic and vascular channels, depending on the nature of the tumour. Occasionally mitoses may be observed in benign tumours such as fibroma. As stated at the beginning of this chapter, further reading on oncology is recommended.

References

1. Fine, G. (1968). Neoplasms of the pericardium and heart. In *Pathology of the Heart and Blood Vessels*. 3rd Edition, p. 851. (Springfield, Ill: C. C. Thomas)

2. Fine, G. (1975). Primary tumours of the pericardium and heart. *Cardiovasc. Clin.*, **5**, 208

3. McAllister, H. A. and Fenoglio, J. F. (1978). Tumours of the cardiovascular system. *Atlas of Tumour Pathology*. Second Series, Fascicle 15. (Washington DC: Armed Forces Institute of Pathology)

4. Doohen, D. J., Greer, J. W., Diorio, N. and Timmes, J. J. (1964). Emergency excision' of a myxoma of the right ventricle which was obstructing the right ventricular outflow tract. *J. Thorac. Cardiovasc. Surg.*, **47**, 342

5. Oliver, G. C. and Missen, G. A. K. (1966). A heavily calcified right atrial myxoma. *Guy's Hospital Rep.*, **115**, 37

6. Landing, B. H. and Farber, S. (1956). Tumours of the cardiovascular system. *Atlas of Tumour Pathology*. Section III, Fascicle VII, p. 13. (Washington DC: US War Department)

7. Hudson, R. E. B. (1965). *Cardiovascular Pathology*. Volume 2, p. 1581. (London: E. Arnold Ltd)

8. James, T. N., Carson, D. J. L. and Marshall, T. K. (1973). De subitaneis morbitus. I. Fibroma compressing His bundle. *Circulation*, **48**, 428

9. Soler-Soler, J. and Romero-Gonzalez, R. (1975). Calcified intramural fibroma of the left ventricle. *Eur. J. Cardiol.*, **3**, 71

10. Olsen, E. G. J. (1980). In *The Pathology of the Heart*. Second Edition, p. 173. (London and Basingstoke: Macmillan Press Ltd)

11. Anderson, J. A. and Fischer-Hansen, B. (1974). Primary pericardial mesothelioma. *Dan. Med. Bull.*, **21**, 195

12. Bisel, H. F., Wroblewski, F. and La Due, J. S. (1953). Incidence and clinical manifestations of cardiac metastasis. *J. Am. Med. Assoc.*, **153**, 712

13. Coller, F. C., Inkley, J. J. and Moragues, V. (1950). Neoplastic endocardial implants. Report of a case. *Am. J. Clin. Pathol.*, **20**, 159

14. Morgan, W. E. and Gray, P. B. (1977). Lymphatic metastasis in the mitral valve. *Br. Heart J.*, **39**, 218

Arterial Diseases

The morphological changes of both common and rarer arterial diseases will be detailed in this chapter. Atherogenesis has already been described in detail in Chapter 5.

Diseases Affecting Predominantly Large Arteries

Marfan's Disease

This is an hereditary connective tissue disease and the criteria for diagnosis are:

> Major criteria
> A positive family history
> Dislocation of ocular lenses

> Minor criteria
> Skeletal stigmata
> Cardiovascular involvement
> Increased urinary hydroxyproline excretion[1].

For a firm diagnosis one major and/or one or two minor criteria at least must be present.

Cardiovascular involvement consists of aneurysmal dilatation of the root of the aorta and aortic insufficiency. The valve leaflets are thin and transparent with a bluish tinge and separation of the leaflet at the commisures may occur.

Histologically, Marfan's disease in the aorta is characterized by fragmentation of the elastic component of the media (Figure 11.1) varying in severity. Accumulation of mucopolysaccharides (Figure 11.2) is common but usually does not attain cystic proportions. Elastic fragmentation is not confined to the areas of mucoid accumulation but may also be found in areas of muscle or collagen degeneration. Dissection of the aorta is a major complication[2]. In the aortic valve leaflets the zona spongiosa is prominent (Figure 11.3), degeneration of fibrosa and fragmentation of the elastic tissue with no increase in vascularity summarizes the histological changes. Secondary thickening due to aortic valve insufficiency may be severe. Marfan's disease may affect other arteries such as the pulmonary and coronary arteries. As fragmentation of the pulmonary trunk is typical in the adult the histological changes are less striking.

Identical macroscopic and histological changes in the aorta and aortic valves have been described in the absence of any stigmata of Marfan's disease. To that condition the descriptions Marfan forme fruste (Figure 11.4) or Marfanoid change or degenerative aortopathy have been applied. Both conditions are seen in the younger age groups (30–40 years)[3,4]

Erdheim's Cystic Medionecrosis

This condition is distinguishable from Marfan's disease or the forme fruste type in that fragmentation of the elastica is confined to foci of mucoid pooling which often accumulate to form cysts (Figure 11.5). It is seen in elderly patients and frequently in dissecting aneurysms.

Dissecting Aneurysms of the Aorta

Dissection is frequently associated with cystic medionecrosis (85%) and in up to 30% in patients with Marfan's disease or the forme fruste type.

Macroscopically, a clear-cut tear, transverse or oblique, frequently situated in the ascending aorta at the point of pericardial reflection is usually identified. A 're-entry' point may or may not be found (Figure 11.6). Separation of the media occurs between the inner two thirds and the outer one third (Figure 11.7a and b). Blood or thrombus is usually present separating true dissection from possible artefactual separation due to preparation of tissue for histological examination. For review of the subject the reader is referred to Hirst et al. 1958[5].

Ankylosing Spondylitis

Cardiovascular involvement includes aortitis and aortic valvulitis characterized macroscopically by thickening of the cusps with rolled margins and separation of the commissures[6] (Figure 11.8). Histology shows an increase in collagen tissue and distortion of the architecture and an increase in vascularity.

In the aorta, fibroelastic intimal thickening may be severe. Fragmentation of the elastic fibres of the media is characteristic with areas of fibrous replacement (Figure 11.9). Adventitial changes include thickening, vessels with severe intimal changes and a chronic inflammatory infiltrate, particularly of lymphocytes, frequently forming cuffs around the vasa vasorum.

Syphilis

Cardiovascular changes occur in the tertiary phase. Macroscopically, aneurysmal dilatation of the aorta is found together with fibrous thickening of the intima. Wrinkling, giving a tree bark effect, is characteristic (Figure 11.10).

Histologically, a focal condensation of elastic tissue is present with areas of vascular fibrous tissue in the media which in the active phase is rich in plasma cells (Figure 11.11). In the later phases fibrous tissue leading to distortion of the medial architecture and folding of the intima results in the tree bark effect noted macroscopically. Adventitial changes include thickening by fibrous tissue, so-called endarteritis of the vasa vasorum and often severe chronic inflammatory cell infiltrates rich in plasma cells, particularly in the active phases, fre-

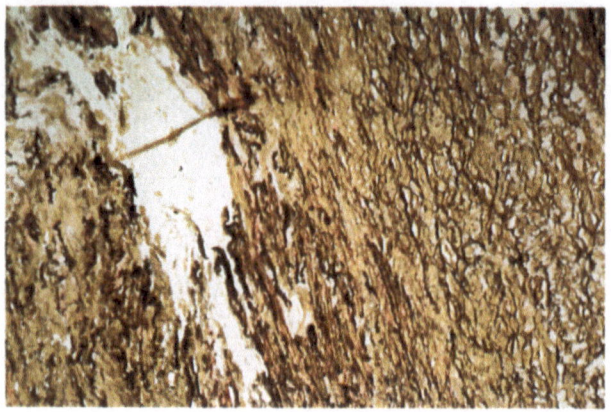

Figure 11.1 Fragmentation of the elastic tissue in the media of the aorta, even in areas away from pooling, is typical in Marfan's disease. Elastic van Gieson × 200

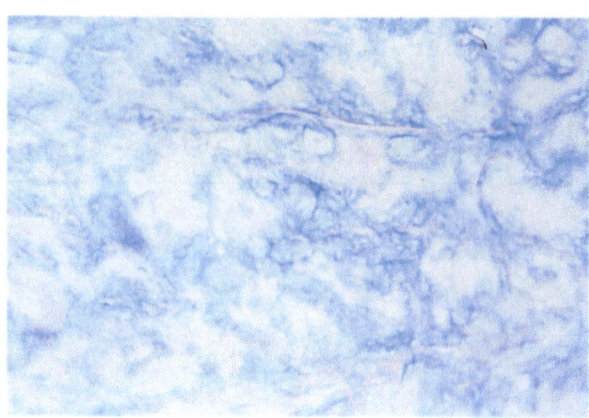

Figure 11.2 Alcian Blue positive material is demonstrated in micropools in this aortic wall from a patient with Marfan's disease. Alcian Blue × 400

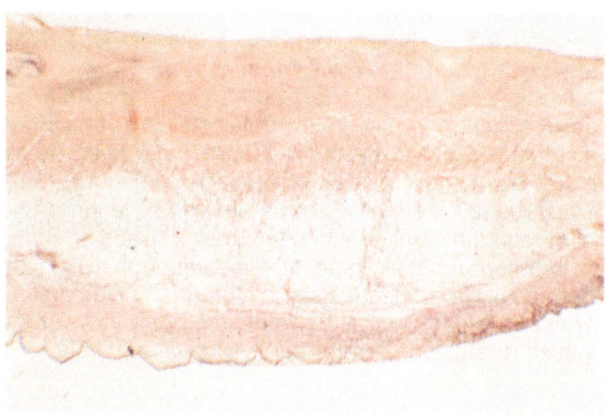

Figure 11.3 Part of the aortic valve leaflet showing a prominent zona spongiosa, a finding frequently encounterd in Marfan's disease. Elastic van Gieson × 50

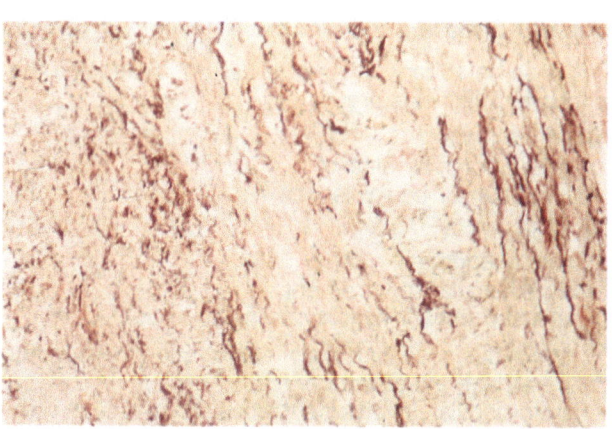

Figure 11.4 Extensive fragmentation of elastic tissue in the aortic media is seen together with areas of some pooling. The changes are identical to Marfan's disease (Figure 11.1) but in view of no other stigmata of that disease having been found in this patient the term Marfan *forme fruste* has been applied. Elastic van Gieson × 200

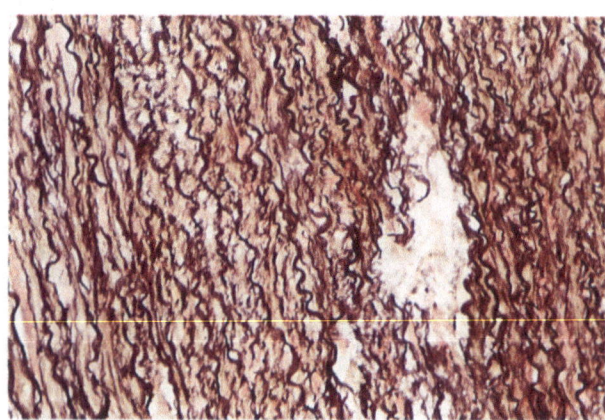

Figure 11.5 Erdheim's cystic medionecrosis is characterized by fragmentation of the elastic tissue of the aortic media confined to areas of pooling. Elsewhere, the elastic pattern is normal. Elastic van Gieson × 200

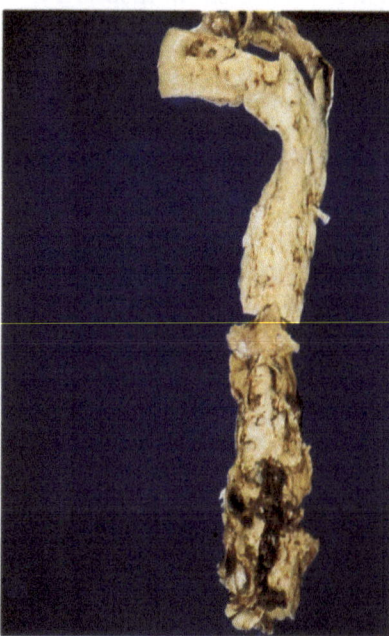

Figure 11.6 Dissecting aneurysm of the aorta showing a transverse tear at the upper end of the vessel. The 're-entry' point can be identified where the thrombus commences in the abdominal part of the aorta

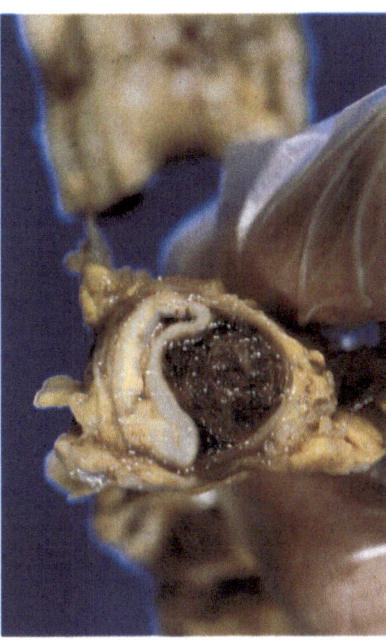

Figure 11.7a Cross-section of a dissecting aneurysm of the aorta. Thrombus is clearly seen between the inner two thirds and outer one third of the aortic wall. The original lumen is collapsed

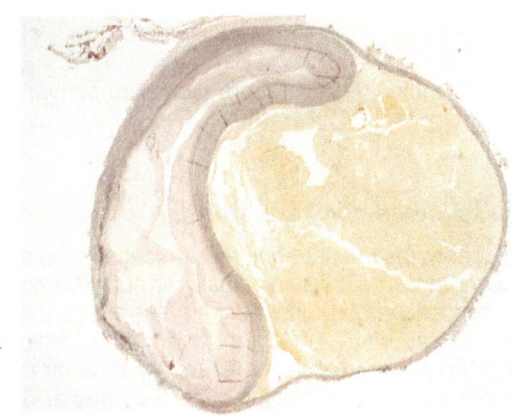

Figure 11.7b From the same case showing only occasional foci of fragmentation of the medial elastic tissue. At other levels of sectioning typical changes of Marfan's disease were found. These abnormalities are, therefore, zonal and may not necessarily affect the entire vessel. Elastic van Gieson × 10

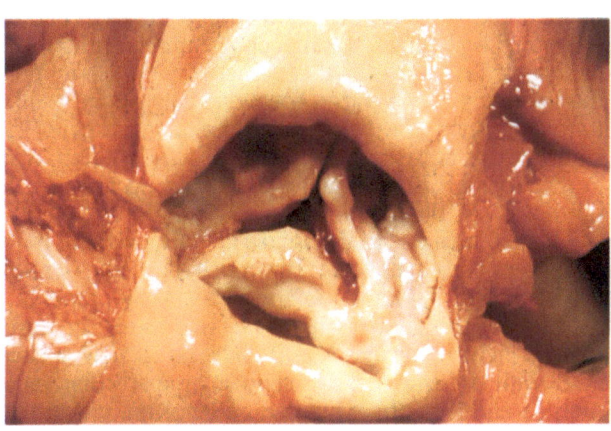

Figure 11.8 The aortic valve in ankylosing spondylitis viewed from above. The valve leaflets are thick and distorted and separation of the commissures has occurred

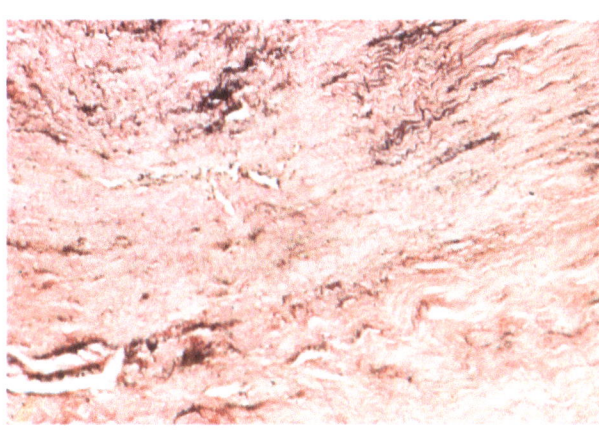

Figure 11.9 Extensive fragmentation of the elastica of the aortic media in areas of mural fibrosis is seen in ankylosing spondylitis. Mucoid pooling does not occur. Elastic van Gieson × 200

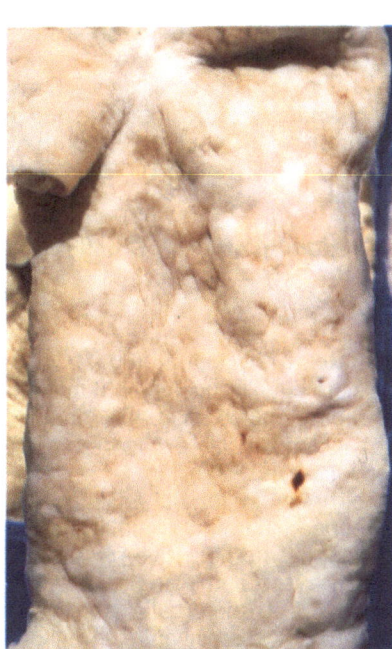

Figure 11.10 Part of the aortic wall showing wrinkling (tree-bark effect) characteristic of syphilis. Fibrous plaques of arteriosclerosis are additionally present

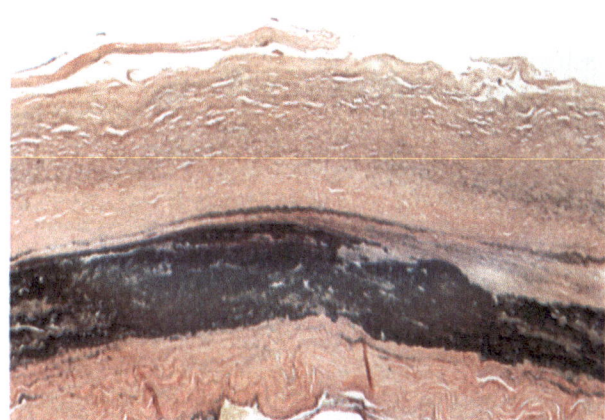

Figure 11.11 Syphilis of the aorta. Condensation of the elastic fibres in which foci of vascular fibrous tissue are interspersed is characteristic. Note the extreme intimal thickening by fibro-elastic tissue (top of the illustration). The adventitia is also fibrotic. Elastic van Gieson × 50

quently surrounding vasa vasorum (so-called perivascular cuffing) (Figure 11.12).

Takayasu's Disease or Primary Aortitis

Other pseudonyms include 'pulseless disease' and aortic arch syndrome[7]. This also usually affects the aorta and its immediate large branches. Females are up to ten times more frequently affected than males. Macroscopically the condition is characterized by saccular aneurysmal dilatations and wrinkling of the intima. The initimal thickening is abrupt, frequently beginning in the sinus of Valsalva and often extending below the renal arteries where intimal thickening ends abruptly (Figure 11.13a and b).

Histologically, the intimal changes consist of loosely arranged connective tissue and mucoid change but it is devoid of any elastic tissue (Figure 11.14a and b). The thickening is usually immense and may greatly exceed the thickness of the media of the vessels affected. The media shows severe disruption of the elastic component, fibrous replacement of the media and chronic inflammatory cells including occasionally giant cells (Figure 11.15a and b).

The adventitia is also immensely thickened, often several times thicker than the media, frequently anchoring the aorta to surrounding tissue, and making removal difficult unless sharp dissection is undertaken (see Figure 11.13a and b).

Pulmonary arteries[8] and smaller arteries such as coronary arteries may also be involved (Figure 11.14a).

Diseases Affecting Predominantly Medium Sized Arteries

Buerger's Disease (Thrombo-Angiitis Obliterans)

Doubt has been cast as to the existence of this disease. There can be no doubt whatever that it exists as a separate entity. It affects younger age groups (25–50 years), predominantly males of all races, resulting clinically in intermittent claudication. The symptoms are aggravated by smoking.

Diagnostic morphological features include an *intact* internal elastic lamina, occlusion by non-retracting thrombus and a panarteritis (or panphlebitis) (Figure 11.16a and b). There must be no other intimal lesion such as arteriosclerosis. Not only are arteries and veins affected but also adjacent nerves, forming the so-called triad (Figure 11.17). Vessels and nerves are affected segmentally so that in a given section an artery only may be involved, whilst in another artery and vein, and in still another the vein only, may be affected. The stages of the disease process may also vary segmentally[9].

The thrombus, apart from non-contraction, shows additional characteristic features. The cellular component includes in the acute phases many neutrophils, occasionally focally aggregated to form micro-abscesses. Eosinophils and giant cells are also identified (Figure 11.18). In the healed phase thick-walled vessels of capillary size are typical (Figure 11.19).

Veins show identical changes. Nerve involvement is usually confined to the epineurium.

Buerger's disease affects medium-sized arteries of the lower and upper limbs, visceral arteries and coronary arteries. Cerebral Buerger's disease is well recognized. Affected small arteries, for example in the toes, have also been described (Figure 11.20).

Mönckeberg Sclerosis[10]

This affects muscular arteries, particularly in adults and progresses with increasing age. It is a benign condition characterized by calcification of the media (Figure 11.21). It may or may not be accompanied by arteriosclerosis. Arteries of the legs and arms and very occasionally temporal or other arteries are involved. The aetiology is unknown but is most likely attributable to vascular spasm.

Giant Cell Arteritis or Temporal Arteritis

This disease affects the temporal arteries and occurs predominantly in elderly females. The condition is characterized by headache, ocular complications which may result in blindness, and systemic complications.

Histologically, the intima is severely thickened and often arranged in two layers. The remainder of the media and the adventitia share in the inflammatory process (Figure 11.22). As far as the intimal thickening is concerned, the inner layer consists of loosely arranged fibrocytes in a mucinous ground substance, whilst in the outer intimal layer more densely arranged collagen fibres are identified (Figure 11.23). Fragmentation of the internal elastic lamina may be extreme and, on the intimal/medial border zone, often a severe inflammatory infiltrate consisting of lymphocytes, mononuclear cells, eosinophils and occasionally plasma cells is identified. Also in that region giant cells of Langhans type are usually but not invariably found[9] (Figure 11.24).

Fibrinoid necrosis of the media is not typical but may, on rare occasions, be seen. Thrombus occluding or partially occluding the lumen is not infrequently present.

Coronary and subclavian arteries and rarely the aorta may be involved (Figure 11.25). Skeletal vessels associated with a fever and resulting in non-articular pain, malaise and loss of weight can be involved, giving rise clinically to polymyalgia rheumatica. Skeletal vascular changes are usually accompanied by changes in the temporal arteries but symptoms referable to the temporal artery may be absent (Figure 11.26).

Infantile Arterial Calcification (Occlusive Infantile Arteriopathy)

This is an uncommon arterial disease affecting infants and is characterized by infantile fibrous proliferation in large and medium sized arteries, elastic degeneration, calcification, and a focal cellular infiltrate at the intimal/medial junction. It has been found that calcification may be scant or absent and when it occurs it is a secondary phenomenon[11]. The coronary artery of a 13-month-old infant is illustrated in Figure 11.27a and b.

Diseases Affecting Predominantly the Smaller Arteries

Polyarteritis Nodosa

This disease typically affects the elderly (60–70 years age group). Both sexes are equally involved but in some series a slight male preponderance has been reported. Clinical characteristics include malaise, fever and loss of weight; the ESR is increased[12].

Histologically, fibrinoid necrosis of the vascular wall accompanied by an intense inflammatory infiltrate rich in neutrophils and eosinophils in the active phases and later replaced by lymphocytes and plasma cells, are typical findings (Figure 11.28). The internal elastic lamina is fragmented (Figure 11.29) and small aneurysmal dilatations may be found. Non-specific intimal thickening may accompany these changes and thrombus may also be present. Rarely, giant cells may be observed.

Small visceral vessels in organs such as gut and kidneys are typically involved but pulmonary and coronary arteries may also be affected.

Thrombotic Thrombocytopenic Purpura (Moschcowitz Syndrome)[13]

This rare, fatal disease is characterized by generalized malaise, severe anaemia, petechiae, fever and pallor affecting small arterioles and venules in the kidney and central nervous system. Small vessels in the myocardium may also be involved.

Histologically, the lumina of the vessels are occluded by fibrin. Fibrinoid necrosis of the vascular walls is frequent but differs from polyarteritis nodosa in that no inflammatory infiltrate is present (Figure 11.30). In the healed phases scarring of the wall, intimal thickening and fragmentation of the internal elastic lamina are recognized.

Rheumatic Vasculitis

This affects the vasa vasorum of the aorta and shows the typical cellular components of Aschoff nodules; nodules themselves are occasionally found (Figure 11.31).

Rheumatoid Arthritis

This disease also affects small vessels. Histologically, localised infiltration of the adventitia with mononuclear cells and occasionally neutrophils are found. The inflammatory process may reach the intima[14]. Intimal proliferation may therefore occur (Figure 11.32) but necrosis, thrombus and aneurysms are usually not evident. Healing occurs without permanent damage.

The heart may be involved in rheumatoid arthritis, rheumatoid granulomas in the valves and valve rings have been recognized. Histologically, they consist of central necrosis, palisading of surrounding histocytes and an outer zone of lymphocytes and plasma cells (Figure 11.33). Rheumatic changes in the heart are well recognized in patients with rheumatoid arthritis.

Vascular Lesions in Hypertension

Pulmonary hypertension is described in Chapter 12. Systemic hypertension can be recognized by an increase in the thickness of the muscular walls of arteries and arterioles, but is difficult to assess accurately due to the absence of an external elastic lamina in these vessels. Diagnostic features are found in the kidneys.

Benign form   Intimal thickening characterized by regular rings of elastic fibres is typical, medial hypertrophy and degenerative changes are found (Figure 11.34).

Malignant form   Fibrinoid necrosis of the media and fragmentation of the internal elastic lamina characterize this condition (Figure 11.35).

Hypersensitivity and Allergic Arteritis

Fibrinoid necrosis of the wall, fragmentation of the internal elastic lamina and an inflammatory reaction are the typical changes. Granulomata may be found to which the term allergic granulomatous angiitis is applied.

Microangiopathy in Diabetes Mellitus

This manifests itself by sub-intimal hyaline change (Figure 11.36) in the small vessels and by thickening of the basement membranes of capillaries and precapillaries (Figure 11.37). Intimal proliferative lesions have also been noted but their specificity is debatable[15].

References

1. Bowers, D. (1969). Pathogenesis of primary abnormalities of the mitral valve in Marfan's syndrome. *Br. Heart J.*, **31**, 679

2. Olsen, E. G. J. (1975). Marfan's disease. *Pathol. Microbiol.*, **43**, 120

3. Olsen, E. G. J. (1975). Cardiovascular System. In Harrison, C. V. and Weinbren, K. (eds) *Recent Advances in Pathology*. Vol. 9, p. 1. (London: Churchill Livingstone)

4. Keene, R. J., Steiner, R. E., Olsen, E. G. J. and Oakley, C. (1971). Aortic root aneurysm – Radiographic and pathologic features. *Clin. Radiol.*, **22**, 330

5. Hirst, A. E., Johns, V. J. and Kime, S. W. (1958). Dissecting aneurysm of the aorta: a review of 505 cases. *Medicine (Baltimore)*, **37**, 217

6. Bauer, W., Clark, W. S. and Kulka, J. P. (1951). Aortitis and aortic endocarditis, an unrecognised manifestation of rheumatoid arthritis. *Ann. Rheum. Dis.*, **10**, 470

7. Ross, R. S. and McKusick, V. A. (1953). Aortic arch syndrome. Diminished or absent pulses in arteries arising from the arch of aorta. *Arch. Intern. Med.*, **92**, 701

8. Singh, D. and Tan. L. (1974). Pulmonary hypertension in Takayasu's arteritis. *Aust. N.Z. J. Med.*, **4**, 581

9. Olsen, E. G. J. (1975). Pathological features of thromboangiitis obliterans and arteritis temporalis and some unusual manifestations. *Pathol. Microbiol.*, **43**, 157

10. Silbert, S., Lippmann, H. I. and Gordon, E. (1953). Monckeberg's arteriosclerosis. *J. Am. Med. Assoc.*, **151**, 1176

11. Witzleben, L. (1970). Idiopathic infantile arterial calcification – a misnomer? *Am. J. Cardiol.*, **26**, 305

12. Rose, G. A. and Spencer, H. (1957). Polyarteritis nodosa. *Q. J. Med. NS*, **26**, 43

13. Bornstein, B., Boss, J. H., Casper, J. and Behar, M. (1960). Thrombotic thrombocytopenic purpura. Report of a case presenting as a chronic neurological disorder and characterized by unusual histological findings. *J. Clin. Pathol.*, **13**, 124

14. Skoloff, L., Wilens, S. L. and Bunim, J. J. (1951). Arteritis of striated muscle in rheumatoid arthritis. *Am. J. Pathol.*, **27**, 157

15. Gotlieb, A. I. (1983). In Silver, M. D. (ed.) *Cardiovascular Pathology*, p. 844. (New York, Edinburgh, London, Melbourne: Churchill Livingstone)

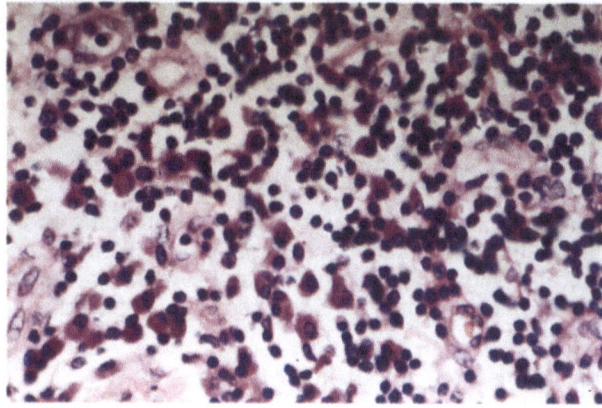

Figure 11.12 A diffuse chronic inflammatory cell infiltrate, rich in plasma cells, in which several vasa vasorum can be identified in this case of syphilitic aortitis. H & E × 400

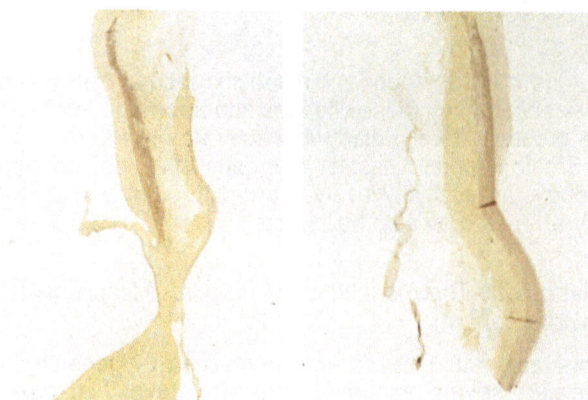

Figure 11.13a (left) The root of the aorta and aortic valve leaflet have been sectioned to show the severe intimal thickening and adventitial thickening of the aorta in this case of Takayasu's disease. Initially, the elastic tissue is normal but progressively diminishes. **Figure 11.13b** (right) At the upper limit of the section no elastic tissue can be identified in the media. As the lower margin is reached the elastic tissue becomes progressively normal.

Figures 11.13a and b are selected from the upper and lower margins of the diseased aorta. Elastic van Gieson × 1

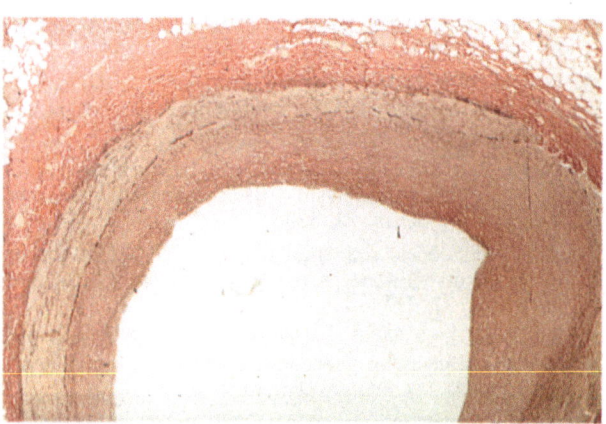

Figure 11.14a Cross-section of part of a large coronary artery involved in Takayasu's disease. Fragmentation of the internal elastic lamina is severe. The concentrically arranged intimal thickening is devoid of elastic tissue. The adventitia is also thick and fibrotic. Elastic van Gieson × 25

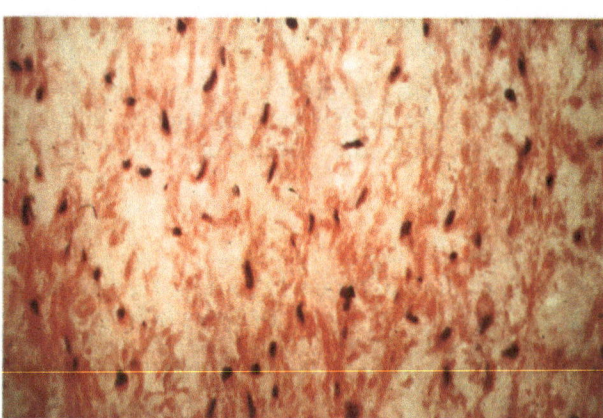

Figure 11.14b A close-up view of the intimal thickening which is composed of loosely arranged collagen tissue and mucoid material. Diagnostically elastic tissue is absent. Elastic van Gieson × 400

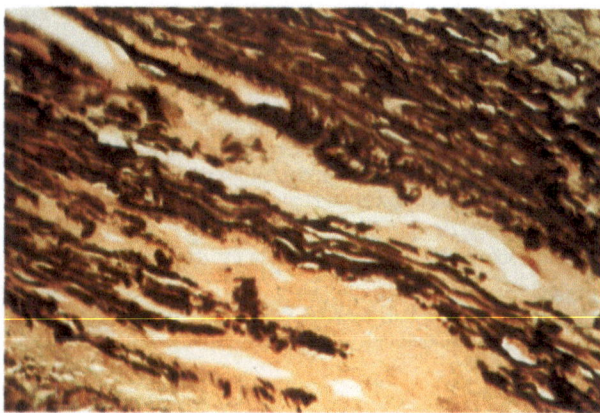

Figure 11.15a Elastic tissue is severely fragmented at the lower right border of the illustration which has been selected from an area where medial changes begin in Takayasu's disease. Elastic van Gieson × 200

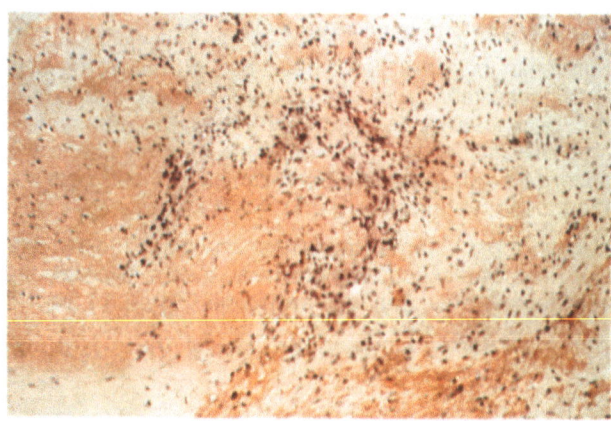

Figure 11.15b This illustration has also been selected from the junction of normal to abnormal aortic media. Chronic inflammatory cells and occasional giant cells are often present. H & E × 50

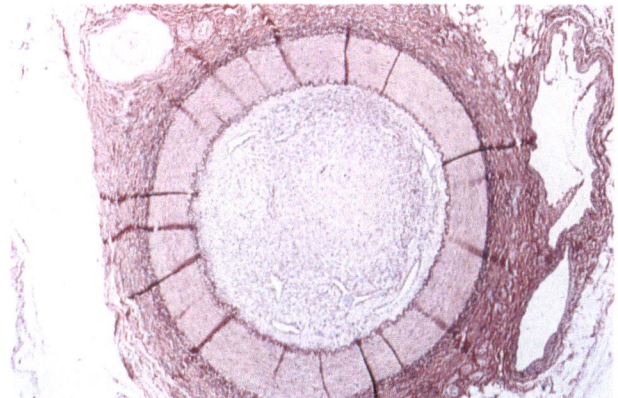

Figure 11.16a Cross-section of the popliteal artery of a case with Buerger's disease. The features are diagnostic consisting of an *intact* internal elastic lamina and a totally occluded lumen filled with *non-contracting* thrombus. Elastic van Gieson × 25

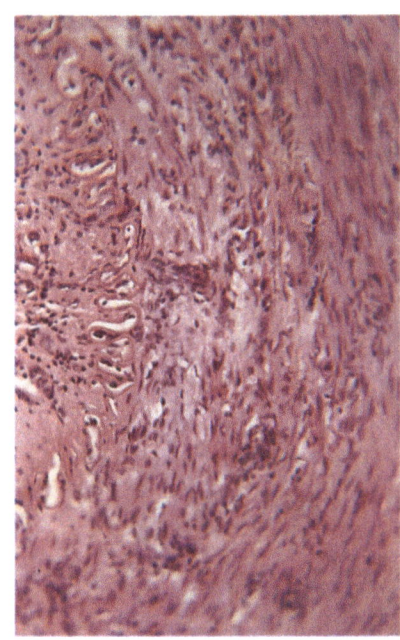

Figure 11.16b From the wall of a medium-sized artery with Buerger's disease showing a panarteritis. The intact internal elastic lamina is thick and convoluted and can even be seen clearly on haematoxylin and eosin staining along the left side of this illustration H & E × 100

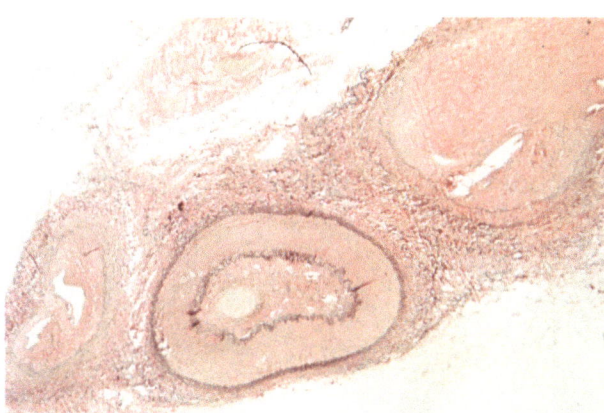

Figure 11.17 An artery and its branch, a vein and a nerve are illustrated. The vessels are bound together by dense collagen tissue. The nerve is also surrounded by collagen tissue. This 'triad' is often seen in Buerger's disease. Elastic van Gieson × 10

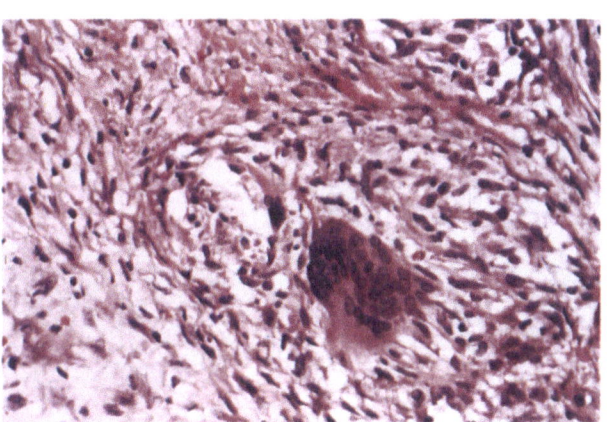

Figure 11.18 Illustration of an area from the centre of an arterial thrombus in Buerger's disease showing a giant cell and aggregation of inflammatory cells. H & E × 200

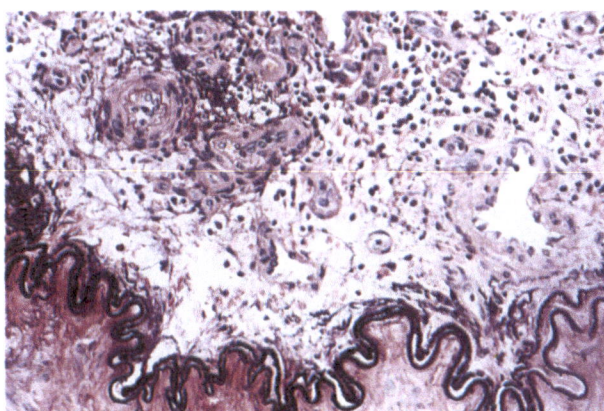

Figure 11.19 In the thrombus, several thick vascular channels, of capillary size but with a thick muscular coat, are also typical of the healed phase of Buerger's disease. Note the intact, thick elastic lamina. Elastic van Gieson × 100

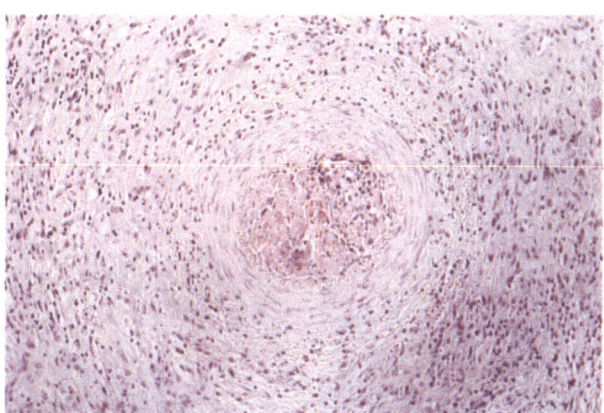

Figure 11.20 Muscular artery from the big toe from a case with Buerger's disease showing all the typical features. H & E × 50

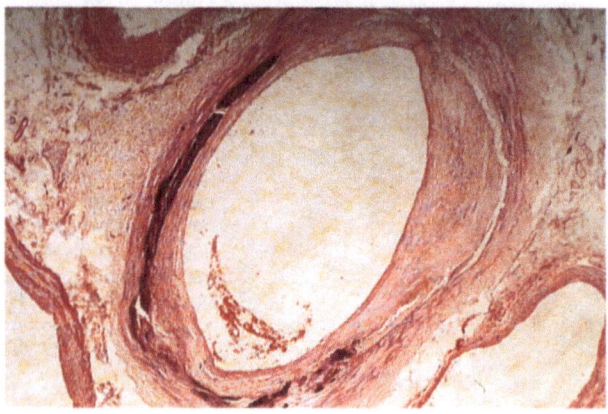

Figure 11.21 Illustrates Mönckeberg's sclerosis of an artery from the arm. The medial calcification is clearly seen affecting approximately half of the arterial media. Arteriosclerosis is also present. H & E × 25

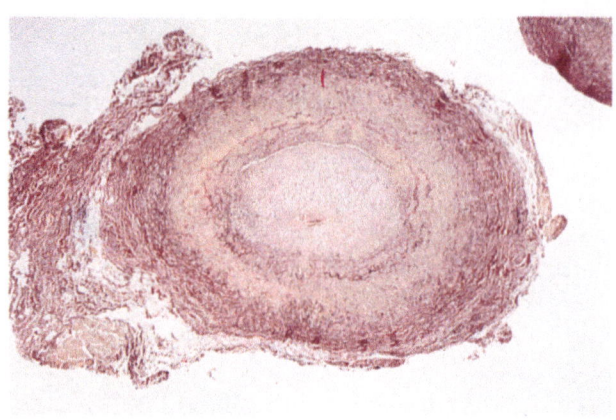

Figure 11.22 Giant cell or temporal arteritis. The photomicrograph shows the features which are illustrated in detail below. Elastic van Gieson × 10

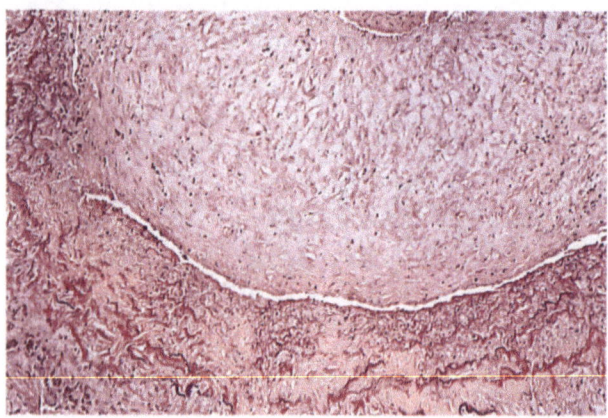

Figure 11.23 Illustration of the intimal thickening in giant cell arteritis often composed in two layers, the inner layer being composed of loosely arranged connective tissue, and an outer layer which is adjacent to the severely fragmented elastic lamina. This outer layer of the adventitia is composed of dense collagen tissue. Elastic van Gieson × 50

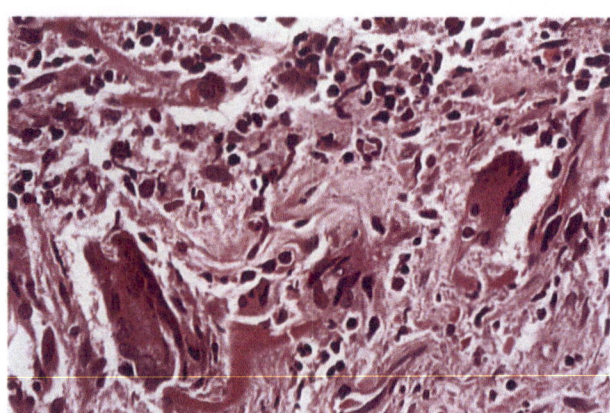

Figure 11.24 A giant cell arteritis from the intimal/medial junction showing giant cells and a mixed inflammatory cell infiltrate. The eosinophilic fragments are elastic tissue. H & E × 200

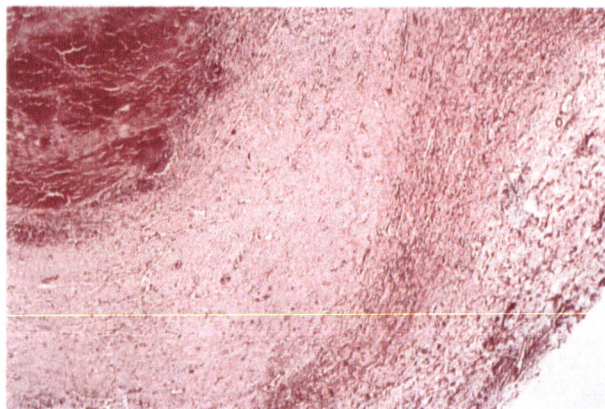

Figure 11.25 A part of the subclavian artery involved in giant cell arteritis. The lumen is occluded by thrombus. Note also the severe intimal thickening and inflammatory cells in the adventitia. H & E × 25

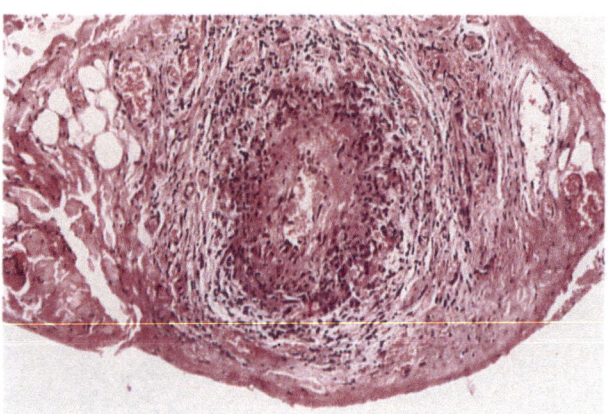

Figure 11.26 Polymyalgia rheumatica. A small artery from the leg showing all the features of giant cell arteritis illustrated in Figure 11.25. The lumen in this vessel is not occluded by thrombus. H & E × 10

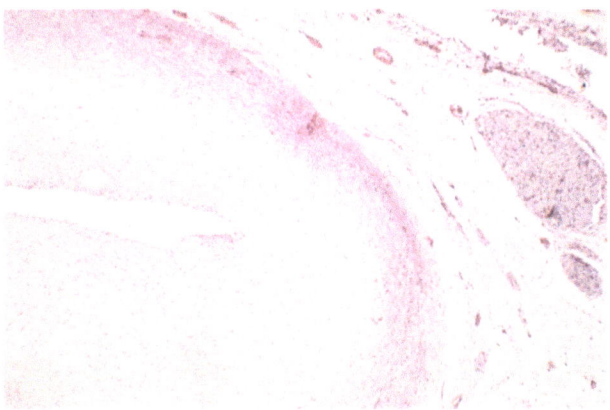

Figure 11.27a Infantile occlusive arteriopathy. Cross-section of a coronary artery (near the ostium) from an infant aged 13 months showing myofibroblastic intimal proliferation, severely narrowing the lumen. Calcification is not present. H & E × 50

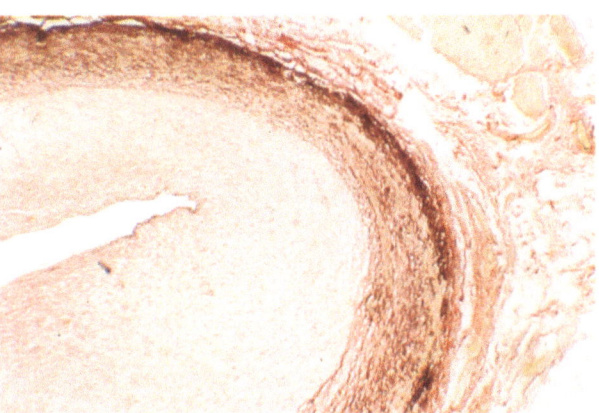

Figure 11.27b From the same artery as Figure 11.27a showing virtual absence of elastic tissue in the intimal proliferation. Elastic van Gieson × 50

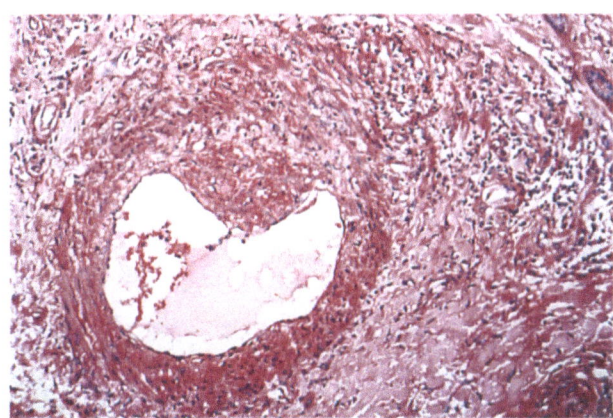

Figure 11.28 Fibrinoid necrosis of the arterial wall and a severe inflammatory infiltrate (predominantly lymphocytic in this illustration) characterizes polyarteritis nodosa. H & E × 50

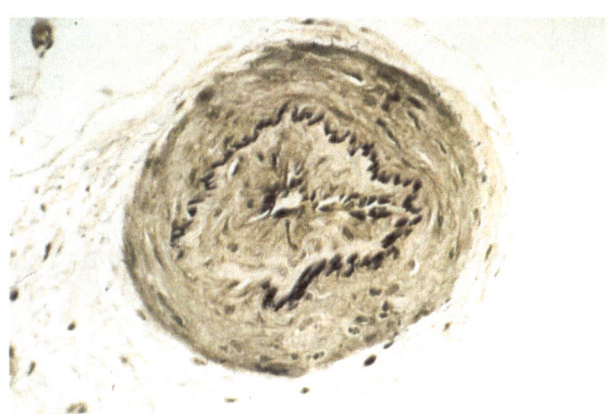

Figure 11.29 A healed small renal artery affected by polyarteritis nodosa. The internal elastic lamina is fragmented and the lumen severely narrowed by organizing thrombus. Elastic van Gieson × 50

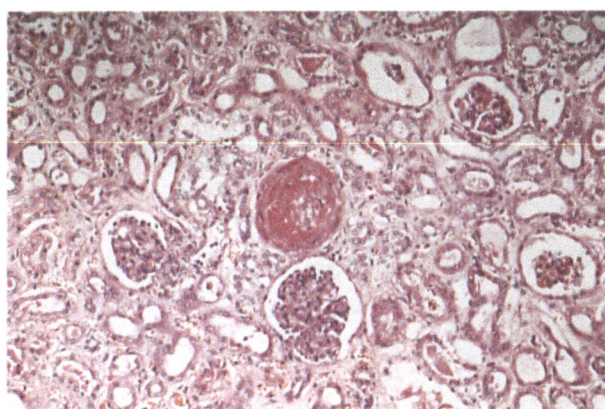

Figure 11.30 Thrombotic thrombocytopenic purpura in a small renal artery. The lumen is occluded by fibrin and the wall shows extensive fibrinoid necrosis. Note the absence of any inflammatory cells surrounding the vessel. H & E × 100

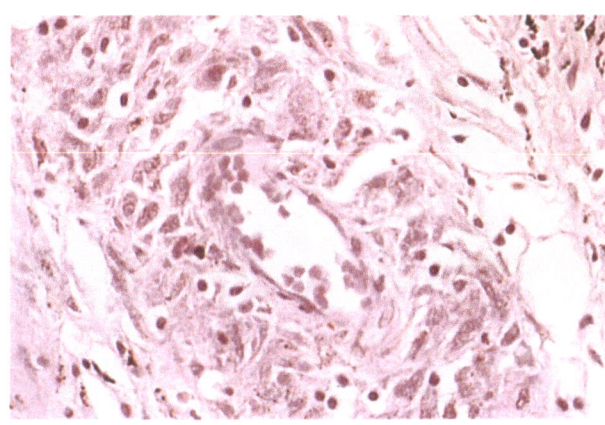

Figure 11.31 Rheumatic vasculitis of vasa vasorum of the aorta showing an Aschoff nodule surrounding the vessel. Aschoff cells, Anitschkow cells and some chronic inflammatory cells are identified. H & E × 200

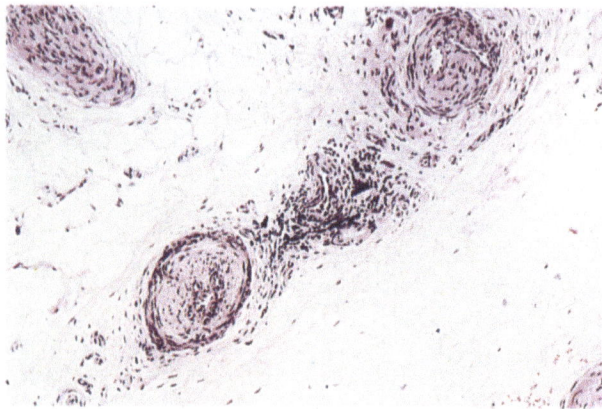

Figure 11.32 Synovial biopsy showing vascular involvement in rheumatoid arthritis. Some adventitial chronic inflammatory cells are seen. Intimal thickening is severe in this case.   H & E × 50

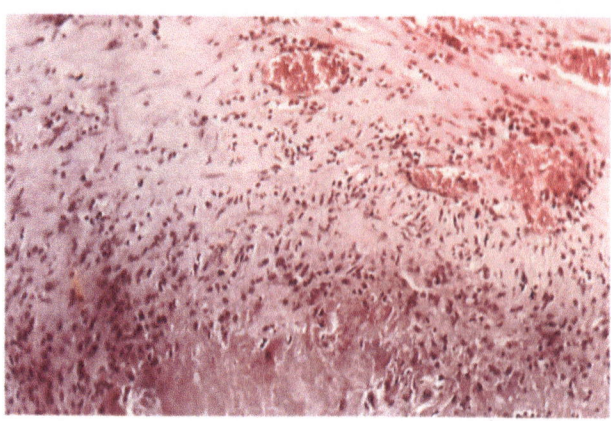

Figure 11.33 A rheumatic nodule is illustrated in this patient with rheumatoid arthritis. A central zone of necrosis, surrounded by histocytes which show palisading, is identified. A few lymphocytes and plasma cells can also be seen.   H & E × 100

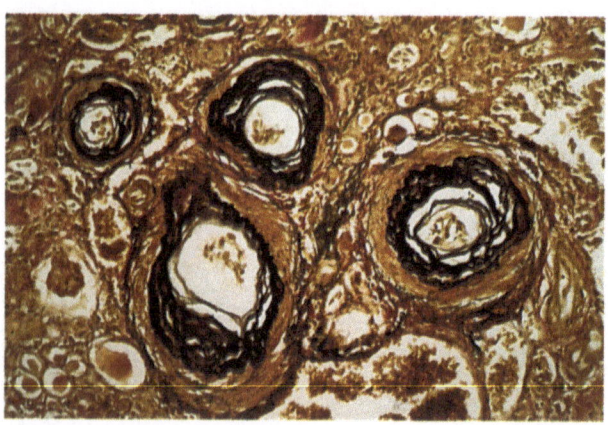

Figure 11.34 Photomicrograph of renal arteries and arterioles in benign essential hypertension. The vascular walls are thick and intimal concentric layering of elastic tissue is characteristic.   Elastic van Gieson × 100

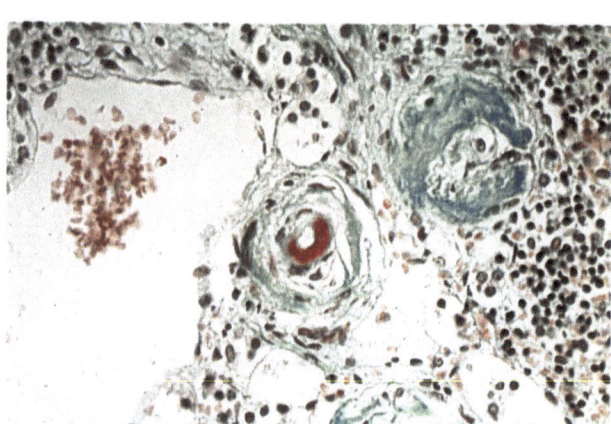

Figure 11.35 Arteriolar changes in 'malignant' hypertension are characterized by fibrinoid necrosis of the wall and fragmentation of the internal elastic lamina.   Martius Scarlet Blue × 200

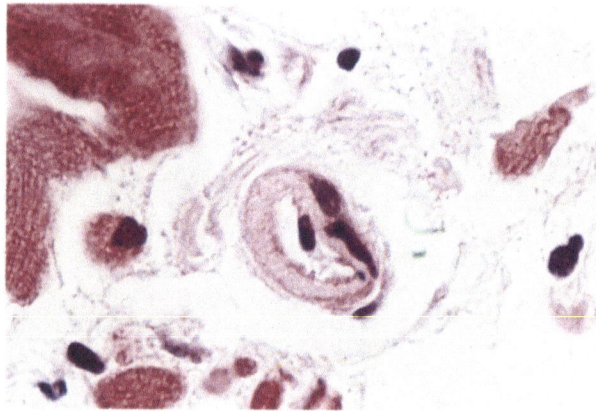

Figure 11.36 Vascular involvement by diabetes mellitus of the heart showing sub-intimal hyaline change (early) of an arteriole. H & E × 400 (By courtesy of Dr G. Lindorp)

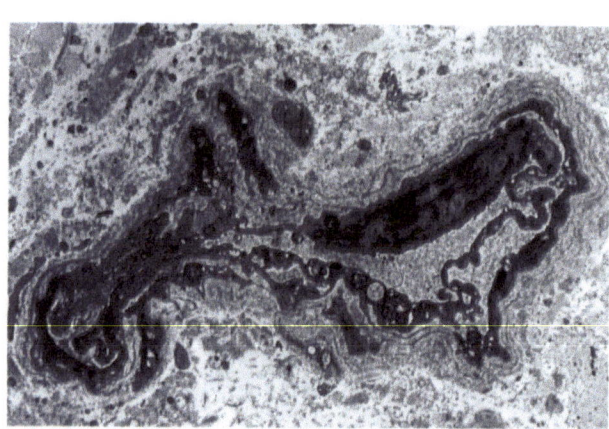

Figure 11.37 Electron micrograph showing thickening of the basement membrane and reduplication in vascular involvement of the heart in diabetes mellitus. Lead citrate and uranyl acetate ×12 000 (By courtesy of Dr G. Lindorp)

To appreciate the changes that occur as a result of pulmonary hypertension it is, perhaps, relevant to consider the normal histology of the pulmonary circulation. For convenience of description the pulmonary vasculature can be divided into:

the extrapulmonary vasculature;
the intrapulmonary vasculature.

Normal Pulmonary Vasculature

Extrapulmonary Vasculature

The pulmonary trunk and the right and left main pulmonary arteries are composed of elastic tissue, smooth muscle fibres and collagen tissue. In the adult the elastic tissue is sparse and fragmented. Clubbing of the terminal portions of the fragmented elastic fibrils can often be identified[1] (Figure 12.1). The smooth muscle fibres are circularly and longitudinally arranged.

In the newborn and up to approximately the age of 11 years, the elastic pattern of the extrapulmonary arteries differs from that of the adult in that up to the age of 2 years the elastic pattern is that of the aorta (Figure 12.2) but thereafter progressive diminution up to the age of 11 years results in the adult configuration.

Intrapulmonary Vasculature

The intrapulmonary arteries down to a level of an external diameter of 1000 μm are designated elastic arteries. Well-defined internal and external elastic laminae are found and, depending on the size of the vessel, regular bands of elastic tissue can be identified in the media (Figure 12.3).

The muscular pulmonary arteries are vessels of 1000 to 100 μm (external diameter). The histological features consist of well-defined internal and external laminae and a thin muscular coat (Figure 12.4)[2]. Frequently, for convenience, separation is made between large and small muscular arteries. Small muscular arteries can be defined as those vessels measuring between 200 and 100 μm external diameter. Furthermore, transitional arteries, 1000–600 μm, have been described and these are vessels of muscular size where, in addition to the smooth muscle, some fragmented elastic fibres can be identified in the media (Figure 12.5).

Arterioles are defined as those vessels measuring 100 μm or less. They are composed of one elastic lamina only (external) but occasionally a smooth muscle fibre can be identified to approximately 70 μm diameter (Figure 12.6).

As far as the adventitia is concerned, this consists of collagen tissue and lymphatic vessels. It is usually less in width than the media in the elastic arteries but is several times thicker around the muscular arteries to about 300 μm external diameter. Thereafter the adventitia becomes progressively less, so that when the small muscular arteries are reached only a few wisps of adventitia are present.

The Pulmonary Veins

These consist of a well-defined internal elastic lamina, fragmented elastic fibrils, smooth muscle and collagen tissue in the media but have no external elastic lamina. The junction between the media and the adventitia is ill-defined (Figure 12.7). Apart from their location, no histological differences between intra- and extrapulmonary veins exist.

The veins of the *systemic circulation* are also identical, histologically, but as far as the arterial system is concerned only the aorta and its immediate large branches are elastic vessels. The elastic fibrils are in regular alignment (Figure 12.8) which – apart from age changes – remains constant throughout life.

The systemic muscular arteries (the bronchial arteries in the lungs) consist of a well-defined internal elastic lamina, a thick muscular coat and no external elastic lamina (Figure 12.9). Not infrequently, at the medial/adventitial junction some fragmented elastic fibres may condense to form a pseudo-external elastic lamina.

The arterioles in this system are also defined as vessels below the size of 100 μm and consist of an internal elastic lamina and a thick muscular coat which is recognizable to the level of approximately 30 μm (Figure 12.10).

The Changes in Pulmonary Hypertension

Definition and Classification of Pulmonary Hypertension

Pulmonary hypertension is considered to be present when the systolic and diastolic pressures of the pulmonary artery exceed 21.5/9.5 mmHg and when the mean pressure exceeds 14.8 mmHg. It should be added that this is the pressure in adults at rest[3].

Pulmonary hypertension can be classified[4] into primary and secondary types.

Secondary Pulmonary Hypertension

(1) *Passive pulmonary hypertension* (due to raised venous pressure). Examples include left ventricular failure following myocardial infarction, myxoma, cor triatriatum and stenosis of the pulmonary veins or any other cause leading to heart failure.

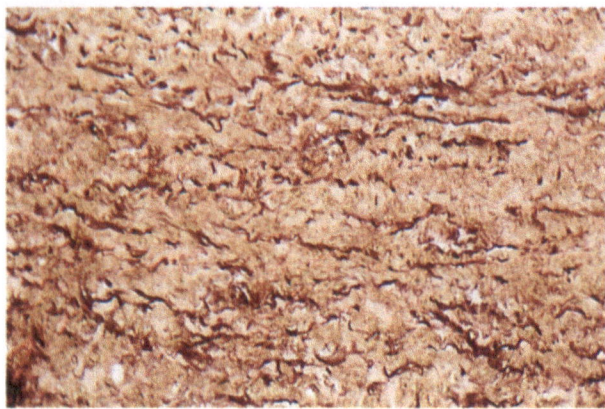

Figure 12.1 Adult pulmonary trunk characterized by fragmented, sparse elastic fibres, many of which show thickening towards their ends which can be club-shaped.   Elastic van Gieson × 200

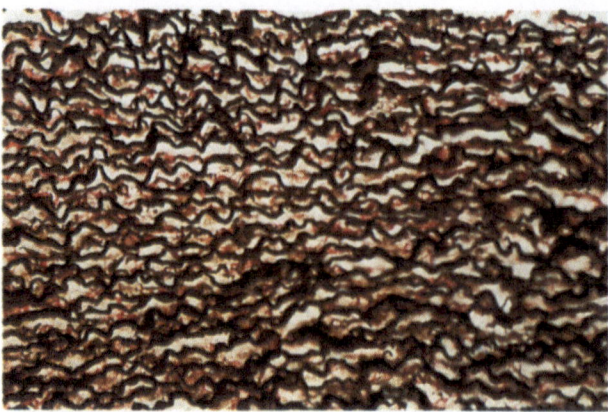

Figure 12.2 Photomicrograph of the pulmonary trunk of a child aged 1½ years. The elastic fibres are in regular, parallel alignment resembling aorta.   Elastic van Gieson × 400

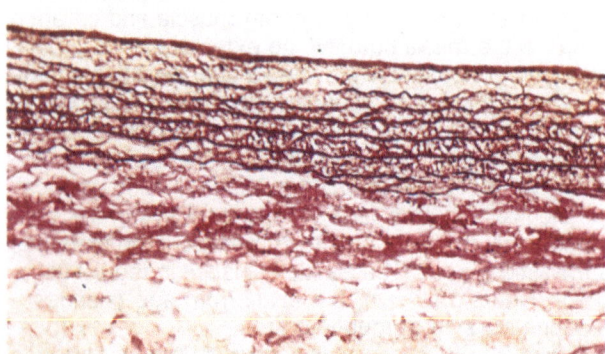

Figure 12.3 Intrapulmonary elastic artery showing, apart from the internal and external elastic laminae, regular bands of elastic fibres. Their number depends on the size of the artery.   Elastic van Gieson × 75

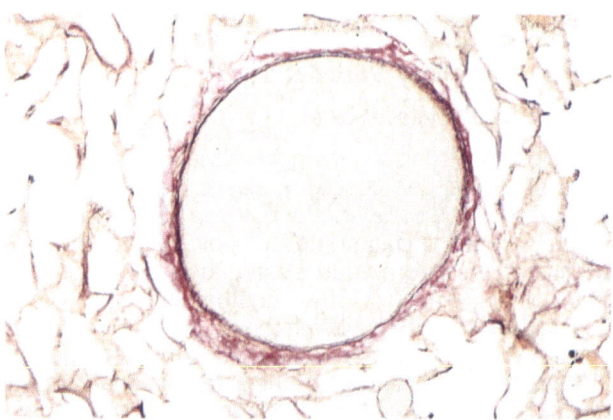

Figure 12.4 Small pulmonary muscular arteries (150 μm diameter) showing well-defined internal and external elastic laminae enclosing a thin muscular coat. The adventitia (in red) is thin. The substance filling the lumen in this and subsequent illustrations is injecting material.   Elastic van Gieson × 100

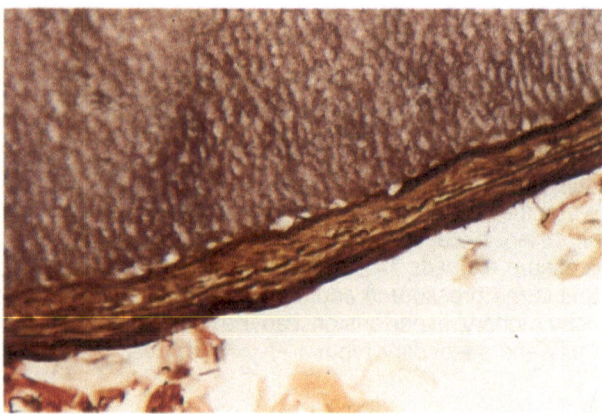

Figure 12.5 Transitional pulmonary artery. In the media some elastic fragments can be seen.   Elastic van Gieson × 50

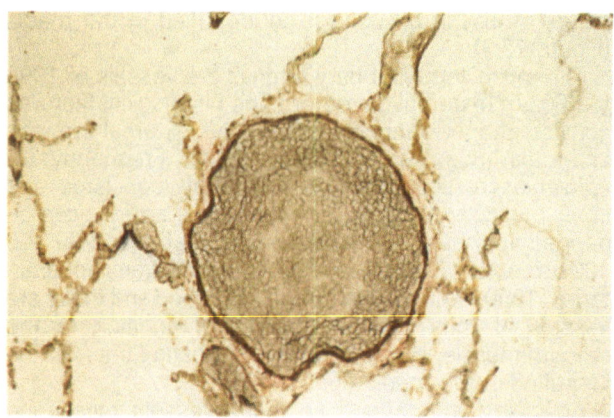

Figure 12.6 A pulmonary arteriole characterized by its size (below 100 μm external diameter) and a single (external) elastic lamina.   Elastic van Gieson × 200

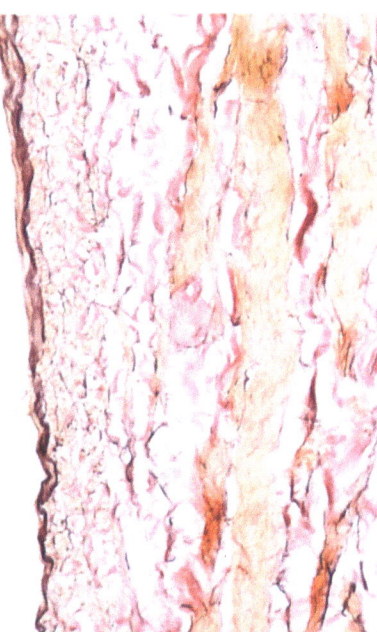

Figure 12.7 Close-up view of the wall of a pulmonary vein showing fragmented elastic tissue throughout the media. Bundles of smooth muscle can be prominent. The medial/adventitial junction is ill-defined. Elastic van Gieson × 400

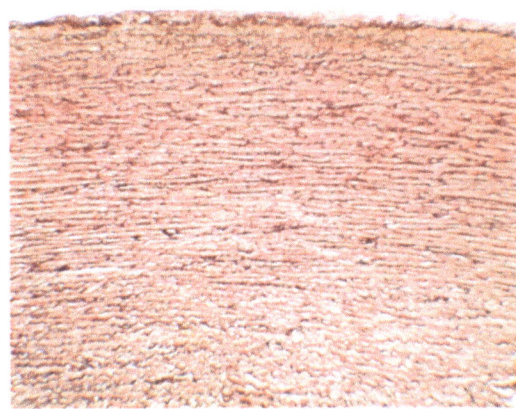

Figure 12.8 Photomicrograph of an aorta. In the media, regularly aligned elastic fibres are seen. Elastic van Gieson × 50

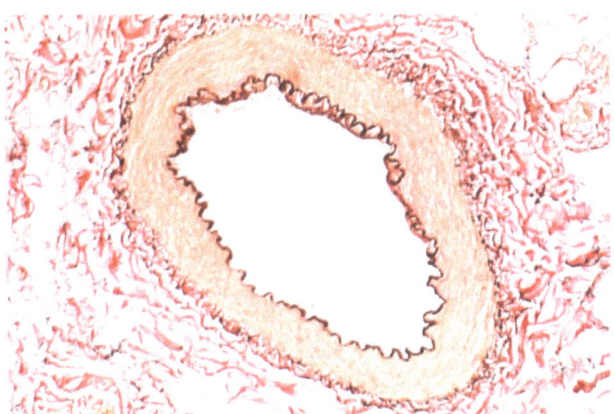

Figure 12.9 Systemic muscular artery (bronchial) showing a well-defined internal elastic lamina, a thick muscular wall and no external elastic lamina. Condensation of adventitial elastic tissue may form a 'pseudo-external elastic lamina'. Elastic van Gieson × 50

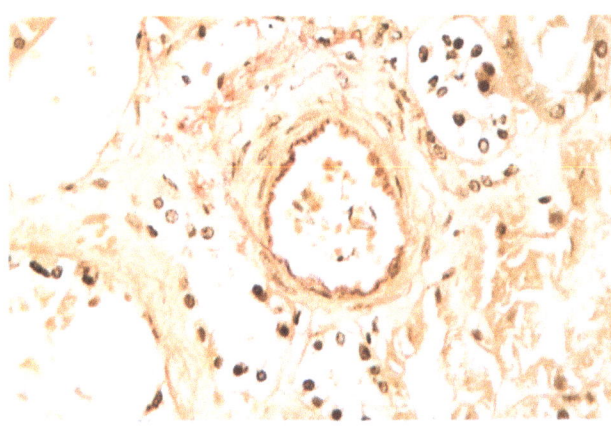

Figure 12.10 Illustration of a systemic arteriole showing an internal elastic lamina and a thick muscular coat. Elastic van Gieson × 400

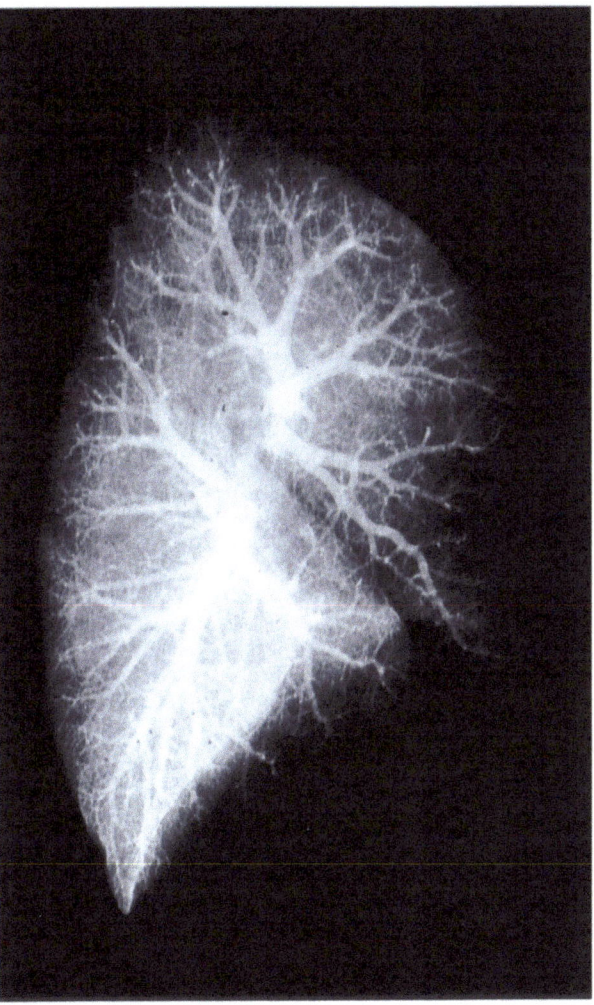

Figure 12.11 Postmortem pulmonary angiogram showing a normal arterial tree. The lumina of the elastic arteries gradually diminishes towards the sub-pleural regions. Good background filling is present (filling of muscular arteries and arterioles). Both zones are equally well filled

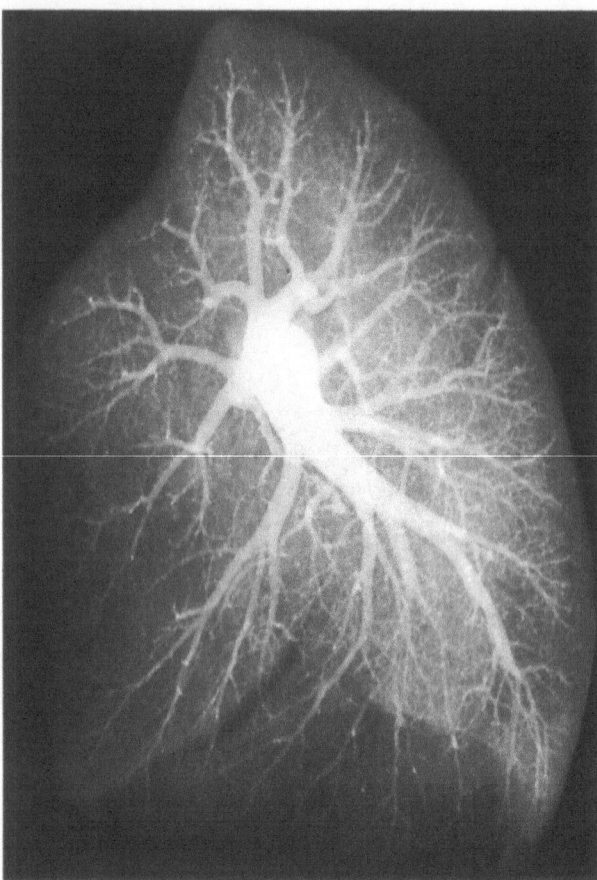

Figure 12.12 Postmorten angiogram of a patient's lung with passive pulmonary hypertension characterized by zonal differentiation which can often be observed in this type of pulmonary hypertension. The upper zone is normally perfused but the lower zone shows diminution of the tertiary branches of the elastic artery and diminished peripheral filling

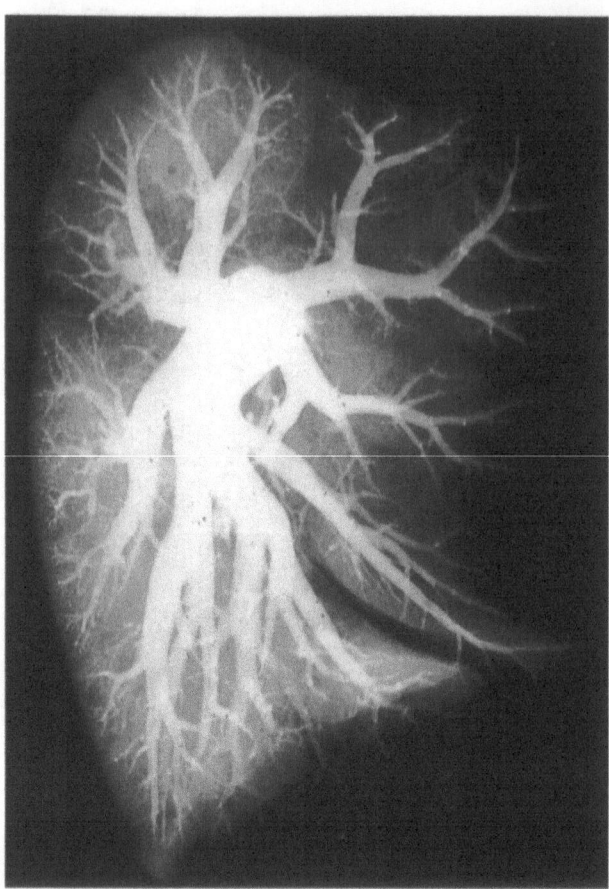

Figure 12.13 Pulmonary hypertension from a patient with an atrial septal defect in the region of the fossa ovalis (Type 2a). Severe dilatation of the elastic arteries and extensive pruning of arterioles and muscular arteries is clearly seen

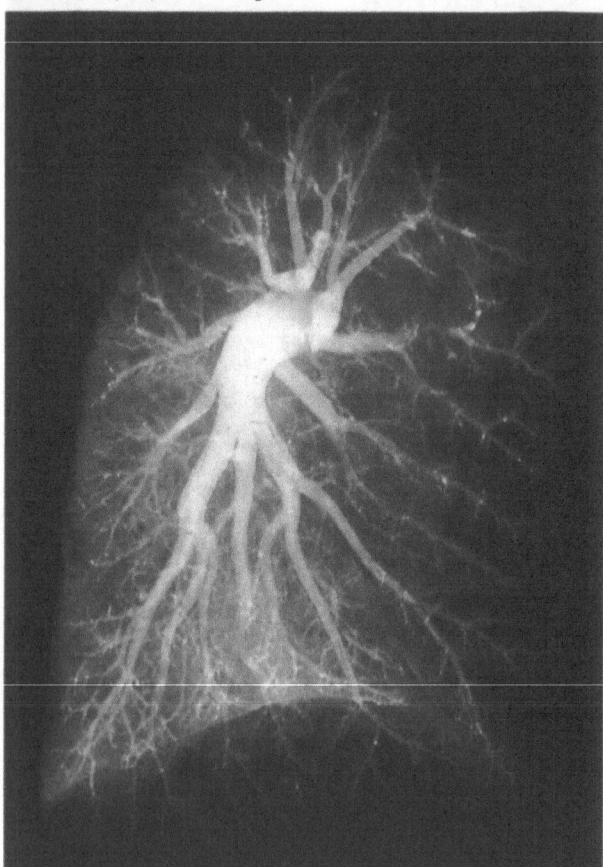

Figure 12.14 Hyperkinetic pulmonary hypertension due to a ventricular septal defect (Type 2b). The features described in the lower zone of Figure 12.12 are also present in the upper zone

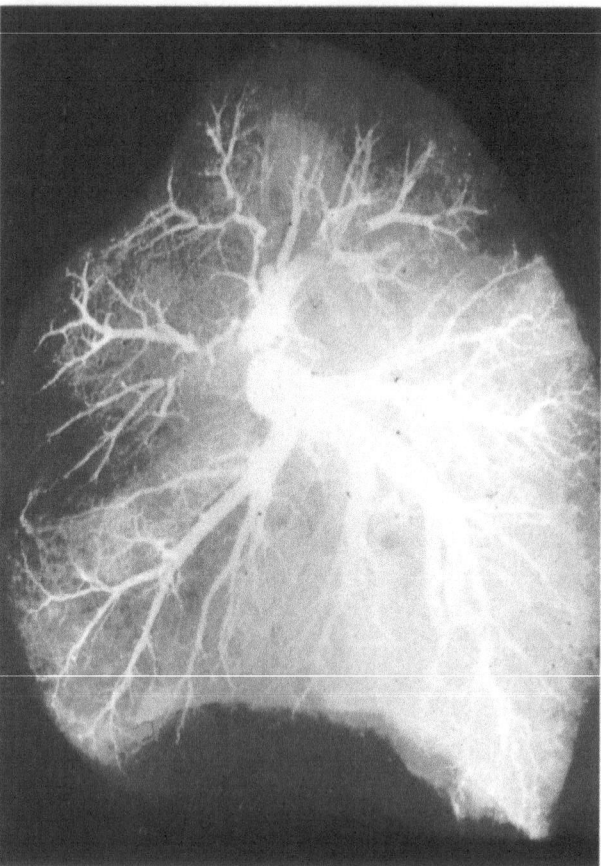

Figure 12.15 Pulmonary angiogram showing several occlusions of the elastic arterial tree, particularly in the apical segment due to thrombo-emboli. The narrow lumina of the elastic arteries, unaffected by thrombo-emboli, and evidence of pruning suggest pulmonary hypertension

(2) *Hyperkinetic pulmonary hypertension*. This can either be due to:
   (a) increased pulmonary flow as in atrial septal defects with left to right shunt; or
   (b) increased force as in ventricular septal defect, patent ductus arteriosus or aorto-pulmonary defect.

(3) *Vaso-obstructive pulmonary hypertension*. This can be:
   (a) luminal as with thrombo-embolism, thrombosis or from non-thrombotic causes such as liquor amnii, tumour or fat embolism;
   (b) in the arterial wall as in polyarteritis nodosa, scleroderma, disseminated lupus erythematosus or Takayasu's disease;
   (c) in the lung parenchyma, which can be due to fibrosis whatever the cause, pneumoconiosis, silicosis, asbestosis or coalminer's lung. Emphysema accompanied by acute bronchitis may also be included.

(4) *Vasoconstrictive pulmonary hypertension*. This is due to increased vascular tonus and may accompany any of the types of pulmonary hypertension mentioned above.

Angiographic Patterns

For good visualization or if morphometric studies are envisaged the pulmonary arterial tree (Figure 12.11) or the venous system can conveniently be injected by means of the apparatus shown in Chapter 1, Figure 1.4 or by manual injection. The normal pulmonary vascular tree shows gradual diminution of the lumina of the elastic arteries and good peripheral filling (i.e. of the muscular arteries and arterioles).

Passive pulmonary hypertension For descriptive purposes the lungs can be divided into zones. The upper zone is defined as the upper lobe and the apical segment of the lower lobe. The lower zone is defined as the middle lobe or lingula and the lower lobe, except for the apical segment.

Zonal differentiation is present in up to 85% of patients with passive pulmonary hypertension[5]. The upper zone is similar in appearance to the normal lung but, when the secondary and tertiary branches in the lower zone are reached, narrowing of the elastic arterial lumina is observed together with underperfusion or 'pruning' of the muscular type of arteries (Figure 12.12). This is due to the changes of pulmonary hypertension becoming manifest (see below).

Hyperkinetic pulmonary hypertension When the flow is increased, as in atrial septal defect, severe dilatation of all the elastic arteries is typical together with extensive pruning of the muscular arteries. There is no zonal differentiation (Figure 12.13).

If pulmonary hypertension is due to excessive force the changes observed in the lower zone in passive pulmonary hypertension are also observed in the upper zone (Figure 12.14). Similar features are also seen in primary pulmonary hypertension.

Vaso-obstructive hypertension Injection with radio-opaque material clearly defines the site of emboli or thrombi that may have caused the pulmonary infarction (Figure 12.15). A tumour embolus is illustrated in Figure 12.16. Organization of thrombo-emboli results in formation of septae (Figure 12.17) or the obstruction may remain in which numerous channels of revascularization can be identified (Figure 12.18).

Histological Changes of Pulmonary Hypertension

If pulmonary hypertension is significant before the age of 2 years, the aortic configuration of the elastic media will remain even if the cause for pulmonary hypertension is removed at a later date. If, on the other hand, pulmonary hypertension becomes significant after the age of 2, then no matter how severe or how long pulmonary hypertension has been present, the elastic of adult configuration will be attained.

For convenience the grading of Heath and Edwards, 1958[6] will be described. As this type of grading was devised for pulmonary hypertension consequent to congenital heart disease with a shunt, it is therefore not applicable to all types of pulmonary hypertension. The striking features are observed in the muscular types of arteries and arterioles.

Grade one
An increase in the medial muscular coat is observed (Figure 12.19). In the arterioles a muscular coat also develops which results in the formation of well-defined internal and external elastic laminae (Figure 12.20). This is referred to as 'arterialization of arterioles'. It is often the first morphological sign that pulmonary hypertension is present.

Grade two
This is exemplified by medial hypertrophy and intimal thickening of the cellular type (Figure 12.21).

Grade three
Medial hypertrophy continues to be observed but intimal thickening, fibro-elastic in type, either concentrically (Figure 12.22) or eccentrically arranged (Figure 12.23), or total occlusion of the lumen characterizes this type of pulmonary hypertension.

Grade four (Grades four to six are severe grades of pulmonary hypertension.)
Grade four is characterized by plexiform and other dilatation lesions. Medial atrophy is found in the parent vessels frequently with an intimal rim of fibro-elastic tissue and, in the cases of plexiform lesions, an outpouching of the vessels is seen with various vascular channels in the pouch (Figure 12.24). Dilatation lesions may take the form of angiomatoid lesions (Figure 12.25) or vein-like dilatations.

Grade five
Grade five consists of haemosiderin deposition throughout the lung. Iron encrustation of the various vascular components such as the elastic laminae. A large number of iron-laden macrophages can be striking (Figure 12.26).

Grade six
Fibrinoid necrosis of the media and an inflammatory infiltrate typifies this grade (Figure 12.27a and b).

It is believed that the plexiform and dilatation lesions are consequent to fibrinoid necrosis of the media (Grade six) and therefore the grading system breaks down as the natural sequence would be Grades one, two and three, Grades six, four and five. For this reason Grades four, five and six are referred to as 'severe pulmonary hypertension'. Grading is also insufficient as far as reporting of pulmonary biopsies is concerned because no indication as to the severity and extent of the lesions is given[7]. It is therefore necessary to evaluate the vessels numerically and to express the result as a percentage, indicating the type of vessel involved and the degree of intimal thickening and other changes that may be present. The stated grade of pulmonary hypertension is

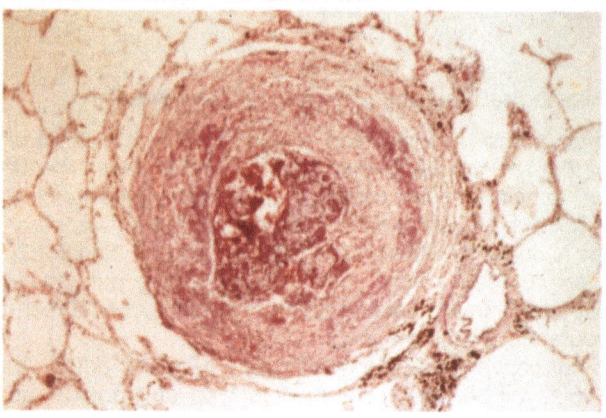

Figure 12.16 Photomicrograph of a muscular artery occluded by a tumour-embolus (chorion carcinoma). Medial hypertrophy is also present. H & E × 100

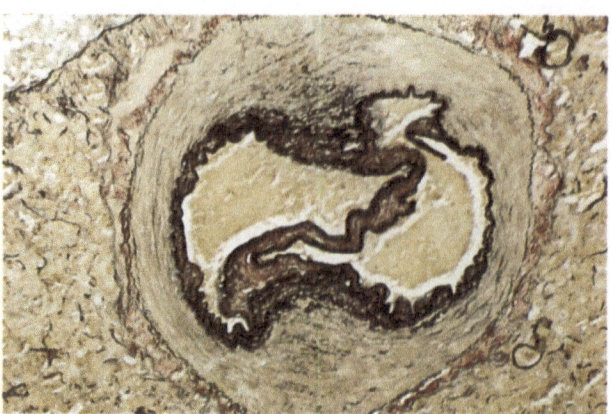

Figure 12.17 Organization of thrombo-emboli often results in septae straddling the vascular lumen. Severe medial hypertrophy is seen indicative of pulmonary hypertension. Elastic van Gieson × 100

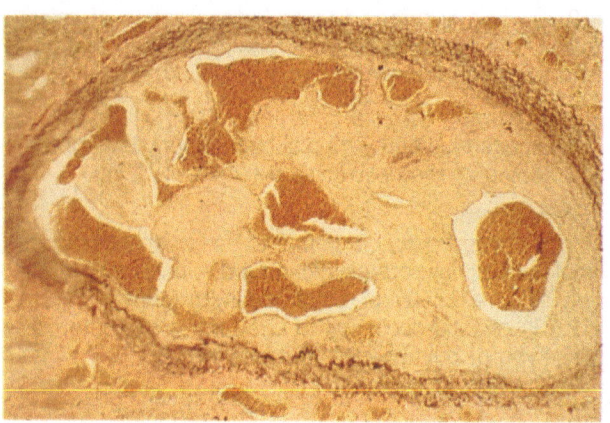

Figure 12.18 Organization of thrombo-emboli may also result in revascularization (capillary-sized channels) within the original thrombo-embolus. Elastic van Gieson × 50

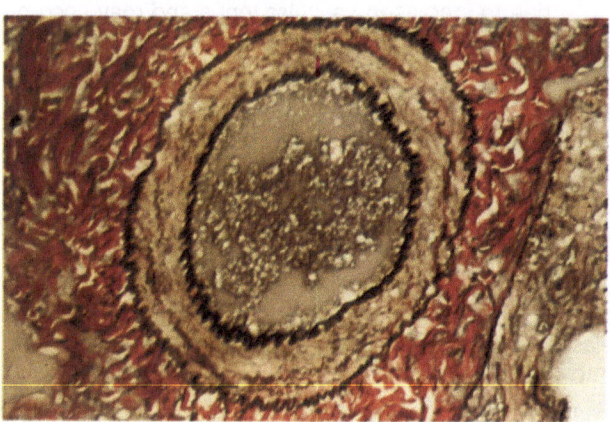

Figure 12.19 Photomicrograph of a pulmonary muscular artery showing a thick muscular coat. Elastic van Gieson × 100

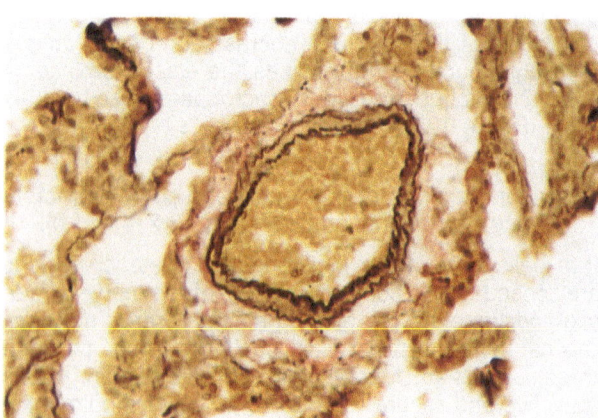

Figure 12.20 Illustration of an arteriole in which two elastic lamina can be identified enclosing a well-developed muscular coat. This is referred to as 'arterialization of arterioles'. Elastic van Gieson × 250

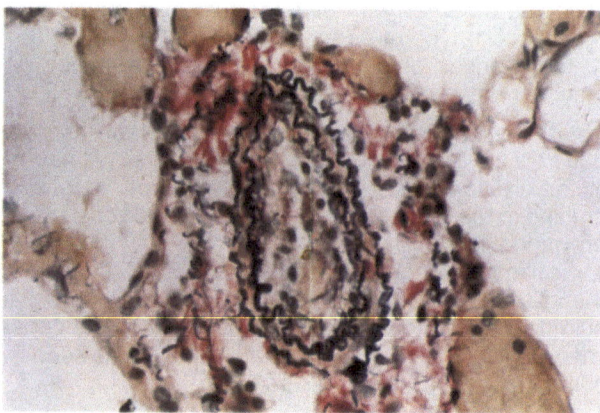

Figure 12.21 'Grade two' pulmonary hypertension in an arteriole showing arterialization and intimal thickening in which several cellular elements, including fibroblasts, can be identified. Elastic van Gieson × 250

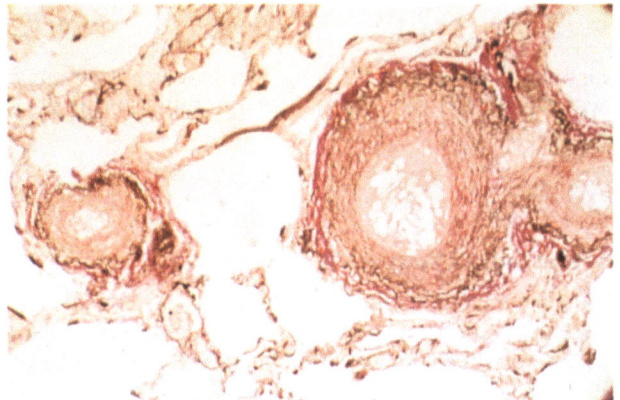

Figure 12.22 Concentric intimal thickening by predominantly collagen tissue in arteries together with medial hypertrophy characterizes 'Grade three' pulmonary hypertension. Elastic van Gieson × 200

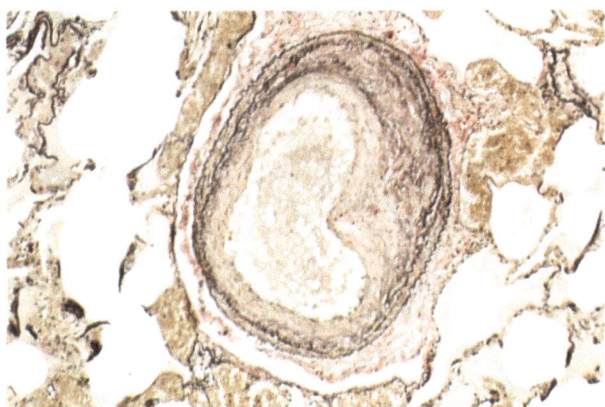

Figure 12.23 The intimal thickening may be fibro-elastic in type and may also be eccentrically placed ('Grade three'). Elastic van Gieson × 150

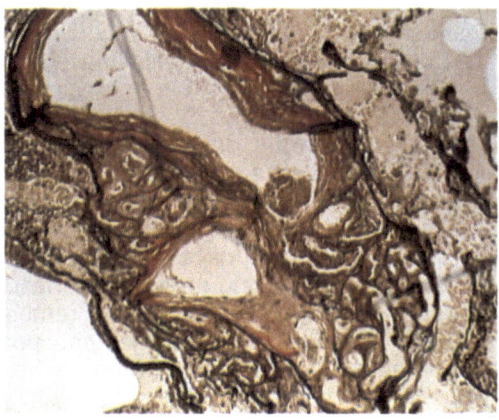

Figure 12.24 Illustration of a plexiform lesion indicative of severe pulmonary hypertension ('Grade four'). Medial atrophy is now seen in the parent vessel which shows fibrous intimal thickening. Elastic van Gieson × 100

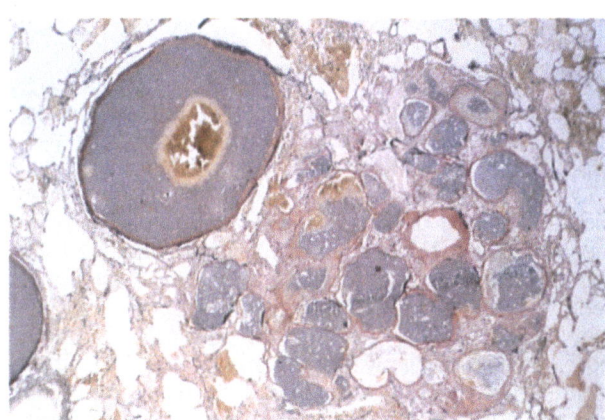

Figure 12.25 Severe pulmonary hypertension showing an angiomatoid lesion characterized by numerous vascular channels of capillary size. Apart from medial atrophy the parent vessel shows, at the level of sectioning, no abnormality. Distal to the sectioning occlusion of the vessel was found on serial sectioning. Elastic van Gieson × 75

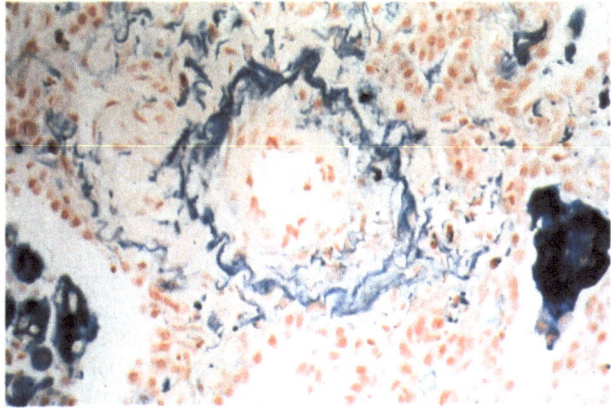

Figure 12.26 'Grade five' pulmonary hypertension showing iron deposition on the elastic lamina, cellular intimal thickening and iron-laden macrophages. Perl's reaction × 400

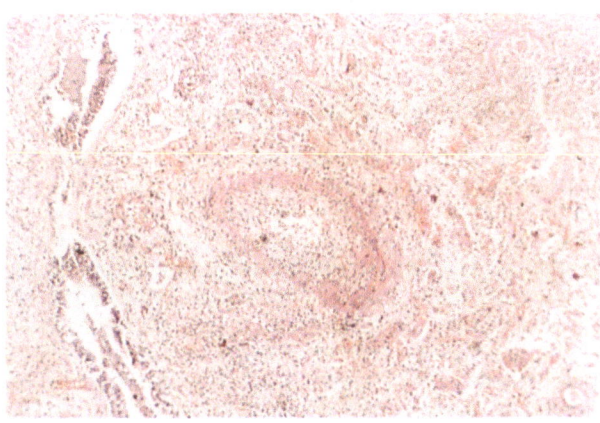

Figure 12.27a Severe pulmonary hypertension 'Grade six'. Fibrinoid necrosis and an inflammatory cell infiltrate are evident. H & E × 50

based on the highest grade of the histological changes found.

The pulmonary veins also show intimal thickening (Figure 12.28) but the assessment of medial hypertrophy or the grade, as described in the arterial system, is not so clearly defined.

In view of the points that have been raised above, Wagenvoort[8] has suggested the following five major forms of pulmonary hypertension:

vasoconstrictive pulmonary hypertension;
chronic embolic pulmonary hypertension;
chronic pulmonary venous hypertension;
chronic hypoxia; and
decreased pulmonary flow.

In decreased pulmonary flow, for example in pulmonary stenosis or tetralogy of Fallot with severe pulmonary stenosis, atrophy of the pulmonary arteries, together with intimal thickening, is found. These are frequently eccentric and referred to as Rich lesions (Figure 12.29). In chronic hypoxia, sub-intimal longitudinal muscle bundles can be identified (Figure 12.30).

Primary Pulmonary Hypertension

By definition the aetiology is unknown but various suggestions have been made including vasoconstriction and repeated small thromboemboli not leading to pulmonary infarction[9]. The severe grades of pulmonary hypertension are usually observed and for this reason a World Health Organization Expert Committee suggested that the term 'primary pulmonary hypertension' should be reserved for the clinical aspects and that from a pathologist's point of view the term 'unexplained plexogenic pulmonary arteriopathy' is more appropriate[10]. Plexiform lesions are by no means always found in cases with this disease.

The condition may be defined as a rare, progressive, usually fatal, chronic elevation of pulmonary arterial pressure of unknown aetiology, sufficient to cause enlargement of the right ventricle. Clinically dyspnoea and chest pain as well as syncope are experienced. Signs include cyanosis, right heart failure and pulmonary systolic murmurs. The prognosis is usually poor but cases of regression of symptoms have been reported. From a pathologist's point of view the severe grades of pulmonary hypertensive changes usually, but not invariably, are evident.

Pulmonary Veno-Occlusive Disease[11]

Clinical features similar to those of primary pulmonary hypertension are identified, but morphologically the small pulmonary veins and venules show severe occlusive intimal thickening and arterialization of the media (Figure 12.31). The arteries are also affected but usually to a minor degree; they may, however, contain thrombi. Oedema, congestion and small foci of interstitial pneumonia as well as fibrosis can be found in the lung parenchyma. These parenchymal changes may be observed in unexplained plexogenic pulmonary arteriopathy and indeed in all other forms of pulmonary hypertension.

Pulmonary Hypertension Associated with Oral Contraceptives

No direct association has been firmly established though

vascular intimal proliferation and severe pulmonary hypertension in the absence of thrombo-emboli have been described[12].

Regression of Pulmonary Hypertension

Once the severe grades of pulmonary hypertension have been reached, removal of the cause does not usually lead to a regression and indeed may worsen the clinical state of the patient prior to surgical intervention, and provided that occlusion of the lung by fibro-elastic tissue (Grade three) is not too widespread. In the lower grades regression of the histological changes may occur following the removal of the cause. It should, perhaps, be noted that, in general, in passive pulmonary hypertension, Grade three is the severest grade observed[10].

Organization of Thrombo-Emboli

The pulmonary circulation lends itself as a convenient experimental model to study the sequence of events of organization of thrombo-emboli. The formation of thrombi in a flowing stream have been mimiced by adaptation of an instrument first described by Chandler in 1958. Blood from a rabbit's ear vein is collected in a sequestrin bottle. The blood is then placed in a non-wettable plastic tube (Figure 12.32) and after reconstituting it with calcium chloride in normal saline it is secured on a turntable which is allowed to revolve at 16 revolutions per minute. After approximately 30 min thrombus is obtained (Figure 12.33a and b). This is finely chopped, washed and re-injected into the same vein from where the blood was drawn. The changes of events that have been observed in a number of rabbits which were killed at intervals varying between 24 h and 10 weeks, will be briefly described.

By 24 h retraction of the thrombo-embolus is already seen (Figure 12.34) and by 48 h disintegration of the cellular elements has begun (Figure 12.35). By 5 days hyperplasia of endothelial cells is becoming manifest; these enter the thrombo-embolus but as these cells reach the centre they assume the histological appearance of fibroblasts (Figure 12.36). By day 10, multinucleate cells can be observed with distintegration of the cytoplasm around which the nuclei become realigned, resulting in capillarization of the thrombo-embolus (Figure 12.37).

By day 14, collagen tissue is observed (Figure 12.38) and by day 21 elastic tissue is seen (Figure 12.39). Progressive retraction continues so that by 6 weeks only a small elevation remains (Figure 12.40). By 10 weeks, some fibro-elastic thickening is all that can be observed[13].

Similar features are observed in man and this was described in 1962–1963 by Irniger[14]. The pulmonary thrombo-emboli in man are similar to those seen in the rabbits, but the changes in the coronary arterial system are slower and therefore once the sequence of events in the lung is known multiplication by three will give the approximate date of the thrombus/thrombo-embolus in the coronary arteries.

As far as sequential changes of organization in the systemic vessels of the extremities are concerned, multiplication by two of the sequence of events in the lungs gives the approximate date of thrombo-embolus in these sites.

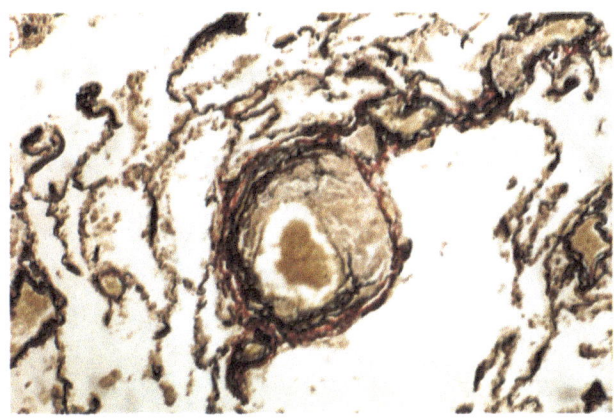

Figure 12.27b Showing 'Grade six' disruption of the internal elastic lamina. Rupture of the vascular wall explains, in this grade and in 'Grade four' (Figure 12.25), haemoptysis which may accompany severe hypertension.　Elastic van Gieson × 150

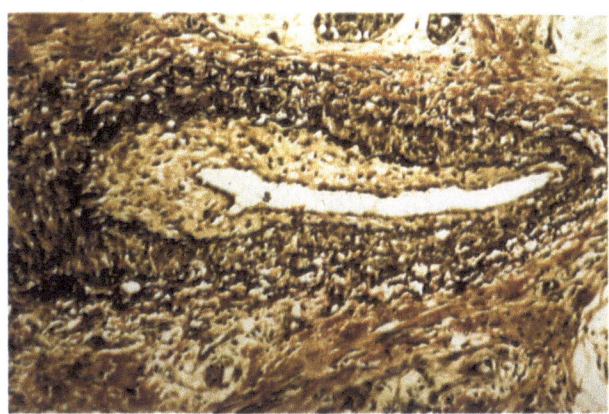

Figure 12.28 An intrapulmonary vein (not injected) is illustrated showing intimal thickening and some medial hypertrophy. The changes in veins are not so clearly assessable as in the pulmonary arterial system.　Elastic van Gieson × 250

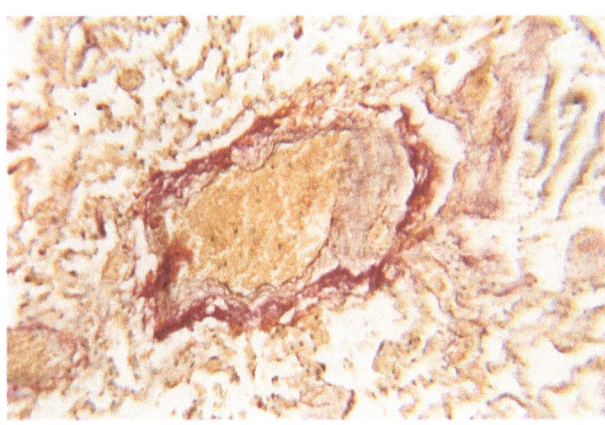

Figure 12.29 Pulmonary arteries with decreased pulmonary flow also show the intimal thickening of 'Grade three', often eccentrically placed (Rich lesions), but atrophy of the arterial wall is present. From a patient with tetralogy of Fallot with a tight pulmonary stenosis and small ventricular septal defect.　Elastic van Gieson × 75

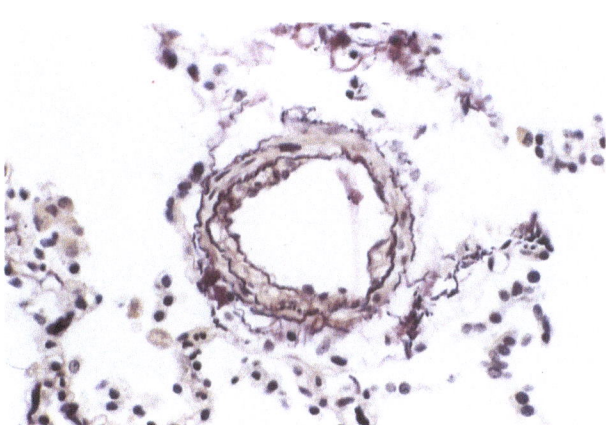

Figure 12.30 Cross-section of a small pulmonary artery showing sub-intimal longitudinal muscle bundles which are typically seen in cases of chronic hypoxia.　Elastic van Gieson × 200 (By permission of Dr B. Addis)

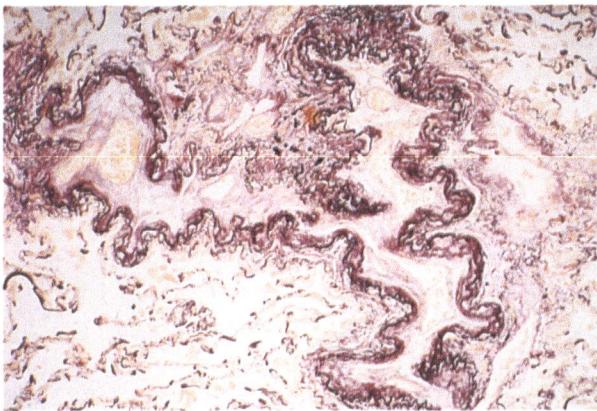

Figure 12.31 Pulmonary veno-occlusive disease showing extensive involvement of the veins which with severe intimal thickening and medial hypertrophy of the smooth muscle may mimic arteries.　Elastic van Gieson × 100 (By permission of Dr B. Addis)

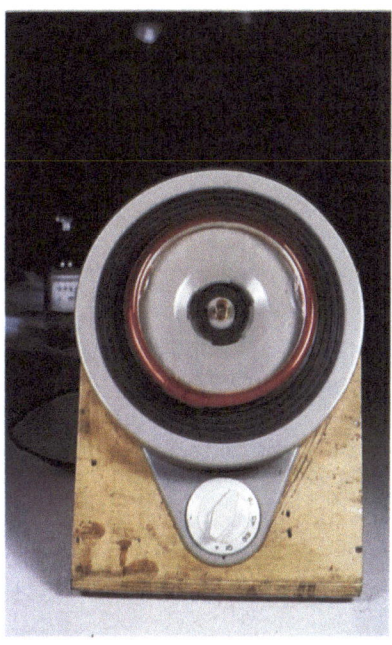

Figure 12.32 Adaptation of Chandler's original apparatus for producing thromboemboli. The apparatus consists of a turntable which is mounted on a box and angled at about 60°. The control knob permits 16 revolutions per minute. The reconstituted blood has been placed in the tubing. After 30 min the thrombus is produced

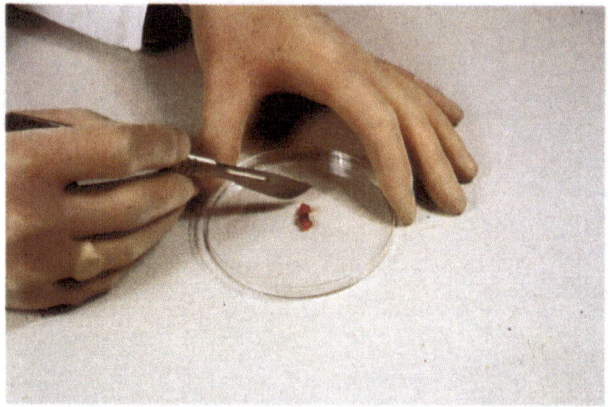

Figure 12.33a The thrombus that has been recovered from the tube (Figure 12.32) is finely chopped, washed in sterile saline and then re-injected into the marginal vein of the rabbit's ear

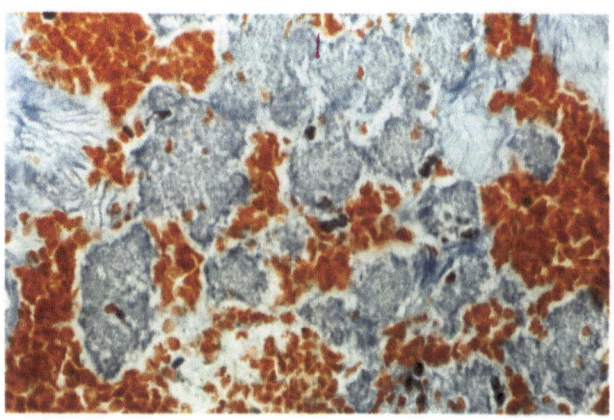

Figure 12.33b Photomicrograph of a thrombus that has been obtained by Chandler's method. Note the organoid structure, clumps of platelets, fibrin, red cells and other constituents of circulating blood. Martius Scarlet Blue × 200

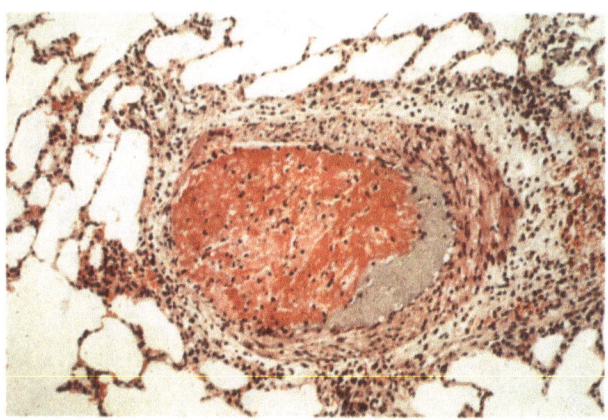

Figure 12.34 Retraction of the thrombo-embolus has already taken place in the pulmonary artery of the rabbit 24 h after injection of the thrombo-emboli into the marginal ear vein. The crescentic-shaped lumen is filled with injecting medium. Endothelialization of the thrombo-embolus has already commenced. H & E × 100

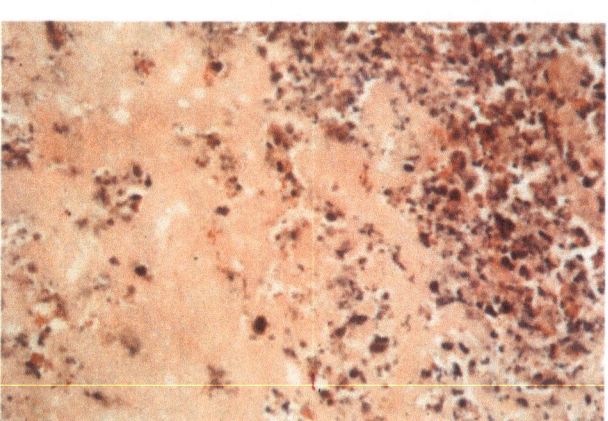

Figure 12.35 At 48 h, disintegration of the cellular elements of the thrombo-embolus is already striking. H & E × 200

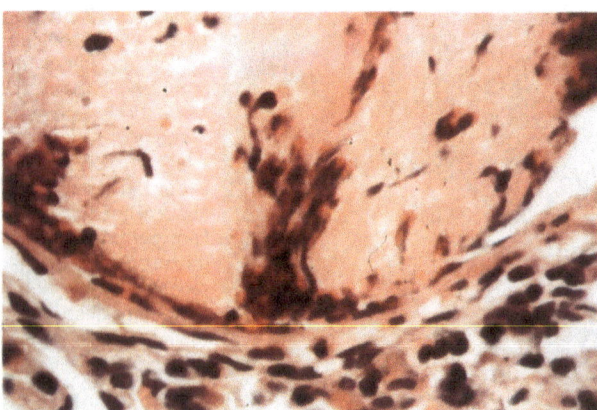

Figure 12.36 By 5 days invasion of the part of the thrombo-embolus in contact with the arterial wall by endothelial cells is well advanced. · H & E × 400

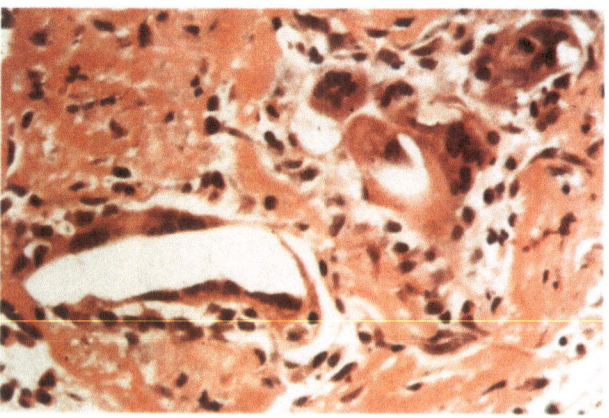

Figure 12.37 Stages of revascularization showing giant cells, the cytoplasm of which disintegrates. Nuclei become reoriented to line the resulting spaces. A capillary can be seen towards the lower left area of the illustration. These features are seen 10 days after re-injection of thrombo-emboli. H & E × 350

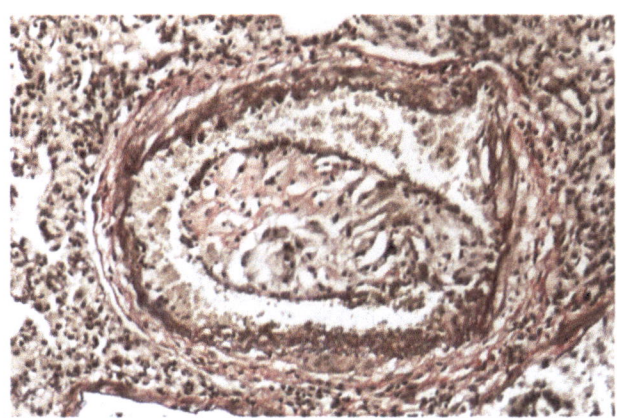

Figure 12.38 By day 14 collagen tissue has appeared. The thrombo-embolus, covered by endothelial cells, is extensively recapillarized. Elastic van Gieson × 150

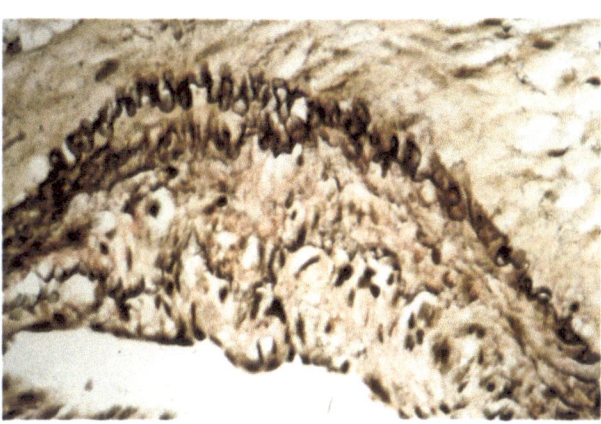

Figure 12.39 Elastic tissue and 'reduplication' of the internal elastic lamina are found. Elastic van Gieson × 400

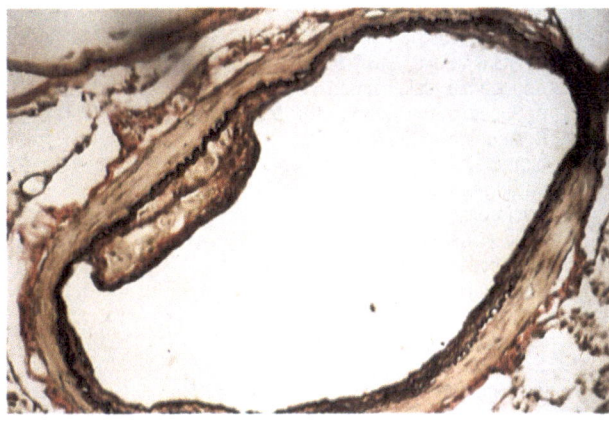

Figure 12.40 Pulmonary thrombo-embolus at 6 weeks. Only a small intimal elevation remains. Elastic van Gieson × 150

References

1. Heath, D., Wood, E. H., Dushane, J. W. and Edwards, J. E. (1959). The structure of the pulmonary trunk at different ages and in cases of pulmonary hypertension and pulmonary stenosis. *J. Pathol. Bacteriol.*, **77**, 443

2. Brenner, O. (1935). Pathology of the vessels of the pulmonary circulation. *Arch. Intern. Med.*, **56**, 211

3. Harris, P. and Heath, D. (1962). *Human Pulmonary Circulation: Its Form and Function in Health and Disease.* p. 48. (Edinburgh: E. & S. Livingstone)

4. Harrison, C. V. (1960). In Daley, R., Goodwin, J. F. and Steiner, R. E. (eds) *Clinical Disorders of the Pulmonary Circulation.* p. 136. (London: J. & A. Churchill Ltd)

5. Doyle, A. E., Goodwin, J. F., Harrison, C. V. and Steiner, R. E. (1957). Pulmonary vascular patterns in pulmonary hypertension. *Br. Heart J.*, **19**, 353

6. Heath, D. and Edwards, J. E. (1958). The pathology of hypertensive pulmonary vascular disease. A description of six grades of structural changes in the pulmonary arteries with special reference to congenital cardiac septal defects. *Circulation*, **18**, 533

7. Wagenvoort, C. A. and Wagenvoort, N. (1973). Hypoxic pulmonary vascular lesions in man at high altitude and in patients with chronic respiratory disease. *Pathol. Microbiol.*, **39**, 276

8. Wagenvoort, C. A. (1974). Classification of pulmonary vascular lesions in congenital and acquired heart disease. *Adv. Cardiol.*, **11**, 48

9. Olsen, E. G. J. (1980). Pulmonary hypertension. In *The Pathology of the Heart*, Second Edition, p. 363. (London and Basingstoke: The Macmillan Press Ltd)

10. World Health Organisation (1975). Primary pulmonary hypertension. In Hatano, S. and Strasser, T. (eds) *Report on a WHO Meeting* (Geneva: WHO)

11. Heath, D., Segel, N. and Bishop, J. (1966). Pulmonary venoocclusive disease. *Circulation*, **34**, 242

12. Masi, A. T. (1976). Pulmonary hypertension and oral contraceptive usage. (Editorial). *Chest*, **69**, 451

13. Olsen, E. G. J. (1974). The production of thrombi and their fate in pulmonary arteries of rabbits. A useful experimental model. *Vasa*, **3**, 256

14. Irniger, W. (1963). Histologische Altersbestimmung von Thromosen und Embolien. *Virchows Arch. Pathol. Anat.*, **336**, 220

Index

Italic type denotes figure numbers